Government and Policy
for U.S. Health Leaders

Raymond J. Higbea, PhD, FACHE
Associate Professor, Health Administration
Program Director, Master of Health Administration
Grand Valley State University
Allendale, Michigan

Gregory Cline, PhD
Assistant Professor, Public and Health Administration
Coordinator, Master of Health Administration
Grand Valley State University
Allendale, Michigan

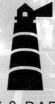

JONES & BARTLETT
LEARNING

World Headquarters
Jones & Bartlett Learning
5 Wall Street
Burlington, MA 01803
978-443-5000
info@jblearning.com
www.jblearning.com

Jones & Bartlett Learning books and products are available through most bookstores and online booksellers. To contact Jones & Bartlett Learning directly, call 800-832-0034, fax 978-443-8000, or visit our website www.jblearning.com.

Substantial discounts on bulk quantities of Jones & Bartlett Learning publications are available to corporations, professional associations, and other qualified organizations. For details and specific discount information, contact the special sales department at Jones & Bartlett Learning via the above contact information or send an email to specialsales@jblearning.com.

Production Credits

VP, Product Management: Amanda Martin
Director of Product Management: Cathy Esperti
Product Manager: Danielle Bessette
Product Assistant: Tess Sackmann
Project Manager: Jessica deMartin
Project Specialist: Kristine Janssens
Digital Project Specialist: Rachel Reyes
Senior Marketing Manager: Susanne Walker
Manufacturing and Inventory Control Supervisor: Amy Bacus

Composition: codeMantra U.S. LLC
Project Management: codeMantra U.S. LLC
Cover Design: Michael O'Donnell
Text Design: Michael O'Donnell
Media Development Editor: Shannon Sheehan
Rights Specialist: Maria Leon Maimone
Cover Image: © lunamarina/Shutterstock
Printing and Binding: Sheridan Books
Cover Printing: Sheridan Books

Library of Congress Cataloging-in-Publication Data
Library of Congress Cataloging-in-Publication Data unavailable at time of printing.

LCCN: 2019039961

6048

Printed in the United States of America
23 22 21 20 19 10 9 8 7 6 5 4 3 2 1

We would like to dedicate this book to our families and GVSU graduate students.

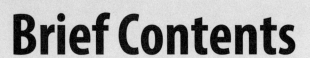

Brief Contents

© lunamarina/Shutterstock

Contents

Chapter 11   Access, the Uninsured, and Health Policy 195

Chapter 12   Payment and Quality 219

Chapter 13   How to Influence the Policy Process 231

Chapter 14   Applied Theory for Professional Advocates 243

Preface

The idea for this textbook began germinating with me (Higbea) in 2013 when I became totally frustrated with the lack of one thorough textbook that covered all of the topics necessary to understand health policy and politics. My first approach was to see if I could get the author of an existing textbook on health policy process to agree to my adding a chapter on political philosophy to his book. Following a couple rounds of communication (emails), he finally stated that what I wanted to do was too big and that I should write my own textbook. I took this as hearty, good counsel and set forth on a path to do exactly as recommended—write my own textbook.

From 2013–2016, I worked on developing the book proposal and chapters on my own only to find that I needed a co-author to help fill in some gaps and spur my thinking on these topics to a deeper level. I was at this point when Greg and I were talking in my office one afternoon and I asked if he would be interested in working with me on this book. It took him less than 30 seconds to say yes. Our partnership as authors has been invaluable on a number of levels since then.

We found that, collectively, we have taught health policy analysis to graduate healthcare administration students for 24 (Higbea 10 and Cline 14) years. During these collective 24 years, we have used reference librarians, five books (up to three at a time), multiple websites, and special speakers to adequately cover the topics of the theories behind policy making, its process, and how healthcare executives can influence the process. While exposure to reference librarians, outside speakers, and websites adds knowledge, interest, and application to the learning process, the necessity and use of five books in order to adequately cover the topic is the driving force behind developing a single book to cover philosophy, history, theory, process, economics, policy outcomes, and advocacy.

This book is designed as a textbook for graduate students and takes a balanced, interprofessional look at several topics, including the need for understanding health theory and policies; political philosophies; the history of health policy; comparative national health systems; policy-making theories; the policy-making process; policy outcomes as framed by cost, access, and quality; and advocacy.

While this book was originally intended for graduate health administration and health policy students, we found that by expanding a few sections, such as public health and personnel, this book would be more applicable to a broader audience of graduate students, such as medicine, nursing, and public health (the last two include graduate courses we teach), as well as to most any clinical profession. We also believe this book could be of value to current private and public organizational and legislative leaders.

Raymond J. Higbea, PhD, FACHE
7 June 2019
Grand Rapids, Michigan

Acknowledgments

Every author quickly realizes that no manuscript comes together without the help of a lot of people who take time to read, comment, and encourage you along the manuscript writing journey. Acknowledging the many family members, colleagues, students, and publishing team always runs the risk of forgetting to name someone so, if we have not listed your name below, it was not by neglect or intent.

We would first like to thank our families who have given up a lot of husband and dad time for book writing time. We would like to call out our boys Miles, Matthew, and Samuel who have spent countless summer hours at the pool while we dads have worked on this text. We would also like to thank our wives Linda and Kelly who have tolerated endless hours of our occupying living rooms as work spaces.

Our colleagues at Grand Valley State University, College of Community and Public Service and our own School of Public, Nonprofit and Health Administration have been very supportive of our efforts to bring this text to fruition. Lara Jaskiewicz has provided detailed feedback following the use of our draft chapters in her class and is responsible for prompting us to include the section on federalism. Our college and school leaders Dean George Grant, Jr., Associate Dean Paul Stansbie, and School Director Rich Jelier have supported this project and encouraged us along the way. Of course, there are also a large group of other GVSU colleagues who have encouraged us whom we would like to thank.

Finally, we would like to thank our publishing team at Jones & Bartlett for taking a risk on us as new authors and agreeing to transform this manuscript into a book. We would like to give special thanks to Mike Brown who, pre-retirement, began this process with us. Next, Danielle Bessette and Tess Sackmann, our editors, have guided the publishing work along with a large group of talented publishing professionals. Without a doubt this book would not have been possible without all of their efforts on our behalf.

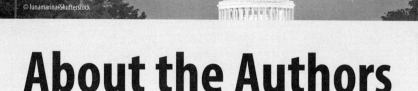

About the Authors

Raymond J. Higbea, PhD, FACHE, is an Associate Professor of Health Administration and Program Director for the Master in Health Administration. Housed in the School of Public, Nonprofit and Health Administration, Grand Valley State University, he joined GVSU in August 2014.

Raymond has 45 years of combined health clinical and administrative experience plus 12 years of teaching graduate students. Over the past 16 years, Raymond has worked on a variety of community-based solutions to community health and policy needs. While he teaches several graduate classes, his focal areas are health ethics, health finance, and public policy.

Gregory Cline, PhD, is an Assistant Professor of Health Administration. Housed in the School of Public, Nonprofit and Health Administration, Grand Valley State University, he joined GVSU in January 2008.

Greg has 22 years of public health and healthcare experience plus 14 years of teaching graduate students. He is the founding editor of the Michigan Journal of Public Health, a successful grant writer, and has consulted with numerous federal, state, and county agencies, private sector healthcare organizations, universities, and as a community-based policy analyst and community-benefit and community-level program evaluator on various projects throughout Michigan.

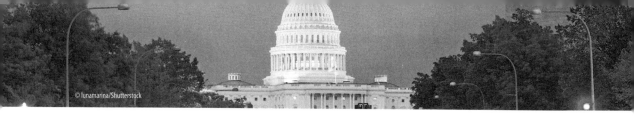

CHAPTER 1

Political Philosophy and Health Policy

This chapter is designed to give healthcare leaders an understanding of political philosophy and health policy by covering the following topics:

- The need for government
- The evolution of U.S. government
- The history of health policy development in the United States
- How political philosophy (left and right) influences the U.S. policy process
- How political philosophy (left and right) influences the U.S. health policy
- The ethics of policy making and public service
  - Social psychology
  - Market and social justice tensions
- Introduction to policy theory and policy analysis

▶ Health

A discussion of health policies must first begin with a discussion of health or how health is defined and how healthcare differs from medical care. A common definition of health is the World Health definition developed in 1948 as part of the World Health Organization (WHO) constitution that states, "Health is a state of complete physical, mental and social well-being and not merely the absence of disease or infirmity."[1] The hallmark of this definition is its recognition that health is more than physical status and includes mental health and social well-being. A limitation of this definition is the idea of physical health being the absence of disease. The concern about "absence of disease" is that it in practice recognizes the absences of acute physical illness at the expense of

---

1 Preamble to the Constitution of the World Health Organization as adopted by the International Health Conference, New York, NY, June 19–22, 1946; signed on July 22, 1946, by the representatives of 61 states (Official Records of the World Health Organization, no. 2, p. 100) and entered into force on April 7, 1948.

chronic illness. A person with a chronic illness, such as diabetes or hyperlipidemia, that is well controlled is not free from disease and they would be considered ill; however, this concept ignores well-controlled chronic illness or as Sartorius states, "Health is a state of balance, an equilibrium that an individual has established within himself and between himself and his social and physical environment" (2006).

Mental well-being also implies the absence of mental illness and the ability to cope with life's daily routine. Two concerns arise with this concept. First, it ignores the individual who has well-controlled mental illness. Second, despite the positive strides we have made as a nation recognizing and treating mental illness, it has only been with the Patient Protection and Affordable Care Act (ACA) and the inclusion of mental health as an essential component of a qualified health plan that mental health has achieved payment parity (PL 111-148, sec 1302 (b)(1)(E)).

Finally, "social well-being" implies a balanced life within the context of an individual's environment (Sartorius, 2006). It also implies that regardless of an individual's state of physical or mental health, one is living a life well-balanced within the context of physical health, mental health, and the environment. The environmental context of social well-being thus embeds the individual's environment, such as public health (sanitation and safe water), public safety, and domestic tranquility, or the lack of it, within her larger community environmental context. All of these environmental concerns (plus many more) are incorporated into the development of each individual's environment and how this environment affects physical and mental well-being.

Scholars and providers have been debating the definition of health for quite some time when consideration is given to the debate that preceded WHO's definition. Dolfman (1974) attempted to develop an operational definition of health in 1974 that considered how individuals functioned within their environment. More recently, Julliard, Klimenko, and Jacob (2006) interviewed a variety of providers regarding health and found similarities in the providers' understanding of health, including (1) the absence of disease, (2) the biopsychosocial aspects of health, (3) environmental influences on health, and (4) a holistic approach to health. Although they found similarities in understanding, they found differences in the culture of practice, stating, "… the culture of various types of healthcare providers may play a stronger role than providers' individual definitions of health in how and which models of health are dominant in their actual practices."

However, in the United States, Shi and Singh (2015) discuss how we practice and pay for a medical model of care focusing on the presence of disease and its treatments as opposed to the more holistic and environmental aspects of health discussed earlier (PL 111-148, sec 1302(b)(1)(I)). While many providers understand the importance of the psychosocial aspects of health and many of the regulatory agencies require providers to address these aspects of care, the practice and payment for medical care in the United States is driven by this medical model. Providers are only paid for providing services if they provide a diagnosis code for the visit. Granted, preventive care has been increasingly paid for by third-party payers and is now required under the ACA as an essential element of a qualified health insurance plan. However, the United States is still functioning under and paying within the structure of a medical model as opposed to a health model. The exceptions to this have been the inclusion of preventive care as one of the essential elements of an ACA qualified health plan and public health policies, such as the clean air (PL 88-206, PL 90-148, PL 91-604, PL 95-95, & PL 101-549) and clean water (PL 80-845, PL 89-234, PL 92-500, PL 95-217, & PL 100-4) acts. Despite all of the aforementioned discussion, the WHO definition still resonates as a fairly reasonable definition due to its holistic view of health as physical, mental, and social well-being.

We will draw on political philosophy to provide a broader context for two explanations of how the United States arrived at this moment in time with this set of health laws and the present healthcare system. The first way is to understand why government exists—beginning with the western European historical basis. This begins necessarily with Hobbes—unless one wishes to describe utopian models.[2] In the second use of political philosophy, we describe the influence of philosophy on policy making with an emphasis on healthcare policy. This approach is separated into two philosophical lenses, the "left" and the "right."

▶ Why Government?

Before examining the evolution of government and governance in the United States, we will start with the "taproot" regarding the purpose of government—someone well known to the early colonists—Thomas Hobbes. In 1651, Hobbes established the basis for government in western political philosophy by asking and answering two questions: "Why does government exist?" and "Why did it come about?" To answer these questions, Hobbes imagined a time when government had yet to be "invented," a time he identified when man existed in nature without government (the state of nature). The state of nature was one of anarchy—the absence of government. In such a state, every human had complete freedom—including the freedom to harm others. Thus, a state of complete freedom paradoxically led to a state of near-constant fear of death and loss of one's property and acquisitions. In such a state, planning for the future was minimal due to the high level of uncertainty synonymous with anarchy.

Hobbes next theorized that humans, recognizing that a state of complete freedom led to anarchy and high levels of uncertainty, ceded some individual freedom to a central authority—government. Government was charged with establishing, monitoring, and enforcing rules that reduced individual freedom while also reducing uncertainty, thus making future planning possible. He termed this ceding of individual freedom "social contract." The social contract is the submission of humans to a sovereign authority, which holds the sole right to make and enforce laws that govern human behavior within a defined territory.

Hobbes also argued that government, in order to be effective, must have a monopoly on the use of force within its territory. Failing to have such a monopoly would, inevitably, lead to arguments when individual (or organizational) behaviors yield negative societal outcomes significant enough to merit government intervention. These arguments, if unresolvable, would lead to armed conflict. Thus, within its territory, effective, stable, long-term government is only possible where the (central) government has this monopoly. Most modern nation-states follow this pattern. The most obvious nation that does not is the United States.

The Founding Fathers fully rejected this portion of the social contract, opting instead for separating the "monopoly" use of force across the central (federal), state, and local government units. This separation of government power (known as federalism) is evident in healthcare policy by the decisions of some states on participating in the expansion of Medicaid and the setting up of state health insurance exchanges.

Today, we largely argue over the scope of government, not its need. Our arguments stem from differences over when individual (or organizational) behaviors yield negative societal outcomes significant enough to merit government intervention. The challenge of democratic governance is balancing government activity for good while limiting as much as possible unnecessary, harmful, and sometimes fruitless intrusions on civil society. A healthy civil society has long been recognized as a necessity for healthy, stable governance (Ehrenberg, 1989). "Civil society"

---

2 This is not meant to minimize the value of the work of Aristotle, Plato, and many other earlier philosophers. Rather, it is a recognition that to understand the answer to "Why government?" in our context, we need to go back no further than the western European–derived context—which begins with Hobbes.

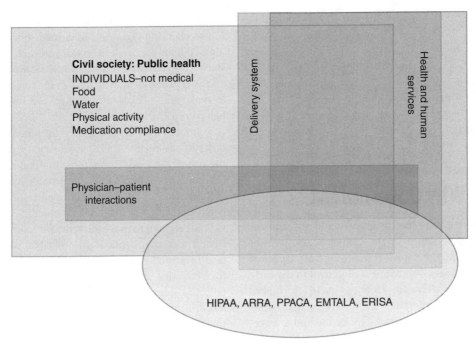

FIGURE 1.1 Civil Society in Public Health and Healthcare Services

Greg Cline, Dissertation for PhD at Michigan State University, May 2001. Courtesy of Greg Cline.

is important as the concept that describes all human associations that occur beyond government's control and influence (**FIGURE 1.1**). This is the source of each society's behavioral norms, which are drawn from cultural norms extant within different social/ethnic/geographic groupings. The ongoing associations keep both norms "alive" and refresh and alter these norms over time. Civil society can be weakened, shrunk, or altered in some fashion by government action. If too much "space" is taken up by government action (for Hobbes, too much individual freedom ceded to sovereign authority), the consequent reduction in associations beyond government control and influence will inevitably weaken civil society in that nation.[3]

The early colonists were influenced by their ancestors who arrived seeking religious freedom and the pursuit of the freedoms championed in Enlightenment thinking perhaps best exemplified by John Locke's thoughts on the natural rights of man. These natural rights include life (the ability to live), liberty (the ability to live as one desires), and property (the ability to control one's acquisitions). Taken together, religious freedoms and natural rights require a government to be strong enough to guard these freedoms but not so strong as to prohibit their practice. This tension led to the debate about the nature of our federal government during the time of the Revolution and development of our Constitution. The weak central government

---

3 This is particularly problematic as the effects on stable governance due to changes in civil society have been found to be unpredictable. The starkest examples remain the variations in conversion to democracies of Warsaw Pact states after the fall of the Soviet Union. Those states with strong civil societies prior to World War II (Poland, Czechoslovakia, the Baltic states) established functioning democracies and market economies with much less strain and in less time than states which had either weak pre-war civil societies (Romania, Bulgaria) or nearly absent pre-war civil societies (Russia) prior to 1939.

established under the Articles of Confederation resulted in a series of coordination and control problems among the 13 colonies (Maier, 2010). In an effort to address these problems, the Federalists sought to replace the Articles of Confederation with a new Constitution establishing a strong central government with three equal but separate branches (Maier, 2010). A series of arguments for a new Constitution and stronger federal government were published by the Federalists in *The Federalists Papers*. Conversely, the Anti-Federalists thought the weaknesses of the Articles of Confederation could be addressed through amendments and a new Constitution was unnecessary. The Anti-Federalists were concerned that a new Constitution would erode the sovereignty of the states and the natural rights of man. This concern and debate about the rights of man (citizens) resulted in the delayed ratification of the Constitution until the drafting of the Bill of Rights as the first amendment to the Constitution.

Although the word "health" does not appear in the Constitution or the Bill of Rights, the founders were aware of the need for strong health laws. The Federalists believed these should emanate from the federal level—however, the Anti-Federalists managed to ensure these powers were left to the states. By 1807, though, President Jefferson had evolved on the need for coordination between states and coordination with federal authorities. When communicating his list of issue areas regarding this coordination, the first and second items on his list were on quarantines and health laws.[4]

While the Federalists and Anti-Federalists were both Republicans who agreed on the need for a representative government, they continued to disagree and debate on the strength of the federal government. Throughout the course of debate, both claimed victory, with the Federalists winning the debate for a new Constitution and the Anti-Federalists winning the debate for a Bill of Rights. The presidency also changed hands between both, with Washington (Federalist), Adams (Federalist), Jefferson (Anti-Federalist), Madison (Federalist), and Monroe (Anti-Federalist), much like it has in recent history between Republicans (weak central government) and Democrats (strong central government). Over the course of history, party names and philosophies have shifted but the debate over a strong versus weak central government has persisted. One author suggests that the argument for a weak central government was a result of many early Americans being "second sons" who had no or limited inheritance in their aristocratic European home and found America as a land where they could build their own identity (Hannan, 2013). Although the United States did not have an aristocratic class, it did have leading families in commerce, trade, and politics and it was from these leading families that many early political and governmental leaders emerged.

The next contest of strong versus weak central government occurred during the Civil War. While the most well-known reason for the war was the abolition of slavery, the southern states saw it as a test of weak central government (state sovereignty) versus strong central government. Although the concepts of "positive" and "negative" liberty had not yet been named as such, President Lincoln clearly articulated both concepts in 1864 and how these two aspects of liberty led to the conflict then underway.[5]

Positive liberty is defined as "freedom to," while negative liberty is defined as "freedom from." While these two aspects of liberty are not always found in opposition, in the United States these two concepts have come to define the two-party system, with each party championing one liberty over the other. In the context of the Civil War, positive liberty led the North to seek the end of slavery—providing those enslaved freedom. The South focused on defending negative

---

4 "For many are the exercises of power reserved to the States, wherein a uniformity of proceeding would be advantageous to all. Such are quarantines, health laws … etc." (Lipscomb & Bergh, 1903).
5 These concepts were first named and defined by Isaiah Berlin in 1958.

liberty—freedom from government interference in the ownership of slaves.[6] Following the culmination of the war, the federal government passed Amendments 14 and 15 defining citizenship and voting rights—strong central government amendments prohibiting states from limiting these rights.

The 20th century witnessed several episodes of strong central government development including World War I (conscription—1914), Prohibition (making illegal the manufacture and transportation of alcoholic beverages—1920–1933), the Great Depression (New Deal economic and social support programs—1933–1938), World War II (conscription and rationing—1939–1945), the Great Society (social support, poverty, and health care—1963–1965), and the Cold War (the first peacetime presence of a large standing Army and the parallel development of the military–industrial complex—1950–1989).

While the size of the federal government grew during each of these episodes, the greatest growth occurred through the implementation of the New Deal and Great Society programs. Throughout this era (1940–1970), the size of the federal workforce grew by 315% (**FIGURE 1.2**) and expenditures as a percent of GDP by 226% (**FIGURE 1.3**).[7] The subsequent 40 years (1970–2010) witnessed relatively flat workforce growth of less than 1% (Figure 1.2) and growth of expenditures as a percent of GDP of 20% (Figure 1.3).[8] Throughout this period, the debate over the size of the federal government was limited, although there was some growing unease that began around the time of the Great Society from the conservative (Anti-Federalist) side with the emergence of politicians, such as Senator Barry Goldwater and commentator William F. Buckley, Jr. This movement to "reign in the size of government" culminated with the election of Ronald Reagan as president in 1980. Reagan championed the idea of a smaller federal government and frequently stated his goal was to "get government off the backs of Americans." Most recently,

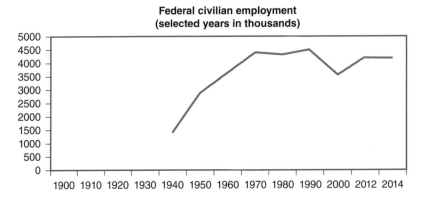

FIGURE 1.2 Federal Employment

Federal Office of Personal Management.

---

6 Today, the clash of these two liberties in healthcare policy may be found in the two sides of the choice/abortion debate, the guarding of a woman's right to choose or the lives of unborn children.

7 It is possible that total defense spending exceeded and still exceeds the costs of the Great Society programs. Arriving at a figure for all U.S. defense spending is difficult, as substantial expenditures for some aspects of national defense are located outside of the Department of Defense, such as some nuclear costs (Department of Energy), military satellite launches (NASA), etc.

8 It should be noted that growth in state and local government markedly increased during this time frame while the federal workforce's growth remained flat.

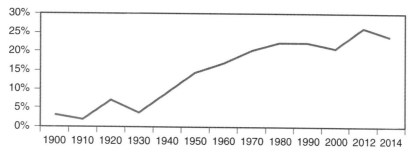

FIGURE 1.3 Federal Spending as Percent of GDP

U.S. Bureau of Economic Development.

the federal government has grown by direct intervention at the end of the George W. Bush administration and throughout the Barack Obama administration through the economic stimulus packages intended to blunt the fall of the credit markets when the real estate market crashed in 2008, the Patient Protection and Affordable Care Act of 2010 (PL 111-148 & PL 111-152), and Dodd-Frank Wall Street Reform and Consumer Protection Act of 2010 (PL 111-203). The first 2 years of the Donald Trump administration have been characterized solely with a focus on deregulation, although with little regulatory change in health care.

▶ The Enlightenment and Political Philosophy

The Founding Fathers of the United States were men of the *Enlightenment*, a period marked by the end of absolute, hierarchical monarchical and religious rule and the emergence of an *enlightened* populace. A great distinguishing characteristic of this period was a recognition that a leader's legitimacy emanated from the people, not from their office or family heritage. This understanding produced various forms of *republicanism*, or representative government. The Enlightenment produced a number of scholars, thinkers, philosophers, and political actors that are too numerous to include in this brief discussion. Thus, two philosophers and political actors have been chosen as representatives of each philosophical side of the debate about the type of Republican government the United States should establish.

▶ Philosophical View from the Left

Two leaders who influenced the development of the left and whose influence continues today are Jean-Jacques Rousseau (1712–1778) and Thomas Paine (1737–1809). As a philosopher, Rousseau influenced American political philosophy through his work on *The Social Contract*, which provided some structure for how a society can develop a government that will work to the benefit of all of its members. *The Social Contract* embraces the idea that there is a balance between rights and duties and that all citizens share these rights and duties equally. Rousseau posited that these shared rights and duties can be achieved through a sovereign and a government. The characteristics of the sovereign include representation of the whole population, representation of the population's general will, and functions as the legislative body for the government. The government is separate from the sovereign and implements the laws. Implied within this model is the idea of representative government that is directly responsible to the citizenry.

Paine influenced American political philosophy through his multiple writings and

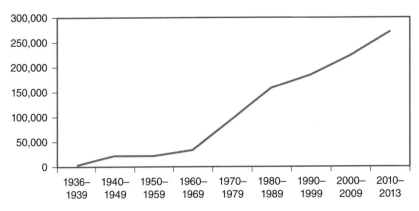

FIGURE 1.4 Total Rules

Federal Register.

speeches. *Common Sense* is his written work that most influenced the Revolution by making a sermon-like argument for the colonies to dissent and free themselves from British rule. Throughout his arguments, he advocated for equality, liberty, and for systems of government that would ensure their existence. His arguments were consistently in favor of big, as opposed to small, incremental changes to government. Thus, he argued that the current relationship with Britain was beyond repair and needed to be abandoned, and a new government needed to be established to protect the colonists' liberty and quality of life.

With these two complementary and foundational philosophies of big changes and maintenance of the *social contract* reinforced by the work of multiple politicians, philosophers, and scholars, modern liberals have developed a political philosophy that embraces a strong federal government intervention and big government programs. Looking back over the 20th century, modern liberals have supported and implemented multiple interventional programs through the New Deal and Great Society programs that sought to support the social contract they believed the federal government had with the citizenry to meet their multiple social and economic needs. During the period from 1930 to 1970, the growth of the federal government increased in physical size as evidenced by the

number of people employed and expenditures as a percent of GDP. From 1970 to current, the physical size of the federal government has been relatively static largely through multiple plans to control expenditures and increase efficiency; however, the number of rules has essentially doubled (**FIGURE 1.4**—several years estimated based on historic trends).

▶ Philosophical View from the Right

Two leaders who influenced the development of the right and whose influence continues today are John Locke (1632–1704) and Edmund Burke (1729–1797). John Locke was a physician and leading philosopher of the Enlightenment period whose writings influenced many of the Founding Fathers of the United States. He is best known for the concept of *separation of powers* and the *natural rights of man*. The concept of separation of powers had its influence on the development of the constitutional monarchies of Western Europe and influenced our founding leaders in how they structured our government into three separate but equal branches with defined responsibilities, checks, and balances on each other. Locke is best known for his work on the natural rights of man and as such is known as the father of classical liberalism. Americans quickly recognize these rights in the second paragraph of the Declaration of Independence, "… that they are endowed by their Creator with certain unalienable Rights, that among these are Life, Liberty, and the pursuit of Happiness …" Locke, however, stated these rights as life, liberty, and property. These rights are held in a hierarchical order, with life the highest right and property the lowest. One does not have the right to property (controlling what we acquire) at the price of another's liberty or life and one does not have the right to liberty (living as one desires) at the cost of another's life.[9]

Edmund Burke was a political philosopher, writer, and politician and a contemporary of our Founding Fathers. While he was not in favor of how the British government treated the American colonies, he was also not in favor of the American colonies separating from Britain and registered his protest of their unfair treatment in his speech "On American Taxation" (1774). He recognized the irreconcilable nature of the conflict as outlined in "Conciliation with the Colonies" (1775) and saw separation as a reasonable, yet regrettable, resolution. Burke had a deep commitment to established institutions and, while he recognized the need for change, favored small, incremental changes that allowed these institutions to maintain their status and function in society while changing enough to meet current societal needs.

These complimentary political philosophies of the natural rights, respect for established institutions (societal and governmental), and incrementalism changes to established institutions have developed into a political philosophy that embraces small or weak central government and small changes to existing institutions or programs without new governmental programs. Thus, modern conservatives insist on the shrinking of existing federal government programs and the regulatory reach of government alongside their embrace of lower taxes, to diminish government's direct role in society. Most recently, this can be seen in the resistance of modern conservatives to the Dodd-Frank (PL 111-203) bill and the Patient Protection and Affordable Care Act (PL 111-148 & PL 111-152).

▶ Philosophical Tensions

After gaining an elementary understanding of how these two philosophical views perceive government and its function and understanding that both political parties passionately believe they have the best answers for America's problems, one has to ask several questions, such as, how can these two groups be so different and bring value to America? Is there any possibility they could ever agree on anything? To these questions we have to answer, "Yes, there is value to their differing views," and "Yes, even though they are currently very polarized, they can agree and get along." Either party left to themselves would produce a society that roughly half of the nation would find onerous and objectionable. The Democrats through their belief in active government intervention in the resolution of social problems could increase the size of government through the provision of additional social services to the point that the government would place higher financial constraints on taxpayers to fund these programs. In contrast, the Republicans through their belief in

---

9   Locke considered property as a gift from God appropriated by individuals through labor to the extent it is useful but not to the extent that it is hoarded or spoiled. Burke built on Locke's principle of personal property ownership and considered property ownership a hedge against the government exercising tyrannical authority over the populace. In contrast, Rousseau considers personal property ownership subordinate to the rights of the community and in Book I, IX states, "For the State, in relation to its members, is master of all their goods by the social contract, which, within the State, is the basis of all rights …"

small government and personal responsibility could limit government interaction in solving social problems, thus leaving some social problems unsolved. These two political philosophies brought together would theoretically yield governmental interventions in social problems that addressed the most serious problems while maintaining a fiscally sound and less constraining government.

Schattschneider (1960) discussed how Americans' view of government has evolved from satisfaction in gaining increased access to government (p. 113) to a belief "… that they have a general power over government as a whole and not merely within government …" (pp. 113–114). An argument could be made that the increasing political polarization and hollowing out of the middle (Figure 1.4) documented by Pew's 2014 Political Polarization survey is a natural result of this evolving attitudinal shift. The unfortunate result of this type of polarization is the lack of meaningful political action and the failure for either side to effectively govern.

Further insights into the political polarization of the American public are gained from the exhaustive analysis of the American public's ideological disposition and voting patterns conducted by Philip Converse in the last half of the 20th century and the continuation of his analysis by Kinder and Kalmoe (2017) (**FIGURE 1.5**). These scholars argue that ideology requires breadth, structure, and stability (p. 21), which is lacking and rare in American voters. Further describing the American voter, Kinder and Kalmoe posit they have "dim understanding of basic ideological categories, weakly structured and unstable opinions, [and] fragmentation … into narrow issue publics" (p. 21). This assessment of American voters is substantiated by analysis of results from the American National Election Survey conducted every 4 years from 1960 through 2012. Analysis of these survey results includes American voter ideological stability, the dissociation of voting from ideology, and voting patterns associated with political party affiliation. These findings align with the work of Haidt (2012), who describes how American voters politically align with their social groups.

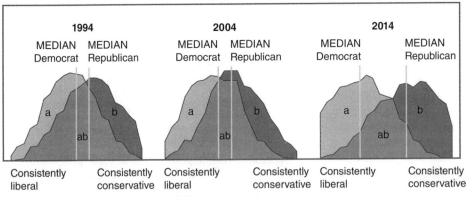

Distribution of Democrats and Republicans on a 10-item scale of political values

Source: 2014 political polarization in the American Public
Notes: Ideological consistency based on a scale of 10 political values questions. The area mentioned as "a" in this chart represents the ideological distribution of Democrats; the area mentioned as "b" represents Republicans. The overlap of these two distributions is indicated as "ab". Republicans include Republican-leaning independents; Democrats include Democratic-leaning independents.

FIGURE 1.5 Democrats and Republicans More Ideologically Divided than in the Past

▶ Social Psychology

Haidt (2012) takes a social psychology approach to describing political-philosophical views and associated predictable social behaviors. Attributes of social behavior are described by six dyadic opposites: care/harm, liberty/oppression, fairness/cheating, loyalty/betrayal, authority/subversion, and sanctity/degradation. *Care/harm* focuses on the provision of compassion or meeting a need as opposed to suffering or intentionally causing harm. *Liberty/oppression* focuses on the ability of individuals to live free and flourishing lives in society without interference of a strong authoritarian figure. *Fairness/cheating* focuses on mutual partnership, mutual benefits, and cooperation that do not culminate in one party taking advantage of another for personal gain. *Loyalty/betrayal* refers to group cohesion, pride, and self-sacrifice as opposed to group shame, desertion, or treason. *Authority/subversion* refers to mutually beneficial hierarchical relationships, not to self-serving authoritarian rule. *Sanctity/degradation* refers to respect of people and personal dignity as opposed to any type of defacement or abuse. The influential strength or intensity of these dyads can be attributed to an individual's political philosophy, moral matrix, and resultant social behavior (**FIGURE 1.6**) and provides another technique for predicting philosophically associated social (moral) behaviors.

▶ Ethics

Even today when we examine ethics we must start with the original Greek philosophers. In Aristotle's *Politics and Ethics,* he writes about exercising *virtue* as the source of happiness. This virtue is who we are at the core, whether personal or professional, and is the source of *integrity* referred to in professional codes of conduct and the source of personal satisfaction. Aristotle argued that values flowed from virtue. Ethics are the behavioral norms that individuals (or groups or societies) follow to

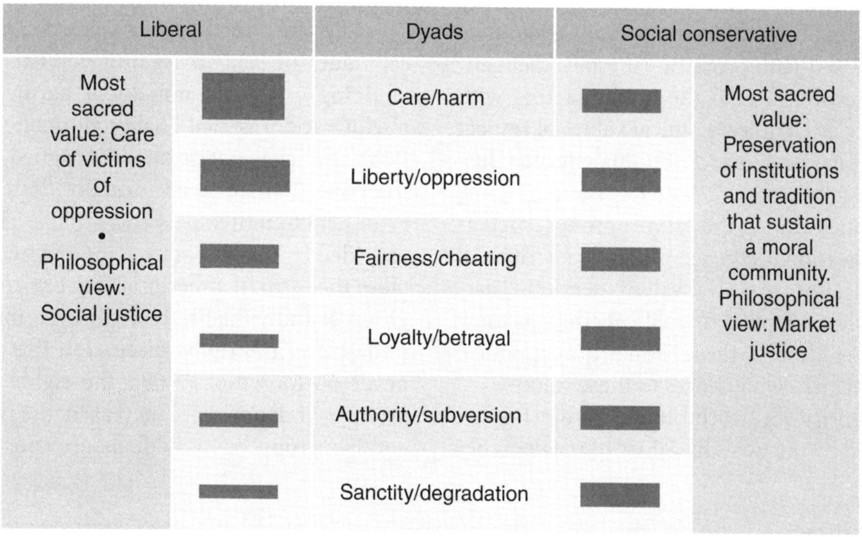

Liberal	Dyads	Social conservative
Most sacred value: Care of victims of oppression • Philosophical view: Social justice	Care/harm	Most sacred value: Preservation of institutions and tradition that sustain a moral community. Philosophical view: Market justice
	Liberty/oppression	
	Fairness/cheating	
	Loyalty/betrayal	
	Authority/subversion	
	Sanctity/degradation	

FIGURE 1.6 Moralistic Social Psychology Dyad

Modified from Haidt, J. (2012). *The righteous mind: Why good people are divided by politics and religion.* New York, NY: Vintage Books.

maintain those values. When virtue is exercised as an expected action, Aristotle considers these actions to be *just*, or in economic and leadership terms, transactional. Conversely, when virtue is exercised for its own sake, Aristotle considers this to be *noble*, or in economic and leadership terms, *transformational*.

While Aristotle posits that we continually hone our ethical virtues of who we are by practicing them, Kant takes a more rationalist approach by positing that our ethical actions are based on analyzing the demonstration of duty through the lens of human dignity. Stated differently, Aristotelian self-governance is achieved through training, whereas Kantian self-governance is achieved through rational suppression of natural appetites and emotions through judgments to duty. Regardless of the source or approach to ethics, the point of congruence that all national citizens and residents agree upon is that politics and policy making must be conducted in an ethical environment and in an ethical manner that places the good of the citizenry above those of the politicians or policy makers.

Political ethics should not be confused with personal ethics that can differ from person to person based on cultural background, values training, and ethical training. Nor should they be confused with professional ethics that generally revolve around the idea of acting with integrity or healthcare ethical values of respect of persons, beneficence, nonmaleficence, justice, veracity, or care.[10] Arguably there are some similarities among these three groups, such as the professional ethical value of integrity. All of the healthcare ethical values mentioned earlier could be applied to political ethics at some level. Yet despite these similarities, political ethics has its own nuances to these values.

Veracity, or truthfulness, is most often depicted by the two sub-values of *transparency* and *conflict-of-interest*. Transparency is the ethical value that most frequently gets politicians into ethical trouble resulting in sanctions ranging from censure to expulsion from office. As a part of public office accountability, politicians and public officials have to publicly disclose their finances, usually accomplished by disclosing their tax returns and public disclosure forms. Public officials are under rigid financial requirements, and irregularities on either of these two documents can trigger an ethics investigation. Veracity is also associated with complete disclosure of documents and information when requested by governmental oversight agencies or through FOIA request by public or private agencies. Finally, transparency is important when discussing policy development and its impact on constituents. The lack of transparency results in public officials being labeled liars, erodes public trust of the official, and can result in the end of a public career. *Conflict-of-interest* results when a public official privately benefits from public action, such as legislation or granting a contract, or when a public official's decision can be influenced by previous decisions or influential relationships.

The two foundational healthcare ethical values of *beneficence* and *nonmaleficence*, of doing good and not doing harm, are an obvious and unstated goal of all public policy. Public policy is not normally designed to hurt someone. Rather, it is normally designed to be of help to individuals and groups. The help provided by public policy solutions frequently takes the form of either granting or protecting group or individual rights; however, there is a trade-off in the rights discussion that should never be forgotten. When the rights of one group or individual are increased, the rights of another group or individuals are constrained

---

10 *Respect of persons* is demonstrated through the attitude of personal dignity, autonomy, confidentiality, and consent. *Beneficence* is bringing benefit to others or doing good. *Nonmaleficence* is to do no harm. *Justice* is the exercise of virtue (Aristotle) or fairness (Rawls). *Veracity* is truthfulness, transparency, or no conflict of interest. *Care* is relationships, compassion, and context.

or diminished. The balancing act resulting from this discussion is a philosophical question of social good versus individual freedom and often evokes a further discussion of *justice*.

Justice is fairness. Rawls (2001), as one of the more prolific writers and thinkers on justice in the past century, asserts that justice as fairness is "… framed for a democratic society …," takes political justice as "…the basic structure of society …," and is a form of political liberalism as evidenced by an individual's relationship "… within the basic structure of society …" (Rawls, 1971, 2001). In light of the earlier, Americans generally agree with the need for fairness and equitability regarding access to opportunities and participation in our government. Access to opportunities is where Americans differ as to their opinions as what these opportunities are and how involved

government should be ensuring them. These differences are framed in their opposing political philosophies that can be crudely framed as a rights versus commodities discussion or in less incendiary terms as market and social justice (Shi & Singh, 2015).

▸ Market and Social Justice

The characteristics delineated in **TABLE 1.1** assist in understating which policy approaches to public and healthcare problems align with each philosophical view and how each side views the government's role in remedying imbalances in health care based on the ethic of fairness or justice. The focus from the right is

TABLE 1.1 Market and Social Justice	
Market Justice	**Social Justice**
Characteristics	
■ Views health care as an economic good	■ View's health care as a social good
■ Assumes free-market conditions for health services delivery	■ Requires active government involvement in health services delivery
■ Assumes that markets are more efficient in allocating health resources equitability	■ Assumes that the government is more efficient in allocating health resources equitably
■ Production and distribution of healthcare determined by market-based demand	■ Medical resource allocation determined by central planning
■ Medical care distribution based on people's ability to pay	■ Ability to pay inconsequential for receiving medical care
■ Access to medical care viewed as an economic reward of personal effort and achievement	■ Equal access to medical services viewed as a basic right

(continues)

TABLE 1.1 Market and Social Justice	*(continued)*
Market Justice	**Social Justice**
Implications	
▪ Individual responsibility for health	▪ Collective responsibility for health
▪ Benefits based on individual purchasing power	▪ Everyone is entitled to a basic package of benefits
▪ Limited obligation to the collective good	▪ Strong obligations to the collective good
▪ Emphasis on individual well-being	▪ Community well-being supersedes that of the individual
▪ Private solutions to social problems	▪ Public solutions to social problems
▪ Rationing based on ability to pay	▪ Planned rationing of health care

Shi, L., & Singh, D. A. (2015). *Delivering health care in America: A systems approach* (6th ed.). Burlington, MA: Jones & Bartlett Learning.

on the individual and the individual's responsibility of maintaining access to healthcare services either through employer-sponsored healthcare coverage or through individually purchased health insurance. The focus from the left is on access to healthcare services as a public good that should be provided by direct government involvement. A third option that bridges these two views considers access to healthcare services as a quasi-public good similar to education. This option guarantees access to a basic level of healthcare services by the federal government, with individuals having the option to obtain an equal level of basic services and any services beyond the basic level through the private market.

▶ Theories and the Need for Theories Overview

Conceptual frameworks, theories, and models are tools used to decrease the complexity of the policy-making process and help predict and describe how the process works. Sabatier (1999) succinctly summarizes Ostrum's distinctions of these three tools.

In her view (Ostrum's), a *conceptual framework* identifies a set of variables and the relationships among them that presumably account for a set of phenomena. The framework can provide anything from a modest set of variables to something as extensive as a paradigm. It need not identify directions among relationships, although more developed frameworks will certainly specify some hypotheses. A *theory* provides a "denser" and more logically coherent set of relationships. It applies to some of the variables and usually specifies how relationships may vary depending upon the values of critical variables. Numerous theories may be consistent with the same conceptual framework. A *model* is a representation of a specific situation. It is usually much narrower in scope, and more precise in its assumptions, than the underlying theory. Ideally, it is mathematical. Thus, frameworks, theories, and models can be conceptualized as operating along a continuum involving increasing logical interconnectedness and specificity, but decreasing scope.

In an effort to simplify the types of conceptual frameworks, theories, and models encountered in the policy-making process, we have simplified them into *process oriented conceptual frameworks, theories, and models* and *interest group–oriented conceptual frameworks, theories, and models* (**TABLE 1.2**). Process-oriented conceptual frameworks, theories, and models explore and describe processes of how policies are developed and adopted by governmental (federal, state, and local) entities. Interest group–oriented conceptual frameworks, theories, and models explore the human factors behind how interest groups are organized and how they seek to influence policy development, implementation, outcomes, and modifications. Neither of these categories completely describe how policies are developed.

TABLE 1.2 Policy Conceptual Frameworks, Theories, and Models and Major Characteristics	
Process-Oriented Conceptual Frameworks, Theories, and Models	**Interest Group-Oriented Conceptual Frameworks, Theories, and Models**
Multiple streams ■ Problems ■ Policies	Social constructivism ■ Positive associations ■ Negative associations
■ Politics ■ Policy window ■ Policy entrepreneur	Institutional rational choice ■ Behavior-based ■ Action arena ■ Values ■ Official and unofficial policies ■ Consensus ■ Punishment
	Network approach ■ Issue action group ■ Policy advocates and experts ■ Values ■ Cohesion
Punctuated equilibrium ■ Stable incrementalism ■ Shock	Advocacy coalition ■ Common belief systems ■ Education ■ Specialization ■ Resources ■ Deal with wicked and difficult problems

Modified from Sabatier, P. A. (Ed.). (1999). *Theories of the policy process.* Boulder, CO: Westview Press.

Rather, these categories should be used to complement each other and more fully describe the policy process. This mixed method of policy analysis is analogous to the use of mixed quantitative and qualitative methods, where quantitative methods are used to describe and predict what will or has happened and qualitative methods describe how or why they happened. Keeping with this analogy, process-oriented conceptual frameworks, theories, and models are analogous to quantitative research methods that describe what is happening in the policy development process. Interest group conceptual frameworks, theories, and models are analogous to qualitative research methods and describe why the influence or power of the group influences the policy development process. Process and interest group conceptual frameworks, theories, and models will be discussed in more detail in Chapter 3.

▶ Policy Analysis

Leaders have two choices when it comes to understanding the content of policies: They (1) can search for the policies, read them, and analyze them to draw their own conclusions or (2) can rely on professional associations and news organizations to summarize, interpret, and analyze policies. If a leader wishes to personally find the policies, there are several websites where the majority of the documents can be found (**TABLE 1.3**). However, by going through professional associations and keeping abreast of the news, the executive can save time and get trusted insight from policy analysts. Whether the leader decides to personally analyze a policy or rely on the analysis of another, the *Policy Analysis Organizational Framework* (Appendix) is a tool that can assist in organizing and understanding policies. Further discussion of policy analysis tools and methods will be covered in Chapter 8.

TABLE 1.3 Websites for Public Policies	
Policy Websites	
http://congress.gov	Federal policies
http://www.govetrack.us	Federal policies that are linked by updates and modifications
http://www.whpgs.org/f.htm	Federal, state, and local sites
https://www.federalregister.gov/articles/search#advanced	Federal rules, regulations, and documents
http://www.senate.gov/reference/common/faq/how_to _committe_hrg.htm	Legislative committee hearings
http://congressional.proquest.com/profiles/gis/search /advanced/advanced	Legislative committee hearings
http://www.loc.gov/law/help/judicial-decisions.php#federal	Federal and state court decisions
http://www.supremecourt.gov/opinions/opinions.aspx	U.S. Supreme Court opinions

References

American Medical Association. (1847). Proceedings of the National Medical Conventions held in New York, NY, May, 1846 and in Philadelphia, May, 1847.

Dolfman, M. L. (1974). Toward operational definitions of health. *The Journal of School Health*, *44*(4), 206–209.

Ehrenberg, J. (1989). *Civil society: The critical history of an idea*. New York, NY: New York University Press.

Haidt, J. (2012). *The righteous mind: Why good people are divided by politics and religion*. New York, NY: Vintage Books.

Hannan, D. (2013). *Inventing freedom: How the English speaking peoples made the modern world* (pp. 135–140). New York, NY: HarperCollins.

Julliard, K., Klimenko, E., & Jacob, M. S. (2006). Definitions of health among healthcare providers. *Nursing Science Quarterly*, *19*(3), 265–271. doi:10.1177/0894318486289575

Kinder, D. R., & Kalmoe, N. P. (2017). *Neither liberal nor conservative: Ideological innocence in the American public*. Chicago, IL: University of Chicago Press.

Lipscomb, A. A., & Bergh, A. E. (Eds.). (1903). *The works of Thomas Jefferson in twelve volumes: Federal edition, volume 10* (pp. 236–237). New York, NY and London: G.P. Putnam & Sons.

Maier, P. (2010). *Ratification: The people debate the constitution, 1787–1788*. New York, NY: Simon and Schuster.

Rawls, J. (1971). *A theory of justice*. Cambridge, MA: Harvard University Press.

Rawls, J. (2001). *Justice as fairness: A restatement*. Cambridge, MA: Harvard University Press.

Sabatier, P. (1999). *Theories of the policy process*. Boulder, CO: Westview Press.

Sartorius, N. (2006). The meanings of health and its promotion. *Croatian Medical Journal*, *47*(4), 662–664.

Schattschneider, E. E. (1960). *The semisovereign people: A realist's view of democracy in America*. Wadsworth, OH: Thomson Learning Academic Resource Center.

Shi, L., & Singh, D. A. (2015). *Delivering health care in America: A systems approach* (6th ed.). Burlington, MA: Jones & Bartlett Learning.

Starr, P. (1982). *The social transformation of American medicine: The rise of a sovereign profession and the making of a vast industry*. New York, NY: Basic Books.

Appendix

Policy Analysis Organizational Framework

▶ Introduction

Public policy is designed to correct a problem that is either (1) easiest for the government to correct or (2) only possible for the government to correct.

Leaders unfamiliar with analyzing policy often struggle to craft clear, well-organized, complete analyses of a policy (whether federal, state, or local). This framework provides an overarching organizational frame for policy analysis and is designed to ensure that a leader can quickly and clearly understand the key components of a law, including (1) who it is meant to help, (2) what the legal changes entail, (3) who is targeted by these changes, (4) the intended outcomes, and (5) the anticipated unintended outcomes.

Policy analyses are often never read all the way through in one sitting and are frequently referred back to by a leader to recall a specific aspect of the analysis. Due to this, ensuring that all major organizational components are completely covered in a clear and careful fashion is critical to the successful use of the analysis.

Getting Started

After identifying a law to analyze, find a copy of the law and read it completely. While reading the law, use the organizational breakdown provided to note the law's components (beneficiaries, targets, instruments, outcomes, and recommendations for advocacy). If the law is too long to completely read in one sitting, identify a component or set of components to analyze and only analyze that component or set of components.

Making Claims

Whenever a claim is made (these will be mostly found in your outcomes and/or recommendations for advocacy section), it *must* be supported. To support a claim, reference scientific research findings or clearly stated and referenced facts. These findings may come from journal articles and research studies published by foundations, trade associations, advocacy organizations, and government agencies.

▶ Introduction

A description of the *policy* being assessed. Depending on the complexity of the policy, this could be as short as one paragraph or as long as a page (or slightly longer).

Policy Beneficiaries

Detail the *policy beneficiaries*. Policies are designed to *benefit* some group that is deemed to need some benefit that is best provided by government. This group (or groups) is identified in this organizational framework as *beneficiaries*. Do not assume that targets are beneficiaries. Frequently, the beneficiaries are hardly mentioned in the language of the law and are often not required to do anything at all.

Policy Targets

Detail the *policy target(s)*. Policies apply *instruments* to clearly identified *targets*. Targets are a group or groups that are identified in the law as being subject to new (or changed) instruments in order to achieve some benefit. Targets are not always the intended beneficiaries of a law.

Policy Instruments

Present and explain the *policy instrument(s)* and how these instrument(s) are expected to affect changed behavior. *Instruments* include any of the following:

New or altered rules or regulations

New or altered incentives or disincentives to encourage or discourage behavior

New or altered penalties or sanctions for breaking rules or regulations

New or altered processes for interfacing with others (individuals, organizations, or government)

Any adjudication procedures specific to the policy

Describe each instrument in enough detail to ensure that a reader knows which of the groups is identified earlier.

Policy Outcomes

Describe the policy's *intended outcome(s)*. These are the stated end goals of the policy as contained in the law and include the intended end goals (outcomes) of the law.

Describe the policy's *unintended outcome(s)*. Both supporters and detractors of a policy frequently provide unintended positive and negative outcomes. First, start by identifying the policy beneficiaries and targets and then by identifying the trade or advocacy organizations that are concerned with the beneficiaries and targets. The relevant trade associations or advocacy organizations frequently conduct or commission studies to prove unintended outcomes that have occurred or potentially will occur.

Recommendation for Advocacy

Explain how the policy could be *reformulated* to be more effective or equitable by altering any or all of the analyzed components: beneficiaries, targets, instruments, or outcomes. Finally, explain why the reformulation is more effective or equitable than the existing policy.

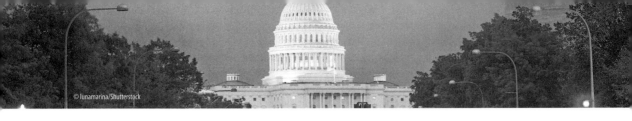

CHAPTER 2

How We Got Here: U.S. Health Policy History

This chapter is designed to give healthcare leaders an understanding of U.S. health policy history by covering the following topics:

- The history of health policy
- How the U.S. health system developed
- How selected major components of the Patient Protection and Affordable Care Act developed

▶ History of Health Policy and Development of the U.S. Health System

The history of health policy development in the United States had its beginnings at the state, as opposed to federal, level, with few exceptions. These exceptions, beginning with the Sailors and Marines Act of 1798,[1] addressed the narrowest of constituencies. State-level action began with a series of medical licensing laws passed circa 1800, abolished circa 1830, and re-established post-Civil War. Prior to post-Civil War era licensing regulations, the practice of medicine lacked standardization, with almost anyone who desired to practice medicine being able to open a practice and assume the title of doctor. With the rise of several alternative options to allopathic medicine, including homeopathic (1796), osteopathic (1874), naturopathic (1895), and chiropractic (1895) medicine in the 1800s, the public was not always certain about what they were getting when receiving treatment from a "doctor." Doctors of Medicine were concerned about distinguishing themselves from alternative practices with the establishment of licensing laws based on ensuring the quality of treatment received from individuals claiming the title of "doctor." While ensuring quality is the claim every trade group uses when seeking licensure, economists view licensure as a restraint of trade

---

1   This laid the foundation for what would become the U.S. Public Health Commissioned Corps.

or a legal method for keeping the "undesirables" out of the business (AMA, 1847). Ironically, there were legal disputes among the alternative forms of medicine, such as the 1907 lawsuit in Wisconsin in which a chiropractor was jailed for practicing osteopathic medicine (*State of Wisconsin v. Morikubo*).

The Bill for the Benefit of the Indigent Insane in 1854 was the second recorded federal healthcare legislation. This bill's intent was for the federal government to provide land for the establishment of asylums for the insane, deaf, and dumb. It was passed by both houses of Congress but vetoed by President Franklin Pierce (D), who viewed this as a federalism issue. He claimed that the states, not the federal government, should be responsible for social welfare concerns. Little, if anything, happened in the United States for another 70 years, with the next mention of federal involvement in healthcare provision being Theodore Roosevelt's presidential platform in 1912. The third piece of federal healthcare legislation was the Promotion of Welfare and Hygiene of Maternity and Infancy Act (1921). Also known as the Sheppard-Towner Act, this progressive piece of legislation, which passed both houses of Congress and was signed by President Woodrow Wilson (D), provided federal funding for maternal and child care.

During this same 70 years, Germany and Britain enacted social support legislation that would eventually be replicated by the modern industrial world and would ultimately influence the United States. In an effort to gain the support of labor, German Chancellor Otto von Bismarck was the first to propose social support legislation and have it passed into law. The Sickness Insurance Law (1883) established sickness funds paid for by the employee (2/3) and employer (1/3); the Accident Insurance Law (1884) was employer-funded and precursor to workers' compensation laws; and Old Age and Disability Insurance (1889) was an old-age pension plan and precursor to Social Security in the United States. About 40 years later, British Prime Minister David Lloyd George sponsored the enactment of several social service policies, including the National Health Insurance Act (1920) that provided laborers protection against illness costs and unemployment.

▶ Brief History of Payment

In the United States, health insurance had its beginnings in the 1860s through the late 1920s in a series of disability insurance offerings (sickness funds) by a variety of insurance companies that were designed to protect laborers from loss of wages, as opposed to payment for medical costs.[2] The Baylor Plan, established in 1929, was the first organized health insurance plan, cost 50¢ per month or $6 per year, started so university professors could pay their hospital bills. The Baylor Plan was soon followed by a flurry of similar plans that were ultimately chartered by state laws as Blue Cross plans. A decade later in 1939, physician payment was organized in a similar manner under Blue Shield plans. While it may seem intuitive to assume that physicians would welcome these insurance products that ensured payment, the opposite was what actually happened. Physicians were vehemently opposed

---

2   The average length of illness during this era was 4–6 weeks, resulting in no income for the employee during this period of illness and convalescence. Thus, the need for income stability or disability payments was provided through sickness funds costing employees 1% of their wages. When the first sickness (medical) insurance was offered through Baylor University Hospital to help university professors pay their hospital bills, it also cost employees approximately 1% of their wages.

to these plans, fearing the payer's intervention between them and their patient, and frequently cited that they were "… opposed to anything that intervened between the physician-patient relationship."

There was quite a bit of administrative and legislative activity during the Franklin Roosevelt (D) and Harry Truman (D) presidencies that sought to enact national health insurance legislation. However, none of it was fruitful. Both Presidents faced considerable and aggressive lobbying efforts against national health insurance by the American Medical Association (AMA), who continued with their campaign regarding the sacredness of the physician–patient relationship saying that no one should intervene in that relationship. President Roosevelt (D) was concerned enough about the aggressive physician lobbying that he dropped his consideration of including health insurance as a part of Social Security legislation, for fear of it causing the legislation to go down in defeat. The quest for national health insurance received its final blow with the defeat of President Truman's (D) Fair Deal (1949). With this defeat, the Democrats realized they needed to change strategies and, while pursuing the ideal of national health insurance in some format, they began to do so on an incremental basis. Three significant healthcare laws passed under President Truman (D): the National Mental Health Act (1946) established the National Institute of Mental Health, the Hospital Survey and Construction Act (1946), also known as the Hill-Burton Act, had a goal of establishing 4.5 beds per 1000 people and required participating hospitals to provide uncompensated care, and the Federal Water Pollution Control Act (1948) provided federal funds for the elimination of waste from tributaries.

Due to post-World War II wages and price freezes, employers were unable to provide their employees with additional cash wages. In an effort to provide some type of pay increase, employers began providing employees with non-cash wage benefits in the form of health insurance coverage. In 1949, the Supreme Court upheld a National Labor Relations ruling allowing benefits to include in collective bargaining, and in 1954, health insurance premiums were declared a tax exemption for businesses.

During the decades of the 1940s and 1950s, the public became aware that healthcare needs of the elderly were often not addressed, or addressed in a limited fashion, due to their lack of financial resources. Thus, the Kerr-Mills bill (1960) was passed to provide funding for states to care for the poor elderly, and although the bill was helpful, it was incomplete. The major healthcare legislation that came from the 1960s is Medicare (1965) and Medicaid (1965). The battle for these two bills was legendary, with the AMA opposing them until after their passage, and was remarkable and exemplary for how President Lyndon B. Johnson (D) managed the legislative and implementation processes. This legislation ushered the United States into the provision of national health insurance for the general population, albeit to limited populations.

The 1970s and 1980s continued to witness a flurry of legislative and administrative activity, with the result of the activity primarily being incremental increases in programs ensuring access and legislation addressing the increasing cost of healthcare services. The most significant of these legislative actions was the Social Security Act of 1983 (Prospective Payment Act) that ushered in bundled payments based on diagnostic and historic data. The hospital prospective payment system was introduced as Diagnostic Related Groups (DRG) in 1983; the Outpatient Prospective Payment System consisting of Ambulatory Payment Classifications (APC) for hospital-based outpatient services and Current Procedural Terminology (CPT) for other outpatient-based services were launched in 2000.

One federal law enacted in the 1970s—not often associated by the public with health care, although it has had profound, long-term effects on state-level healthcare reform efforts—is the Employee Retirement and Income Security Act (ERISA). ERISA was intended to accomplish (in addition to many other goals) two healthcare goals: to establish a legal requirement for basic health insurance portability and to preempt state insurance regulators from oversight of "self-insured" health plans. Although ERISA established a legal basis for health insurance portability, it was found to be ineffective in practice. Today, we refer to this health insurance portability as "COBRA" after the 1985 Consolidated OmniBus Reconciliation Act (COBRA) that strengthened the requirement for insurers to offer portability at a stable price for a set time period.

The long-term effect of ERISA that most affected healthcare reform efforts at the state level (prior to Chapter 58 of Acts of 2006 of the state of Massachusetts) was the preemption of state insurance commissions from oversight of self-insured health plans. Prior to ERISA, state insurance commissions were believed to hold regulatory oversight over these plans. This was due to the phrasing used to describe these employer benefit plans as "self-insured." The term is a layperson's phrase that means the absence of an actuarially determined financial instrument. The high capital requirements necessary to operate self-insured health plans restrict this option to medium or large firms. The preemption of state oversight of these "health insurance" plans removed the richest source of employer-based covered lives from healthcare coverage risk pools. It was not until the 2006 Massachusetts healthcare reform that a state found a path around this preemption (see Section PPACA).

The 1990s were noteworthy for continued activity addressing cost and access to care with four remarkable additions. The first of these additions was an administrative act, with President George H.W. Bush (R) establishing the National Committee on Quality Assurance (1990) that broadened the federal government's list of concerns from access and cost to include quality.

One of the healthcare system's greatest obstacles has been defining quality. Providers do not seek to provide poor care, yet they have trouble defining quality care. Most recently, quality has been defined by adherence to evidence-based practices and the patient's perception of the care episode. The next noteworthy action was the attempt by President Bill Clinton (D) to establish a national health system through this Health Security Plan (1993). This plan was burdened with a number of political problems and, ultimately, never made it to legislation.

The third noteworthy action was the Health Insurance Portability and Accountability Act (HIPAA) (1996) that was passed by both houses of Congress and signed into law by President Clinton (D). This law, which was designed to provide portability of health insurance and administrative simplification, updated the confidentiality law of 1970. The fourth activity was an attempt to control healthcare costs by a shift from fee-for-service payment to capitated payment under managed care companies. While the managed care companies were successful in controlling costs, the treatment restrictions they implemented to achieve those cost savings were so draconian that they resulted in over 1000 state laws that essentially said, "You can't do that." As a result of this backlash, managed care companies greatly moderated their approach and introduced Preferred Provider Organizations (PPO) that have become the most common type of health insurance over the past 20 years.

The year 2000 to the present saw a continued activity on the access, cost, and quality themes with three major legislative actions. The first was the Medicare Drug Improvement and Modernization Act (2003), signed into law by President George W. Bush (R), primarily known for providing prescription drug coverage for Medicare recipients. The second legislative action was the American Recovery and Reinvestment Act (2009) that included the Health Information Technology for Economic and Clinical Health Act (HITECH) (Title XIII) that provided incentives for the implementation of electronic medical records throughout healthcare organizations in a meaningful fashion. The third legislative action was the Patient Protection and Affordable Care Act (PPACA) (2010) that sought to increase access for uninsured individuals, decrease cost, increase incentives for quality, and provide incentives to test innovative care delivery and payment models. This act has been noted for the polarizing politics that surrounded its development and passage (no Republicans voted for it) and the ineptitude and variability, demonstrated in its aggressive implementation (e.g., health insurance exchanges), and the substantive legal challenges it has endured. The HITECH and PPACA are noteworthy for the coercive negative reimbursement associated with several of their programs (e.g., meaningful use, value-based purchasing, ACO negative risk sharing).

Undoubtedly, the past 100 years have witnessed a flurry of administrative, legislative, and judicial action regarding how health care is delivered in the United States. The United States has moved from President Franklin Pierce, who in 1854 stated that social support matters were the responsibility of the state, to legislation that has shared that responsibility with the states (Medicaid), to moving more aggressively toward federal responsibility

(PPACA). As evidenced by current political turmoil, this journey is not over and will certainly continue through national shifts in political aptitude and power.

▶ PPACA[3]

The passage of the Patient Protection and Affordable Care Act (PL 111-148 and PL 111-152) was an attempt by Congress to increase access, increase quality, and decrease the cost of healthcare services. Its subsequent signing into law by President Barack Obama (D) on March 23, 2010, was the natural culmination of over 100 years of iterative policy decisions and development (see Chapter 1, Table 1.1). Upon close examination of the PPACA, it is clear that there is nothing new in this law. Every policy idea in this law has either been tried at a lower level of government or been discussed in policy circles for decades. For a quick summary of the title names and numbers of subtitles, parts, and sections, see **TABLE 2.1**. In the following sections, we provide three policy development examples: first, how states worked as innovators leading the way on coverage of children up to 26 years of age; second, how a policy progresses through iterative steps with the concept of an individual mandate and health exchange beginning with the Republicans during the Nixon (R) administration and ending up as a Democratic concept in the PPACA; third, how the administrative branch used Medicare waivers as a tool for testing innovative ideas during the George W. Bush administration

---

3 Republicans have vowed since the passage of this law to repeal it and replace it with "something better" that has yet to be defined. After taking control of the presidency, Senate, and House of Representatives in 2016, they attempted numerous times to repeal and replace this law and have not been able to bring their caucus to agreement on what a repeal and replacement would look like. Congress was successful in repealing the tax penalty for not complying with the individual mandate through tax reform (PL 115-97) legislation. We believe that it is unlikely they will achieve this goal and that the PPACA will follow the pattern of other legislation by being continually revised and updated to accommodate the needs of the populace and nation. Due to unsuccessful legislative repeal, the executive branch is attempting to weaken the PPACA through the administrative rules process.

TABLE 2.1 Titles Within PPACA and HCEARA

PL 111-148—Patient Protection and Affordable Care Act

Title	Topic	Subtitles	Parts	Sections
I	Quality, Affordable Health Care for All Americans	7	11	72
II	Role of Public Programs	11	0	41
III	Improving the Quality and Efficiency of Health Care	7	6	95
IV	Prevention of Chronic Disease and Improvement of Public Health	5	0	27
V	Healthcare Workforce	8	0	48
VI	Transparency and Program Integrity	8	2	49
VII	Improving Access to Innovative Medical Therapies	2	0	8
VIII	CLASS Act	0	0	2
IX	Revenue Provisions	2	0	20
X	Strengthening Quality Affordable Health Care for All Americans	8	2	84
PL 111-152 Health Care and Education Reconciliation Act of 2010				
I	Coverage, Medicare, Medicaid, and Revenues	6	0	31
II	Education and Health	2	2	19

Congress.gov.

that resulted in the CMS Innovation Center and Accountable Care Organizations (ACOs).

Coverage of Dependent Children up to 26 Years Age

Title I (A)(II)(2714) of the PPACA provides for the coverage of children "... until the child turns 26 years age." As with many other sections of the PPACA, this idea was adopted from similar statutes enacted by 31 states (NCSL, 2016). These states had a variety of requirements for children to be between the ages of 19 and 25 years and to be either single, dependent, in college, or some combination of these three. In contrast, the PPACA allows any child between the ages of 19 and 25 years to continue to get coverage through their parent's health insurance regardless of marital status or dependency. The restrictions of this plan include limitation of the coverage to the child and do not include coverage of a grandchild (child of the child) or spouse. Levine, McKnight, and Heep (2011) found that the state plans resulted in an increase in insurance coverage for the 19–25 years age group of approximately 3%. Meanwhile, the PPACA has demonstrated an increase of this same age group of 10%, or 3.2 million young adults, resulting in decreasing the uninsured rate for this age cohort from 30% in 2010 to 14.9% in 2016 (Gallop, 2016; NCSL, 2016).

Health Insurance Exchanges

A major premise of the U.S. health system is that access to healthcare services is linked to payment and payment is linked to possession of health insurance. In an effort to address the uninsured, Congress mandated that all Americans have health insurance or pay a penalty (tax), unless the purchase of health insurance posed a significant hardship, defined as 8% of gross adjusted income. Congress also provided expanded Medicaid for individuals under 138% of the poverty level and an individual market health insurance exchange for individuals between 133% and 400% of the federal poverty level. In an effort to blunt the financial impact to low-income families, Congress provided premium subsidies, with the largest of the subsidies going to individuals and families between 133% and 250% of the federal poverty level.

The concept of an exchange for the purchase of health insurance was alluded to by Butler (1989) in his discussion of a conservative plan for healthcare reform that advocated for a transfer of the tax credit to individuals, including a mandate for coverage and some type of purchasing alliance, and described by Enthoven (1993) in his discussion of managed competition. Just prior to the enactment of the PPACA, the Massachusetts Health Plan (2006) included a mandate for the possession of health insurance coverage and the Massachusetts Corridor (exchange) for the purchase of individual policies. One lesson learned from the Massachusetts Plan was the need for counselors to assist individuals in the sorting out of insurance needs and options (AHRQ, 2013). This resulted in the PPACA provision of grant funding to train navigators to provide this assistance to individuals seeking policies on the Health Insurance Exchange (Marketplace; PL 111-148 (III)(F)(3510)).

Implementation of the Health Insurance Marketplace was challenged by a number of barriers, including Supreme Court challenges to the individual mandate, Medicaid expansion regulations, vendor performance, management oversight and involvement, and time. Within hours of President Obama signing the PPACA into law, lawsuits were filed by state attorney generals and industry groups to block the law and to question the constitutionality of portions of the law, such as the individual mandate. These lawsuits were combined *in National Federation of Independent Businesses et al. v. Sebelius, Secretary of Health and Human Services, et al. (No. 11–393) including Department of Health and Human Services et al. v. Florida et al. (No. 11–398), and Florida et al. v. Department of Health and Human Services et al. (No. 11–400)*; argued: March 26, 27, and 28, 2012, and decided: June 28, 2012. In this case, the Supreme Court ruled in part for the United States that the individual mandate and the tax (penalty) were constitutional and in part against the United States that the requirement of the states expanding Medicaid or losing all Medicaid funding was too coercive. This ruling had several practical implementation ramifications, including at minimum, a loss of 2 years of preparation time for development of the exchange and a flurry of legislative activities in the states as they debated if or how to expand Medicaid.

When the Health Insurance Marketplace opened in the fall of 2013, 24 states had developed their own exchanges and 36 defaulted, either completely or in some type of hybrid fashion, to the federal exchanges. The initial debut of federal health insurance marketplaces was bereft of technical and design precision, resulting in multiple consumer delays and frustrations. The Department of Health and Human Services (HHS) immediately began a process of addressing and remediating these problems with changes in vendors and CMS managers that addressed these problems. Unfortunately, the negative consumer experiences had already sullied the exchange, despite continuously improved technical performance during the initial and subsequent years. Development of the federal health insurance exchange was a complex process that included the functions of linking the various private insurance options with income verification through the IRS and citizenship

through the Department of Homeland Security. One argument in favor of the vendors is that due to the legal challenges, they were deprived of adequate time to appropriately develop and test this IT infrastructure. The counterarguments include vendor incompetence, lack of CMS management supervision, and political unwillingness to delay implementation to provide additional time for IT development. Regardless, the functionality of the exchanges has steadily improved and is now working fairly well (from a consumer lens), although not all of the intergovernmental department links have been established.

The prime rationale for the health exchanges was to allow a greater number of individuals the option, although a mandatory option, to gain access to healthcare services via the purchase of a health insurance policy meeting a predefined minimum standard. There is no doubt that the uninsured rate has dropped since the implementation of expanded Medicaid and the Health Insurance Marketplace (see **TABLE 2.2**); however, the increase in

TABLE 2.2 Uninsured Rate, Health Insurance Exchange Estimates, and Actual Enrollment

Year	Uninsured Rate Q1 (%)	CBO Estimates (millions)	Enrolled (millions)
2010	16.0	–	–
2011	15.7	–	–
2012	17.3	–	–
2013	16.3	–	–
2014	15.6	13.0	8.0
2015	14.0	20.0	11.7
2016	11.0	25.0	12.0

ASPE Issue Brief Health Insurance Marketplace Premiums for 2014, 2015, 2016, and 2017.

the number of individuals possessing health insurance policies has underperformed estimates by the CBO, while the number of individuals added to the Medicaid roles has exceeded expectations. Two reasons (one negative and one positive) have been frequently cited as the cause for the under enrollment in the health insurance exchanges: (1) under enrollment of the 18- to 35-years age group and (2) an unexpected number of small businesses continuing health insurance to their employees as opposed to dropping coverage, paying the penalty for not offering coverage, and sending their employees to the Health Insurance Marketplace.

Finally, the insurance product defined by the PPACA has a set of 10 requirements, a set of actuarial values for consumers to choose from, and a requirement that rate increases be approved by both the state insurance regulatory agency and CMS. The actuarial values are 90% (platinum), 80% (gold), 70% (silver),

and 60% (bronze). What the actuarial value means is that the insurance plan would pay for the actuarial value and the consumer would be responsible for the remaining portion. Another requirement written into the PPACA was that these plans had to be based on a community rating that included age, gender, and smoking history, with a 1:3 spread being the maximum allowed difference in premiums. The factors of a new product, narrow allowable actuarial rating knowledge, and competitiveness resulted in these products having very low initial prices. The result of these low prices and the effect of adverse selection resulted in large annual losses for insurance companies. Due to the large losses, several insurance companies exited selected unprofitable markets, completely exited the health insurance exchange, or requested large annual premium increases that have frequently been approved. **TABLE 2.3** demonstrates the national averages and increases for these insurance plans.

TABLE 2.3 Insurance Plan Averages and Increases

| Year | 27-Year-Old Before Tax Credit | | | | 27-Year-Old with Income of $25,000 | | Family of Four with Income of $50,000 | |
	Lowest Bronze	Lowest Silver	Lowest Gold	Lowest Catastrophic	Second Lowest Silver Before Tax Credit	Second Lowest Silver After Tax Credit	Second Lowest Silver Before Tax Credit	Second Lowest Silver After Tax Credit
2014	$165	$204	$222	$149	$208	$145	$753	$282
2015	$265	$336	$382	$439	$222	$143	$803	$407
2016	$294	$359	$406	$550	$240	$143	$896	$405
2017	$366	$433	$538	$674	$303	$142	$1090	$405

ASPE Issue Brief Health Insurance Marketplace Premiums for 2014, 2015, 2016, and 2017.

Accountable Care Organizations

Accountable Care Organizations (ACOs) appear in Section 2706 Pediatric Accountable Care Organization Demonstration Project and Section 3022 Medicare Shared Savings Program of the PPACA. In both of these sections, the ACOs must "… be willing to become accountable for the quality, cost, and overall care …" (Sec. 1899 (2)(A)) of their assigned beneficiaries. This accountability for the care of these beneficiaries is achieved through deliberately planned coordination of beneficiary care.

ACOs can best be understood by first gaining an understanding of "Care Organizations" and then a discussion of "Accountability." Care Organizations have been around for a long time and refer first to a group of physicians who have agreed to work through a network concept to provide coordinated care for a group of beneficiaries. Care Organizations can take the organizational form of highly organized business models, such as large multispecialty group practices (e.g., the Mayo Clinic or Cleveland Clinic) or a network of independent physician practices that have agreed to work together in a coordinated manner. Two federal examples of Care Organizations are HRSA-sponsored rural networks and the Geisinger Cardiac Trial (Medicare Waiver). In both of these examples, the act of coordination of care and fluid communication that accompanied it has resulted in greatly reduced fragmentation of care, increased quality of care and health outcomes, and financial savings of several million dollars.

The initial literature on ACOs described groups of physicians that would come together as a legal entity and then enter into additional network agreements with other institutional providers, such as hospitals (Bard & Nugent, 2011). As this concept matured, physician groups found themselves to be undercapitalized and underprepared as professional managers needing to establish and manage these complex organizations. While organizing a network of physicians remains the core concept of ACOs, the organization and management of them has been absorbed by health systems that have greater capital and managerial resources. Since 2010, hospitals and health systems have embarked on a process of vertical integration that has included the purchase of physician practices, allowing them to develop the organizational depth necessary to develop ACOs and positively respond to many other PPACA care coordination and payment provisions. Once a care organization has become a legal entity, it can begin to bill Medicare for services and take on the "accountability" role for the "… cost, quality, and overall care …" of Medicare beneficiaries.[4]

ACOs are an organizational model still under fee-for-service payment, but with risk component associated with the quality of patient outcomes. CMS has a very detailed process for ACOs to determine their performance benchmarks and an equally detained process for determining quality performance. Under the Shared Savings Program, ACOs can agree to a one-sided (positive risk) option with payment ranges of 2%–3.9% or two-sided (positive and negative risk) agreements with payment options of 2%. CMS recommends that organizations with limited to no experience managing care coordination, quality, and patient outcomes choose the one-sided risk option until they gain adequate experience. The two-sided (risk) shared savings program is only suitable for organizations that have extensive experience managing patients in a coordinated manner,

---

4   In the current environment, "Accountable Care Organization" is a legal term used by CMS for Medicare payment, whereas "Clinically Integrated Network" is an equivalent care coordination and payment model associated with non-Medicare beneficiaries.

including robust tracking of patient quality and outcomes. For example, two-thirds of the initial ACO programs (CMS referred to these as Pioneers) have left due to their inability to absorb the negative risk. All of the "exited" organizations from the Pioneer ACO program are well-developed and well-managed healthcare organizations. These organizations remain committed to the ACO model but are simply not yet able to sustain the risk associated with the Pioneer ACO program. For CY 2015, the mean shared savings for the remaining Pioneer ACOs was $3 million, with a range of savings from $24.5 million to $1.6 million.

▶ Physician Payment: Usual, Customary, and Reasonable to MACRA

The federal government entered into the realm of physician payment with the passage of Medicare and Medicaid in 1965. Medicare was patterned after the 1960s-era Blue Cross and Blue Shield program. Thus, physician payment followed suit, patterning physician payment on these same plans and paying physicians based on usual, customary, and reasonable charges. Usual, customary, and reasonable charges paid physicians whatever they billed, so long as it was in line with similar bills for physician services or procedures within the geographic area.

Due to the lack of payment controls built into this payment model, physician payments grew at a steady and rapid pace, resulting in Medicare Part B (75% payment for physician services) becoming the largest domestic program funded through general revenues by the mid-1980s. Congress addressed this rapid physician payment growth in the Omnibus Reconciliation Act of 1989 (PL 101-239) by establishing a physician fee schedule based on the value of physician services provided.

The model for valuing physician services was established through Resource-Based Relative Value Scale (RBRVS), which considers "… the relative value of the work, practice expenses, and malpractice risks associated with each physician service" (PL 101-239), and took into consideration geographic variation, inflation, changes in demand, service-related technology, and inadequate access. This bill also sought to cap payment for physician services by setting the increase in unit service inversely proportional to past increases in service quantity. This rationale resulted in the establishment of Medicare Volume Performance Standards (MVPS) in 1992 that initially decreased the growth rate in payment for physician services. Eventually, surgeons and primary care physicians found these caps to be disadvantageous, petitioned Congress, and received separate surgical and primary care caps.

Decreased growth in physician payment did not last long, causing Congress to address rapidly growing physician payment again in the Balanced Budget Act of 1997 (PL 105-33). This legislation replaced the Medicare Volume Performance Standard with the Sustainable Growth Rate (SGR). The SGR calculation included (1) the estimated percentage change in fee for physician services, (2) the estimated percentage change in the average number of Medicare fee-for-service beneficiaries, (3) the estimated 10-year average annual percentage change in real gross domestic product per capita, and (4) the estimated percentage change in expenditures due to changes in regulations (Spilberg, 2014). As with MVPS, the SGR initially controlled physician expenditures; however, beginning in 2002, the SGR resulted in a negative increase of 4.8%, with the subsequent 12 years of negative increases culminating in a 2014 negative increase of 20%. Congress did not allow any of these negative increases to proceed, and, as a result of physician lobbying, passed legislation every year from 2002 to 2014 to reverse the negative increase and provide for a modest annual increase of no more than 2%. Finally, in 2015, both parties in Congress and the physicians had enough of this annual event and passed the Medicare Access and CHIP Reauthorization Act of 2015 (MACRA).

MACRA is a bipartisan statute commonly referred to as the permanent doc fix that passed by wide margins in both chambers of Congress (House R-212 & D-180; Senate R-46, D-44, & I-2) and was signed into law on April 16, 2015. MACRA consolidated physician reporting and payment into either the Merit-based Incentive Payment System (MIPS) or the Alternative Payment Models (APM). MIPS consolidated reporting by replacing Physician Quality Reporting System, Meaningful Use, and the Value-Based Modifier and adding Improvement Activities. The Physician Quality Reporting System (PQRS) was established in 2006 as part of the Tax Relief and Health Care Act (PL 109-432) to provide incentives for reporting quality data to Medicare. These quality data were based on a list of quality measures that were chosen by and appropriate for the type of practice. Meaningful Use came out of the American Recovery and Reinvestment Act of 2009 (PL 111-5) and incented physician practices and other healthcare organizations for acquiring and using an electronic medical record in a meaningful way. Meaningful use incentives were staggered over a series of years, with reporting requirements increasing in number and complexity over time and the rewards of participation more generous to the voluntary early adopters and coercive to those who resisted. The Value-Based Modifier is applied to the physician fee schedule and rewards physicians for providing high-quality care at a low cost. Finally, Improvement Activities reward physicians for providing care focused on care coordination, patient engagement, and patient safety. Alternative Payment Models (APMs) are programs such as ACOs that provide physicians with 5% additional incentive for assuming some risk in

the provision of high-quality care for patients with specific clinical conditions, episodes of care, or populations. Of note, CMS does not recommend physicians choose this option without previous experience with risk-based contracts.

Since 1965 when the federal government entered the realm of physician payment, they have consistently sought to pay physicians appropriately for the services they have provided. What has changed over the years has been the desire to control the growth and predictability of payments. Since 2006, additional measures associated with payment have included quality of care, patient safety, and use of an electronic medical record in a meaningful way. Stated otherwise, we have moved from paying for cost to paying for value (quality/cost).

▶ Legislation 2010 and Forward

Since passage of the Patient Protection and Affordable Care act in 2009, there have been numerous unsuccessful attempts by Republicans to repeal the PPACA, such as the American Health Care Act (House—passed), Better Care Reconciliation Act (Senate—failed), Health Care Freedom Act (Senate—failed), and American Health Care Act (Senate—failed). These bills all failed due to the inability of the Republican caucus to coalesce around support for a replacement bill that maintained their principles of small federal government, while not taking away healthcare access that many of their constituents deemed important. The Republicans were successful in passing tax reform legislation (PL 115-97) that repealed the tax penalty for not possessing health insurance (Part VIII, Sec. 11081).

The other noteworthy healthcare legislation passed during this period was the 21st Century Cures Act (PL 114-225). This is a lengthy piece of legislation with 18 titles, 24 subtitles, and 228 sections. As the bill is lengthy, it can be divided into three main sections: 5 titles and 116 sections address research funding, leadership, and reporting requirements; 9 titles and 87 sections address mental health programs, payment, and access; 4 titles and 25 sections address Medicare and Medicaid access, continuation of services, and payment.

▶ Federalism

Unitary, confederation, and federal are three common models of national or central government. Unitary central government is an approach used by the British, in which a central authority controls all levels of government and makes laws that are administered locally. Confederation is an approach where a voluntary group of states choose to associate with a central government. Within this model, if the states are weak, the central government is strong, and if the states are strong, the central government is weak. Federalism is an approach to governance that attempts to balance the power between a central or federal government and its provinces or states. In the United States, the need for this form of governance was driven by a lack of trust and a history of negative experiences with a strong British central government. This lack of trust resulted in our founders adopting the Articles of Confederation in 1777 (see **TABLE 2.4**) that provided for an extremely weak central government and strong state governments. The Articles of Confederation eventually proved to be untenable due to states acting like their own countries, performing acts such

TABLE 2.4 Articles of Confederation, Constitution, and Bill of Rights		
Document	**Action**	**Date**
Articles of Confederation	Adopted	November 1777
Articles of Confederation	Ratified by all 13 states	March 1781
Articles of Confederation	Congress approved a convention for revision	February 1787
Constitutional Convention	U.S. Constitution written	May–September 1787
U.S. Constitution	Adopted	September 1787
U.S. Constitution	Ratified by 9 of 13 states	July 1788
Bill of Rights	Approved by Congress	September 1789
U.S. Constitution	Ratified by all 13 states	May 1790
Bill of Rights	Ratified by 10 of 14 states	December 1791

Library of Congress.

as printing their own currency and charging tariffs on goods and merchandise crossing state borders. Ultimately, these actions caused Congress to approve a constitutional convention in 1787 to address its weaknesses and provide recommendations to strengthen it. This constitutional convention convened in Philadelphia from May to September of 1787. Much to the dismay of Congress, it found the Articles of Confederation beyond repair and produced a new U.S. Constitution. Following some acrimonious debate about the members of the constitutional convention exceeding their charter, Congress adopted the U.S. Constitution in September 1787.

The new U.S. Constitution first addressed the separation of powers by assigning legislative responsibilities to Congress (Article 1), executive responsibilities to the President (Article 2), and judicial responsibilities to the Supreme Court (Article 3). Article 4 delineates the federal government's responsibility to the states and citizens including: assurance of public acts, proceedings, and judicial records (section 1), citizen rights (section 2), admittance of new states (section 3), and a Republican form of government (section 4). Additionally, the Constitution provided for the approval of amendments to the Constitution (Article 5) and assurances that debts and legal agreements will be honored as the supreme law of the land and that all governmental officials will be bound by oath to support the Constitution (Article 6), and that nine states are required to ratify the Constitution (Article 7).

Over the next 10 months, the Constitution was heatedly debated in the public and 13 state legislatures, with most of the debate focused on the absence of individual and states' rights. Several states were only ameliorated when a bill of 12 rights was produced (only 10 passed) and included in the debate. In September 1788, nine states had ratified the Constitution, and 1 year later, in September 1789, Congress approved a bill of 10 rights. While the Constitution delineated federal responsibilities and powers, the limits of their encroaching powers on the states are only ensured by the Tenth Amendment that states:

> The powers not delegated to the United States by the Constitution, nor prohibited by it to the States, are reserved to the States respectively, or to the people.

Once the Bill of Rights was approved by Congress, the remaining four states ratified the Constitution by May 1790. Since the Bill of Rights were amendments to the Constitution, they had to be ratified by two-thirds of the states, with that threshold reached in December 1791.

While the Constitution and Bill of Rights balances federal and state responsibilities, there is a level of ambiguity to these responsibilities that allows this balance to adapt to different times and situations (Holahan, Weil, & Wiener, 2003). In the United States, we have experienced at least seven eras of federalism (see **TABLE 2.5**). The first era, Dual Federalism (1789–1933), was the longest and included the most distinct roles for the federal and state governments that later came to be known as layer-cake federalism. The next two eras, Cooperative Federalism (1933–1960) and Creative Federalism (1960–1968), ushered in a time when the federal government developed programs that were implemented at the state and local levels with federal funding and policy guidance. The intergovernmental exchange initiated by these two eras, and the subsequent ones that followed, became known as marble-cake federalism, with the most well-known and successful of its programs being Medicaid. Finally, the last four eras, New Federalism (1968–1980), New New Federalism (1980–1993), Devolution (1993–2008), and Deep Devolution (2009–2016), are all characterized by progressively providing states with

TABLE 2.5 Federalism Eras	
Era	**Characteristics**
Dual Federalism (1789–1933)	Distinct federal and state roles
Cooperative Federalism (1933–1960)	New deal programs; federal grants-in-aid to address state and local needs
Creative Federalism (1960–1968)	Great society programs; doubling federal grants-in-aid amount with increased number of more narrowly focused programs
New Federalism (1968–1980)	Provided states federal funds with more policy-making discretion
New New Federalism (1980–1993)	Less federal money to states with more control given to states and increased unfunded mandates
Devolution (1993–2008)	Return of power and legislative authority to states for development of policies addressing local problems
Deep Devolution (2009–2016)	More federal aid to states and cities with increased federal control

Modified from Starling, G. (2011). *Managing the public sector* (9th ed.). Boston, MA: Wadsworth Cengage Learning.

fewer federal funds and greater control over policy and program development details. These eras are well known for considering states as laboratories for the experimentation of social programs and the waivers allowing the use of federal funds for programs tailored to state needs.

▶ Federal Executive Branch Roles

Executive branch agencies implement the policies enacted by Congress and signed into law by the President. Executive branch agencies at all three levels of governance carry out the day-to-day government operations. Approximately 2000 positions across all federal agencies are appointees, that is, are filled directly by presidential nominations and are not civil service positions. Of those 2000, almost 500 require Senate confirmation before being filled. Despite the large number of appointed positions, most of those filling these positions are careerists.

HHS contains all of the healthcare agencies, along with most components of public health (see organization chart in **FIGURE 2.1**).[5] For health administrators, the most important

---

5 The Environmental Protection Agency houses the environmental health component and the Food and Drug Administration, within the Department of Agriculture, houses the food safety components of public health.

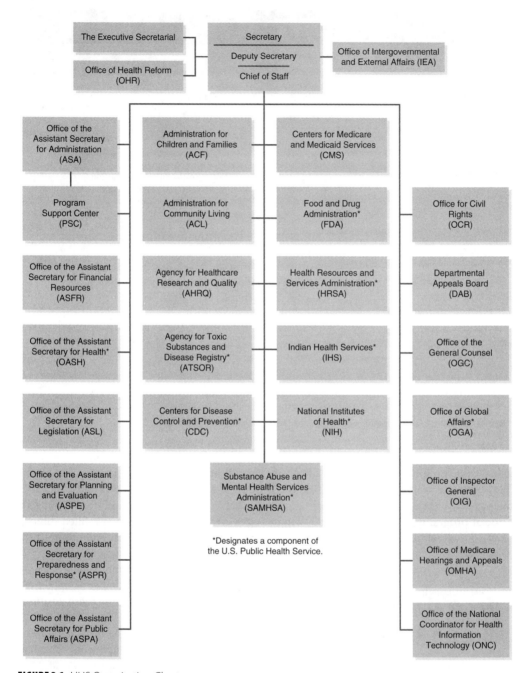

FIGURE 2.1 HHS Organization Chart

https://www.hhs.gov/about/agencies/orgchart/index.html#

agencies within HHS are the Centers for Medicare and Medicaid Services (CMS), the Health Resources and Services Administration (HRSA), the Agency for Healthcare Research and Quality (AHRQ), the Substance Abuse and Mental Health Services Administration (SAMHSA), and the Centers for Disease Control and Prevention (CDC).

Referring to **FIGURE 2.2**, it is easily discernible that the largest of these is the CMS, with over three-quarters of the budgetary outlays for all of the HHS.

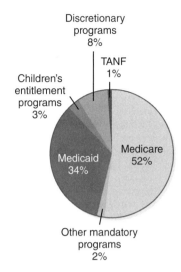

FIGURE 2.2 Federal Healthcare Spending

U.S. Department of Health & Human Services. Federal Tax Policy Center. Retrieved from https://www .taxpolicycenter.org/briefing-book/how-much-does-federal-government-spend-health-care

References

AHRQ Research Activities. (2013, November–December). Based on the Massachusetts experience, consumers will need help navigating health insurance exchanges. Retrieved from http://www.ahrq.gov /news/newsletters/research-activities/13nov-dec /111213ra13.html

American Medical Association. (1847). *Proceedings of the National Convention.* Retrieved from http://ama .nmtvault.com/jsp/viewer.jsp?doc_id=ama _arch%252FAD000001%252F0039PROC&view _width=640.0&rotation=0&query1=&collection _filter=All&collection_name=6863b9b4-a8b5-4ea0 -9e63-ca2ed554e876&zoom_factor=current& search_doc=license&sort_col=publication+date& highlightColor=yellow&color=&CurSearchNum =-1&search_doc1=license&submit.x=0&submit .y=0&page_name=&page_name=

ASPE Issue Brief. Health plan choice and premiums in the 2015 health insurance marketplace. Retrieved from https://aspe.hhs.gov/sites/default/files/pdf/77176 /healthPremium2015.pdf

ASPE Issue Brief. Health plan choice and premiums in the 2016 health insurance marketplace. Retrieved from https://aspe.hhs.gov/sites/default/files/pdf/135461 /2016%20Marketplace%20Premium%20Landscape%20 Issue%20Brief%2010-30-15%20FINAL.pdf

ASPE Issue Brief. Health plan choice and premiums in the 2017 health insurance marketplace. Retrieved from https://aspe.hhs.gov/sites/default/files/pdf/212721 /2017MarketplaceLandscapeBrief.pdf

Bard, M., & Nugent, M. (2011). *Accountable care organizations: Your guide to strategy, design, and implementation.* Chicago, IL: Health Administration Press.

Blumenthal, D., & Monroe, J. A. (2009). *The heart of power: Health and politics in the oval office.* Berkeley: University of California Press.

Butler, S. M. (1989). Assuring affordable health care for all Americans. *The heritage lectures.* Washington, DC: The Heritage Foundation.

CDC. (2016). Social determinants of health—Definitions. Retrieved from http://www.cdc.gov/socialdeterminants /Definitions.htm

Enthoven, A. C. (1993). The history and principles of managed competition. *Health Affairs, 12,* 24.

Friedman, M. (2014). 'Any willing provider' returns. *Arkansas Business, 31*(13), 48. Retrieved from http://search.proquest.com.ezproxy.gvsu.edu /docview/1524650432?accountid=39473

Furman, A. B. (2004). Federal versus state regulation of insurance: An update. *The Investment Lawyer, 11*(12), 21.

Gallop, Well-Being Poll. (2016). Retrieved from http:// www.gallup.com/topic/category_wellbeing.aspx

Holahan, J., Weil, A., & Wiener, J. M. (2003). *Federalism, health, and policy*. Washington, DC: The Urban Institute Press.

HRSA Health Workforce Analysis. (2013, November). Projecting the supply and demand for primary care practitioners through 2020. Retrieved from https://bhw.hrsa.gov/health-workforce-analysis/primary-care-2020

Levine, P. B., McKnight, R., & Heep, S. (2011). How effective are public policies to increase health insurance coverage among young adults? *American Economic Journal: Economic Policy, 3*, 129–156.

McCarthy, D. (1997, Spring). Narrowing provider choice: Any willing provider laws after New York Blue Cross v. Travelers. *American Journal of Law & Medicine, 23*(1), 97–113. Retrieved from http://go.galegroup.com/ps/i.do?p=HRCA&sw=w&u=lom_gvalleysu&v=2.1&it=r&id=GALE%7CA19552665&sid=summon&asid=4d9b921618f64a972146c71e965962b7

Medicare.Gov. (2015). Linking quality to payment. Retrieved from http://www.medicare.gov/hospitalcompare/linking-quality-to-payment.html?AspxAutoDetectCookieSupport=1

National Conference of State Legislatures. (2014). Any willing or authorized providers. Retrieved from http://www.ncsl.org/research/health/any-willing-or-authorized-providers.aspx

National Conference of State Legislatures. (2016). Dependent health coverage and age for healthcare benefits. Retrieved from http://www.ncsl.org/research/health/dependent-health-coverage-state-implementation.aspx

Occupational Safety & Health Act—PL 91-596.

Safe Drinking Water Act—PL 93-523.

Spilberg, G., Nicola, G. N., Rosenkrantz, A. B., Silva, E., III, Schirmer, C. M., Ghoshhajra, B. B., . . . Hirsch, J. A. (2018). Understanding the impact of 'cost' under MACRA: A neurointerventional imperative. *Journal of NeuroInterventional Surgery, 10*(10), 1005–1011. doi:10.1136/neurintsurg-2018-013972

Starling, G. (2011). *Managing the public sector* (9th ed.). Boston, MA: Wadsworth Cengage Learning.

Ungar, R. (2011). Congress passes socialized medicine and mandates health insurance—In 1798. *Forbes*. Retrieved from https://www.forbes.com/sites/rickungar/2011/01/17/congress-passes-socialized-medicine-and-mandates-health-insurance-in-1798/#7ec0c3b553ff

WHO. (2015). Social determinants of health. Retrieved from http://www.who.int/social_determinants/sdh_definition/en/

Appendix

Patient Protection and Affordable Care Act

The Patient Protection and Affordable Care Act (PL 111-148 & 111-152), signed into law on March 23, 2010, is a comprehensive health reform act with 10 titles.

Title I has 7 subtitles, 11 parts, and 72 sections. Subtitle A seeks to increase access to health insurance coverage by expanding existing coverage, such as to adult children up to age 26 years, ensuring coverage of preventative services, or limiting health insurers from discriminating against coverage through tactics such as recessions or lifetime coverage limits. Other actions include efforts to decrease the cost of care and ensure high-quality care delivery. Subtitle B seeks to ensure coverage by not allowing denial of health insurance coverage due to preexisting illness, reinsurance for early retirees, and consumer assistance in locating an affordable health insurance plan. Subtitle C focuses on topics such a nondiscrimination in health insurance, guaranteed issuance, and guaranteed reissuance. Subtitle D provides a detailed description of the essential elements of a qualified health plan, provision of consumer choice in health plans through health insurance exchanges, state flexibility in establishing health alternative programs through waivers, and topics related to reinsurance and risk adjustment. Subtitle E provides criteria for premium tax credits and cost-sharing reductions, eligibility, and small business tax credit. Subpart F details individual and employer responsibility for maintaining minimum health insurance coverage. Subtitle G provides a variety of sections ensuring access to services either by positively stating a protection or by negatively stating how individuals or therapies may not be excluded.

Title II has 11 subtitles, 0 parts, and 41 sections. Subtitle A provides several eligibility requirements including income requirements based on modified gross income, extended coverage to young adults graduated from the foster care system, and payment increases to territories. Subtitle B increases Federal Medical Assistance Percentage and makes technical corrections to the CHIP Reauthorization Act of 2009. Subtitle C provides for enrollment coordination with the health exchanges and allows hospitals to make presumptive Medicaid determination. Subtitle D allows for payment to freestanding birth centers, concurrent care and payment for children under hospice care, and payment to non-physician providers. Subtitle E broadens home care eligibility based on the Pepper Commission Call to Action for Elder Care and State determined plan. Subtitle F increases requirements for pharmaceutical rebates and adds to the list of nonexcludable drugs. Subtitle G provides rationale for calculating the reduction in DSH payments based on the reduction of the uninsured over the previous and current fiscal years. Subtitle H provides for a demonstration project to improve the coverage of Medicare dual eligible and establishes the CMS Federal Coordinated Health Care Office. Subtitle I requires the implementation of core quality measures and a compilation of never events that Medicaid will not pay for, plus three payment demonstration projects. Subtitle J revises Medicaid and CHIP Payment and Access Commission (MADPAC) membership, review and evaluation topics, utilization, and financial performance and requires coordination, as appropriate, with the Medicare Payment Advisory Commission (MEDPAC). Subtitle K provides for increased access to Medicaid for American Indians and makes permanent Indian hospital and clinic full Medicare Part B reimbursement. Subtitle L provides for maternal, infant, and early childhood home visits and support, education, and research on several maternal health concerns.

Title III has 7 subtitles, 6 parts, and 95 sections. Subtitle A links payment for services to patient outcomes through value-based purchasing payment effective for and tailored to all providers that bill Medicare and provides criteria for risk-adjusted reduction in payment to hospitals. Subtitle A also directs the Secretary of HHS to develop a national strategy for the improvement of patient care delivery, outcomes, population health; a process for the evaluation of patient outcome data; and collection, aggregation, and analysis of patient outcome data. Lastly, Subtitle A established the CMS Innovation Center for the testing of payment and care delivery models that enhance the effective and efficient coordination and delivery of care in a cost-effective manner. Subtitle B provides for several technical payments and care delivery technical corrections that focus on increasing beneficiary access to services through extension or enhancement of payment provisions. Subtitle C provides the Secretary of HHS the authority to expand services covered, decreased cost-sharing for beneficiaries, and increased accountability for Medicare Advantage insurers. Subtitle D provides the Secretary of HHS with the authority to increase beneficiary access to pharmaceuticals while extracting cost concessions from pharmaceutical companies and drug plans.

Subtitle E provides criteria for market basket updates and establishment of a Medicare Advisory Board to provide recommendations for maintaining solvency, reducing costs, and increasing quality of care delivery. Subtitle F provides for the funding of healthcare delivery system research determining process and approaches that improve patient care delivery and outcomes; establishment of several delivery models focused on improving patient care access, delivery, and outcomes; improvement in drug promotional literature; and establishment of the Office of Women's Health. Subtitle G ensures that Medicare benefits (including Medicare Advantage) will not be reduced and Medicare solvency will be maintained while improving access and quality of care and reducing costs.

Title IV has 5 subtitles, 0 parts, and 27 sections. Subtitle A, through the establishment of councils and task forces, seeks expert recommendations on preventive health, chronic health prevention and management, integrative practices, and health promotion, and funds programs focused on improving public health and restraining private and public health costs. Subtitle B increases access through the establishment of school-based clinics and oral health services to underserved populations; removes beneficiary costs for U.S. Preventive Services Task Force recommended preventive services; and provides for tobacco-use cessation, weight control or reduction, cholesterol reduction, blood pressure reduction, and avoidance or improved management of diabetes. Subtitle C provides funding for population health programs, negotiation with vaccine producers, restaurant nutritional labeling, and a demonstration project to determine if wellness plans reduce health risks, and requires employers with more than 50 employers provide nursing mothers with a private area to express breast milk. Subtitle D provides funding for evidence-based practices for areas identified through the National

Preventive Strategies or *Healthy People 2020*, disparities research, wellness program efficacy, pain management, and childhood obesity. Subtitle E provides a sense of the Senate and Congress on the need to work with CBO on scoring preventive programs and directs the Secretary of HHS to evaluate federal health and wellness initiatives.

Title V has 8 subtitles, 0 parts, and 48 sections. Subtitle A assesses the need for an increased healthcare workforce to meet the healthcare needs of the population and provides a variety of definitions. Subtitle B provides for the establishment of a national commission to study the need for and training of healthcare workers. Subtitle C provides for a variety of healthcare workforce development grants and student loan repayment programs. Subtitle D provides training grants for individuals preparing for careers in primary care, gerontology, and mental and behavioral health and preparing to become dentists and alternative dental providers, nurse midwives, and baccalaureate nurses and promotes positive health through community health workers and public health professionals. Subtitle E provides for the establishment of Healthcare Centers of Excellence and grant funding for the establishment or modification of health education programs and bridge programs for the accelerated advancement of associate and diploma nurses to baccalaureate level training. Subtitle F increases funding to primary care providers, provides enhanced revisions to primary care residency training, and provides grant funding for the development of new and improvement of existing advanced nurse practice programs. Subtitle G provides for enhanced access for underserved populations through Federally Qualified Health Centers and directs the Secretary of HHS to define medically underserved populations and health professional shortage areas, provisions for the location of primary care practices within community mental health practices, and the establishment and monitoring of key national health indicators. Subtitle H directs the need for annual reports from funded agencies.

Title VI has 8 subtitles, 2 parts, and 49 sections. Subtitle A focuses on physician transparency regarding hospital ownership, hospital admission when the physician is not present, alternatives to office-provided diagnostic procedures, and drug sample reporting. Subtitle B provides criteria for conflict of interest declaration by nursing home leadership, development of compliance and ethics programs, development and maintenance of a Nursing Home Compare website, and development of a complaint resolution process. Subtitle B also provides guidelines for reduction in civil monetary penalties for self-reporting deficiencies with a resolution plan, demonstration projects for monitoring large nursing home providers and development of best practices, and notification of residence upon nursing home closure. Subtitle B includes agency and contract personnel in ongoing, dementia management and patient abuse training. Subtitle C provides for the development and evaluation of a program performing background checks on all caregivers coming in direct contact with long-term patients. Subtitle D provides for the establishment of the Patient-Centered Outcomes Research Institute for the purpose of conducting patient-centered outcomes research and funded by the Patient-Centered Outcomes Research Trust Fund. Subtitle E provides criteria for screening all providers and suppliers to Medicare, Medicaid, and CHIP; enhanced oversight of new providers; establishment of a compliance program; and enhanced coordination, collection, and maintenance of fraud and abuse data. Subtitle E also requires providers ordering items on Medicare-covered beneficiaries to be enrolled in Medicare and additional enforcement mechanisms, including expansion of the Recovery Audit Contractor plan to Medicaid. Subtitle F specifies provider exclusion criteria, disallows claims for services provided outside the United States, extends time for collections, and requires use of the National Correct Coding Initiative or a similar program. Subtitle G clarifies ERISA, adds association prohibitions, directs the Secretary of HHS to develop a uniform national fraud and abuse reporting system, and enhances fraud and abuse enforcement authority. Subtitle H provides for the establishment of a council, advisory board, and forensic center for the provisions of recommendations and training on elder justice abuse, fraud, and exploitation issues. Subtitle I indicates that the Senate recognizes this is an optimal time for states to experiment with malpractice reform.

Title VII has 2 subtitles, 0 parts, and 8 sections. Subtitle A provides criteria for submission of biosimilar licensure, patent, and evaluation and requires the Secretaries of Treasury and HHS to determine associated savings and to apply any savings to debt reduction. Subtitle B expands options for previously excluded providers through use of the 340B discount option, tighter price oversight by the Secretary of HHS, and potential 340B discount expansion based on program evaluation by the U.S. Comptroller.

Title VIII is the CLASS (Community Living Assistance Services and Supports) Act with 0 subtitles, 0 parts, and 2 sections. The CLASS Act provides criteria for establishment of a national voluntary program for the purchase of long-term care insurance that allows individuals with functional limitations to secure necessary care while maintaining financial independence and prices based on actuarial analysis. This act was repealed based on a recommendation from the U.S. Actuaries Office that it was too unstable to price. Based on Multiple Streams (Kingdon, 1984 and 1995) and Multiple Streams (Baumgartner & Jones) theories, the time between when policy ideas are raised to a national level is 20 years. The first time the policy idea of long-term care

insurance was introduced was in 1988 in the Medicare Catastrophic Act that was repealed a little over 1 year later. In 2010, or 22 years later, this same idea was introduced in the Patient Protection and Affordable Care Act and subsequently repealed about 1 year later. We predict that the idea of long-term care coverage will be introduced and passed around 2030 when Baby Boom retirees are projected to peak, thus providing an enhanced political will for action.

Title IX has 2 subtitles, 0 parts, and 20 sections. Subtitle A includes a large variety of taxes, deduction limitations, charge and collection criteria, and fees and mandates an insurer medical loss ratio of 85%. A tax that has received a large amount of public attention is the 40% excise tax on Cadillac health plans. Other taxes include an increase in taxes on nonmedical withdrawals from HSAs and Archer HSAs for 15% to 20%. For nonprofits, this section includes the need to complete and act on a community needs assessment, the charging of uninsured emergency patients the lowest amount charged to those with insurance, and the disallowance of extraordinary collection activities reasonable actions have been taken to determine if the individual qualifies for financial aid. Finally, there are criteria for fees to companies providing branded and imported pharmaceuticals and durable medical equipment providers and the requirement that insurers maintain an 85% medical loss ratio. Subtitle B includes exemption benefits criteria for Indian tribal governments, criteria for the establishment of cafeteria plans by small employers, and criteria for the provision of a therapeutic discovery tax credit of 50% of the annual investment.

Title X has 8 subtitles, 2 parts, and 84 sections. This title consists of a list of amendments per section necessary to enact the Patient Protection and Affordable Care Act. Subtitle A includes actions to increase access by disallowing insurers from discriminating or placing limits on beneficiaries, ensuring a medical loss ratio of 85% for large insurers or 80% for small insurers or ensuring that most premiums are used to pay for beneficiary claims, ensuring that beneficiaries have transparent cost information and a process for appealing disputes, expanding primary care providers to include pediatricians and OB/GYN physicians, and several other actions focused on increasing beneficiary access and choice. Subtitle B focuses on increasing access to and finding for Medicaid and CHIP. Part II focuses on increasing material, social support, and educational opportunities for pregnant and parenting teens and women. Part III allows the use of a certified dental health aid or midlevel dental health provider when allowed under state law. Subtitle C includes 36 sections that focus on improving quality accountability, linking quality with payment, and cost efficiency. Subtitle D—provisions relating to Title V amendments—includes several technical revisions increasing access to services; 100% coverage for recommended preventative services and small business wellness initiatives; and provides criteria, program for young women diagnosed with breast cancer, and development of a national congenital disease surveillance system. Subtitle E includes increases in individuals qualifying for health insurance coverage; multiple incentives increasing the number of primary care providers by broadening primary care qualifications and several educational, practice placement, and financial incentives; the establishment of a National Diabetes Prevention Program; and the establishment of a Community Health Center Fund. Subtitle F includes clarification of access and data use for patient-centered outcomes research, allows midlevel providers working in collaboration with a physician to make face-to-face home visits, increases penalties for healthcare fraud convictions, and

allows states to experiment with tort reform litigation. Subtitle G provides several technical language revisions to program information. Subtitle H includes several technical revenue and tax clarifications.

Title I has 6 subtitles, 0 parts, and 31 sections. Subtitle A includes technical revisions for healthcare premium tax credits, individual responsibility, and individual penalties; provides several technical calculations and definitions including modified gross adjusted income; and establishes the Health Insurance Reform Implementation Fund. Subtitle B closes the Medicare Part D donut hole and makes several technical payment corrections and clarifications. Subtitle C defines federal funding for states and territories that agreed to expand Medicaid; defines primary care and physician payment; and provides criteria for reduction of DSH payments. Subtitle D provides technical language revisions expanding the reach of community health centers; repeals Medicare payment review limitations; provides additional funding to fight fraud, waste, and abuse; and allows the Secretary of HHS to hold DME payments for 90 days if there is a determination of the potential of fraudulent activity. Subtitle E provides several technical tax revisions and adjustments and delays the start of several tax and revenue programs. Subtitle F establishes grants for community and career training programs.

Title II has 2 subtitles, 2 parts, and 19 sections. Subtitle A addresses student loans and loan repayment options. Subtitle B adds provisions regarding excessive waiting periods and lifetime limits; extends dependent coverage to grandfathered health insurance plans; provides a technical correction, striking "covered drugs" and inserting "covered outpatient drugs"; and increases the funds available to community health centers.

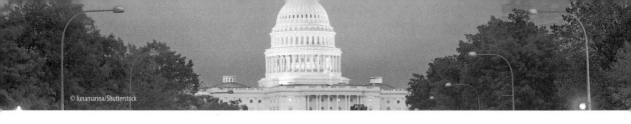

CHAPTER 3

The Rest of the Story: Policy and Power Dynamics, Social Determinants, and the Role of States

This chapter is designed to give healthcare leaders an understanding of the influence of the federalist structure on health policy history in the United States by covering the following topics:

- Federalism and state roles in health policy
- Social determinants
- The dynamics of policy and power in the United States

▶ State Reforms and Roles

Insurance Market Regulation

The basic concept of insurance is that a group of people who have a similar risk, pool their resources together to hedge against a large financial loss associated with their common risk. Three probabilistic assumptions of this concept are (1) the unlikelihood of everybody in the pool suffering the same loss; (2) the greater the size of the pool, the smaller the risk and financial

exposure; and (3) solvency of the risk contract holder (insurance company) and ability to pay claims (see **TABLE 3.1**). During the 1800s, states understood the need to regulate insurance contracts as their responsibility and an exercise of state sovereignty (U.S. Constitution, Amendment 10), since this responsibility was not expressly delegated to the federal government in the U.S. Constitution (Fouse, 1904). States considered their responsibility two-fold: (1) protecting their citizens against fraud potentially associated with these very complex contracts and (2) ensuring the solvency of insurance companies and their ability to pay claims. The argument for states, as

TABLE 3.1 Health Insurance Consumer Protections

Prior to the PPACA, the Following Consumer Protections and Health Plan Affordability Measures Were Left to the States. Some States Enacted All of These Measures, While Others Enacted Only Some or None

Guaranteed issue	Requires insurers to underwrite a plan for anyone wishing to purchase. Depending on the state, there may be no cost limits on these plans. Goal is to prevent residents from being "uninsurable."
Guaranteed renewal	Prevents insurers from dropping individual from coverage due to recent high costs. If insurance is employer-based, it protects employer if community-rating laws are also in place.
Community rating	State-level insurance law requiring health plans to develop plan costs for employers based on cost of insuring a representative sample of a community, rather than the insurance experience of each firm. Generally lowers costs for all, although some firms experience high costs.
Exclusions for pre-existing conditions	Eliminates clauses opting insurers out from covering any or all pre-existing conditions.
Coverage for specific conditions	States have passed laws mandating coverage of costs for "emerging" conditions, the best known being Florida's 2008 mandate requiring reimbursement for healthcare services to persons living with autism.
Risk pools	The concept that a large pool of individuals will spread the risk of costly health events across the group, making it financially viable to insure all at a high level and low cost. States have tried building these by offering subsidies. To date, no state-level risk pool plan has succeeded.

opposed to the federal government, to exercise these responsibilities was rooted in state sovereignty (U.S. Constitution, Amendment 10), and their proximity to the consumers and insurance companies allowed them to more closely monitor insurance activities. States exercised several actions, establishing themselves as regulators of insurance from 1835 to 1861 (see Table 6) through the establishment of the first insurance department (1835), first insurance commissioner (1851), and a standardized process for valuing insurance (1861) (Cooper, 2009; CRS, 1990; Fouse, 1904; McCray, 1993).

Despite state actions to establish themselves as the regulators of insurance, there was action on the federal level to pull this responsibility from the states. The first of these actions was an attempt to shift the argument from state sovereignty (U.S. Constitution, Amendment 10) to the regulation of interstate commerce (U.S. Constitution, Article I, Section 8) that is explicitly a responsibility of the federal government. In *Paul v. Virginia*, the U.S. Supreme Court ruled ". . . issuing a policy of insurance is not a transaction of commerce . . ." Over the next 75 years, Congress attempted and failed to pass legislation stating that issuing insurance was commerce (1897), reaffirmed they had no Constitutional power to regulate insurance (1906), and sponsored but failed to pass a Constitutional amendment giving them power to regulate insurance (1914–1915). Finally, in 1944, the faction seeking federal government regulatory control gained traction when the U.S. Supreme Court ruled in *U.S. v. South-Eastern Underwriters Association* that the issuance of an insurance policy was interstate commerce (U.S. Constitution, Article I, Section 8). Members of Congress were not pleased with this decision, and in 1945 they passed the McCarran-Ferguson Act (PL15) reaffirming that states have the primary responsibility to regulate insurance. The other notable associated activity is the protection of states' rights and federal guidance to the states (Cooper, 2009; CRS, 1990; Fouse, 1904; McCray, 1993).

Throughout the second half of the 1900s and into the 2000s, the federal government incrementally chipped away at state insurance regulatory power through the Employee Retirement Income Security Act (ERISA) (PL 93-406) in 1974, which established self-insured medical plans were not insurance, rather they were a method for paying medical claims that absolved the plan of state regulatory oversight (Wooten, 2014). In 1985, the Consolidated Omnibus Budget Reconciliation Act (COBRA) (PL 99-272) amended ERISA for group plans and the Public Health Service Act, requiring the plans to provide the ability to elect continued coverage to "qualified employees" who lose their health insurance coverage due to a "qualifying event." A federal-state regulatory scheme giving the federal government preemptive rights (HR 2190) was introduced and failed. Next, the Financial Modernization Act of 1999 (Gramm-Leach-Biley or PL 106-102) was passed to loosen financial regulations and reaffirmed the states' role as insurance regulators (Pickens, 2003). In 2009, the Consumer Financial Protection Agency Act (HR 3126) that attempted and failed to establish a Federal Consumer Protection Agency also reaffirmed state regulation of insurance. Finally, the Patient Protection and Affordable Care Act (PPACA) (PL 111-148 & PL 111-152) preempted state minimum insurance standards with minimal federal health plan requirements (Title I, Subtitle D, Part 1, Sections 1301-1304) and, five times throughout the bill, reaffirms the states' role as insurance regulators (see **TABLE 3.2**).

TABLE 3.2 History of Insurance Market Regulation	
Year	**Actions**
1752	Benjamin Franklin instrumental in establishment of household fire insurance through the Philadelphia Contributionship
1835	Massachusetts established the first state insurance department
1851	New Hampshire appointed the first state insurance commissioner
1861	Massachusetts standardized valuation of policy liabilities
1869	U.S. Supreme Court ruled in *Paul v. Virginia* that ". . . issuing a policy of insurance in not a transaction of commerce . . ."

(continues)

TABLE 3.2 History of Insurance Market Regulation	*(continued)*
Year	**Actions**
1869	Bill introduced in Congress stating that insurance companies doing business outside of their state were engaged in interstate commerce—failed
1897	Bill introduced in Congress stating that insurance companies doing business outside of their state were engaged in interstate commerce—failed
1906	House & Judiciary Committees stated Congress did not have the constitutional power to regulate the business of marine, fire, and life insurance
1914–1915	House & Senate bills proposed a Constitutional amendment giving Congress the power to regulate insurance—failed
1944	U.S. Supreme Court ruled in *U.S. v. South-Eastern Underwriters Association* issuing a policy of insurance as interstate commerce
1945	McCarran-Ferguson Act (PL 15) gave states the primary responsibility for regulating insurance
1974	ERISA (PL 93-406) legislation established that self-insured plans were not insurance and, thus not under the authority of state regulators
1985	COBRA (PL 99-272) amends ERISA for group health plans and the Public Health Service Act to require that qualified beneficiaries who lose coverage due to a qualifying event be allowed to elect continued coverage
1993	HR 1290 introduced the establishment of a federal–state insurance regulatory scheme with the federal government having preemptive rights—failed
1999	Financial Modernization Act of 1999 (Gramm-Leach-Bliley—PL106-102) provided for affiliation among banks, security firms, and insurance companies and reaffirmed state regulation of insurance
2009	HR 3126 (Consumer Financial Protection Agency Act of 2009) proposed state regulation of insurance—introduced but failed
2010	PPACA (PL 111-148 & 111-152) established a minimum health insurance standard while maintaining state regulation of insurance

This dynamic exchange is an example of our government working as designed and at its best, with each branch and level of government involved and each branch and level arguing for their authority and checking the others' challenges. Insurance regulation is an executive function, managed by states, that the federal government would prefer to manage,[1] with the judicial branch called upon to resolve successive Constitutional challenges. This one-and-a-quarter-century dynamic seems bound to continue in the future, with one recent proposal being federal legislation allowing insurance companies to sell policies across state lines. If this proposal passes, it would again erode state regulatory power primarily over solvency requirements and dispute resolution.

▶ Any Willing Provider and Freedom of Choice Legislation

Any willing provider (AWP) and freedom of choice (FOC) legislation date back to 1937 and have targeted a variety of provider groups throughout their history, including non-institutional providers (physicians, 33%), institutional providers (hospitals, 29%), and pharmacies (38%). Managed care plans have traditionally contracted with narrow networks of providers, extracting price discounts from them in exchange for access to large panels of patients. Conversely, AWP and FOC laws have not allowed managed care plans to exclude providers from a network if the provider is willing to accept the terms and conditions of the contract. Currently, 27 states have AWP or FOC laws, with 67% of the laws enacted from 1990 to 2009 (**TABLE 3.3**) during the managed care growth era (NCSL, 2015).

Arguments against AWP and FOC legislation by managed care plans were that by the elimination of selective contracting, their ability to secure deep price discounts would be limited and, as a result of screening and monitoring more physicians, their cost of doing business would increase (Morrisey & Ohsfeldt, 2003). With regard to the financial impact of AWP and FOC legislation, Morrisey and Ohsfeldt (2003) document that AWP and FOC states spend $35–$50 more per person, resulting in a managed care disadvantage. Hellinger (1995) demonstrates how AWP and FOC laws increase total managed care operating costs by 1.3%. Despite these documented increased business costs, Carroll and Ambrose (2002) contend the increased costs are minimal and only have a limited impact on managed care financials.

Other groups that sided with the managed care plans in opposition to AWP and FOC laws include: National Governors Association (concerned about loss of cost savings yielded through Medicaid Managed Care plans), American Hospital Association (viewed selective contracting as necessary to reform the national health system), and the business

TABLE 3.3 Public Health Eras	
Prior to 1850	Battling Epidemics
1850–1949	Building State and Local Public Health Infrastructure
1950–1999	Filling Gaps in Medical Care Delivery
After 1999	Preparing for and Responding to Community Health Threats

---

1 Every time the U.S. Congress reaffirmed the state's responsibility to regulate insurance, they also told them they were not doing a very good job of regulating insurance and they needed to tighten up their regulatory actions.

community (concerned AWP and FOC would increase their insurance costs). Oddly, the American Medical Association has been equivocal toward these laws and not voiced a strong opinion for or against them (Hellinger, 1995).

Arguments for AWP and FOC laws come primarily from the insured, who argue that access to a larger provider pool gives them access to higher quality care. Legislators who are empathic toward AWP and FOC laws frequently backed legislation after hearing hardship stories from constituents who had to travel great distances or endure other hardships to use network providers for their medical needs (Hellinger, 1995; Morrisey & Ohsfeldt, 2003). Additionally, the courts have ruled on AWP and FOC plans. The U.S. Supreme Court in *Kentucky Association of Health Plans v. Miller* (2003) ruled in favor of AWP and FOC plans. The eighth U.S. Circuit Court of Appeals in *Prudential Insurance company v. HMO Partners* ruled that ". . . the Arkansas PPA (Patient Protection Act) is saved from preemption under ERISA . . . except with regards to self-funded plans." In summary, AWP and FOC laws have been debated for 80 years, with the largest surge of laws and court rulings occurring since 1990 and deciding for consumer choice and against managed care narrow provider networks.

Linked to AWP and FOC laws is the national movement to ensure patient autonomy. This movement evolved in the latter quarter of the 20th century and was a result of the unintended consequence of the advances of medical technology that resulted in the ability to artificially keep people alive through the use of technology. These end-of-life scenarios culminated in the life-sustaining case of Karen Cruzan in *Cruzan v. Commissioner, Missouri Department of Health*, 497 U.S. 261 (1990), in which the court ordered that life support should be removed from Karen Cruzan and that she should be allowed to die naturally. This court action was followed by the Patient Rights and Self Determination Act, as part of the Omnibus Reconciliation Act of 1990 (HR 5835, Part IV, Part 3). Finally, this action was followed by a variety of state-level actions that made provisions for individuals to make end-of-life decisions in advance through mechanisms such as living will and durable power of attorney for healthcare decisions. The earlier actions resulted from a variety of issue action groups that ranged from international, national, and state levels of government to citizen and professional groups focusing on values or, specifically, the value of life.

▶ Public Health

Born in the mid-1800s, public health focuses on threats to the health of the general population. In the 1800s, especially in the aftermath of the Civil War, many states organized "Boards of Health" to oversee the implementation of rules regarding safe water and sanitation. To this day, the biggest gains in life spans of Americans are attributable to the efforts of this sector. Beginning with control established over water sources and sanitation in the late 1800s to early 1900s, public health broadened its role into immunizations, health statistics, education and promotion, and implementation of portions of low-income social support programs (**FIGURE 3.1**).

▶ Certificate of Need

Once the rise in healthcare costs showed signs of persisting, states searched for policy instruments to restrain the rise. Beginning in 1964, New York State enacted the first Certificate of Need (CON) program. CON programs were enacted in many states based on the belief that the development of expensive services increases the overall cost of health care as systems try to recover the resources invested in the expensive services. The Nixon administration fueled state CON programs with a statute in 1974 requiring all states to enact CON programs. This statute was removed in 1987, leaving states to assess its value. States either maintained, scaled back, or

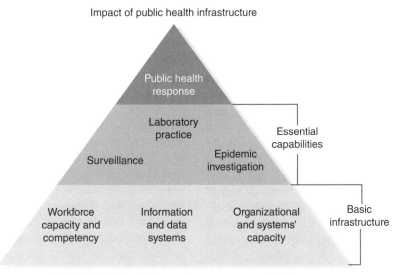

Impact of public health infrastructure

Public health response

Laboratory practice

Surveillance

Epidemic investigation

Essential capabilities

Workforce capacity and competency

Information and data systems

Organizational and systems' capacity

Basic infrastructure

Public Health Infrastructure—the resources needed to deliver essential public health services to every community

FIGURE 3.1 Public Health Infrastructure

Impact of Public Health Infrastructure, Courtesy of Public Health Foundation.

eliminated CON, leaving 35 states still employing the program (NCSL, 2016).

CON tends to cover similar things across those states (e.g., hospital beds, MRIs, cardiac surgery centers, emergency Life Flight helicopters). The commonality is driven by services and/or equipment with initially high capital costs (e.g., purchase of a "Big Bore" MRI) and/or with high ongoing costs for maintaining (e.g., emergency Life Flight helicopters). It has also been argued that CON was solely created to reduce competition on behalf of established market actors.

▶ Scope of Practice, Licensure, and Certification

As mentioned at the beginning of this chapter, state legislatures are the arbiters of scope of practice for healthcare providers. Scope of practice is the legal definition of which

practitioners may "diagnose" patients and then "prescribe" a course of treatment.

The most common inroads on physician scope of practice are being made by nurse practitioners (NPs) and specialties within nursing (e.g., certified registered nurse anesthetists [CRNAs], physician assistants [PAs], certified nurse midwives [CNMs], and pharmacists [PharmDs]). Some or all of these practitioners—often referred to as "physician extenders"—are found on care teams. Care teams are also sometimes defined under scope of practice laws (NCSL, 2015). Lower level "extenders" (e.g., licensed practical nurses, nurse assistants, community health workers) are making inroads in terms of care provision standards, with these lower cost certified professions replacing higher cost "extenders."

Closely tied to scope of practice are professional licensure and certification. Both state legislatures set standards (determined in consultation with professional organizations) for education requirements and experiential requirements of healthcare professions.

▶ Medicaid/CHIP Implementation

State legislatures implement two federal health-care coverage programs: Medicaid and the Children's Health Insurance Program (CHIP). Within the federal regulations defining both programs, states have varying levels of room for the expansiveness of offered coverage (what is paid for) and eligibility (who may obtain coverage). The federal rules for Medicaid permit less variation across coverage offerings and eligibility than the rules for CHIP, and the federal matching funds for CHIP are more generous than for Medicaid. Both programs come with federal matching funds that cover a percentage of program cost. The federal match varies each year based on a state's socioeconomic status. The formula includes, but is not limited to, unemployment rate and mean family income.

▶ Mental Health and Substance Abuse

Historically, individuals with substance abuse issues or other mental illnesses were institutionalized indefinitely in state "asylums" of mental health institutions. President Kennedy ended this practice by deinstitutionalizing mental health treatment through the Community Mental Health (CMH) Act of 1963 (PL 88-164) and moving mental health treatment to local Community Mental Health organizations for community-based or outpatient treatment. CMHs are funded through grants administered through the National Institute of Mental Health and Medicaid, and compete for Substance Abuse and Mental Health Services Administration (SAMHSA) grants.

The Substance Abuse and Mental Health Services Administration was established by Congress in 1992 with the mission "to reduce the impact of substance abuse and mental illness in America's communities." SAMHSA has worked to fulfill its mission through states by providing funding through the Substance Abuse Prevention and Treatment Block Grant and the Community Mental Health Services Block Grant. The legal authority for these block grants is promulgated through the Public Health Services Act, Title XIX, Section 1921 that requires states to (1) provide a plan, (2) conduct a program and services evaluation, and (3) "provide planning, administration, and education activities related to providing services under the plan." These block grants are administered through a variety of provider and community service organizations that allow states to tailor substance abuse and mental health service to the needs of their communities.

Currently, substance abuse and mental health treatment are provided by public and private providers and paid for through public and private grants and public and private insurance. Traditionally, payers have provided greater funding for physical illnesses, resulting in (1) a lack of mental health payment parity, (2) tension between physical and mental health providers and patients, and (3) a considerable amount of payment parity debate in state and federal legislatures. The outcome of these debates has been the enactment of substance abuse and mental health parity laws in all 50 states and U.S. territories, and federal mental health parity laws in 1996, 2008, and 2010. Most of these laws have been feckless and ineffective at gaining mental payment parity, with the implementation of the 2010 law (implemented in 2014) too recent to evaluate.

▶ Social Determinants of Health

The World Health Organization defines social determinants of health as, ". . . the conditions in which people are born, grow, live, work and age" (WHO, 2015). While this definition is a good starting point, the CDC brings some additional clarity to this definition by recognizing five social determinants of health: (1) biology and genetics, (2) individual behavior, (3) social environment, (4) physical environment, and (5) health services (CDC, 2015). Social determinants of health relate to many of the environmental concerns of health care and contribute to an individual's social well-being. Administrators and legislators have a limited ability to influence an individual's biology and genetics, although they can influence the remaining four social determinants through legislation and community development.

Individual behaviors can be influenced by how lifestyle activities are incented or disincentivized. Examples of incented behavior include workplace wellness plans that incent healthy lifestyle choices, and preventative medical care, such as age-appropriate screening, weight loss, and smoking cessation. Participation in both workplace wellness plans and preventive care is frequently rewarded (incented) by discounted health insurance premiums and other financial incentives, resulting in organizational premium savings and positive return on investment (Baicker, Cutler, & Song, 2010; Baxter, Sanderson, Venn, Blizzard, & Palmer, 2014). Fronstin and Roebuck (2015) found that, despite significant increases in health risk assessments (HRAs) and biometric screenings as one large employer, health expenditures increased in the first year primarily due to increased pharmacological spending and secondarily due to HRA and biometric screening findings. Other examples include providing healthy meals in cafeterias and other food venues, providing walking and biking paths, and encouragement of community gardens. Disincentives can be just the opposite, such as banning smoking and higher insurance premiums for individuals not actively seeking to develop healthy lifestyles.

Social and physical environments include developing safe areas for people to work (PL 91-596) and live and ensuring the presence of public health measures, such as sanitation and safe water (PL 93-523). Education has been linked to decreased mortality, decreased incidence of chronic illness, and increased self-reported health status (Cutler & Lleras-Muney, 2007; Telfair & Shelton, 2012). Cutler and Lleras-Muney (2007) also note several social factors that contribute to the education-health paradigm, including poorer health resulting in lower levels of schooling, family background and individual differences in learned skills yielding differing health results (mixed), and increased education directly increasing health. Healthcare leaders who are interested in enhancing the health care of their community could use international examples (Bradley & Taylor, 2013; Squires & Anderson, 2015) to encourage legislation (federal, state, and local) that enhances their community's social, physical, and educational environments.

▶ Policy Process Overview

The policy process consists of policy formulation, implementation, and modification and was originally described by the theories heuristic. The theories heuristic served the policy research community for several years, describing the policy process. However, in recent years, this theory has fallen into disfavor largely due to its unidirectional, or flat directional, process and failure to recognize the dynamism associated with the policy process. Regardless of the criticisms, this theory still helps novice policy researchers understand the steps through which a policy must go to become a law. An enhanced diagram of the policy process, developed by Higbea (see **FIGURE 3.2**), is helpful in describing the steps of the policy process.

Policy formulation is a phase that consists of agenda-setting and policy development. The agenda-setting phase begins with the identification of a problem or the germination of an idea, includes debates of the various policy solutions, and culminates with the development of a policy. This phase of the

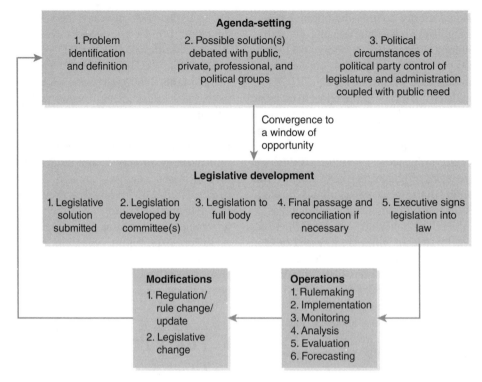

FIGURE 3.2 The Policy Process

policy process is the longest, averaging 20 years, although it can range from as short as 10 years to as long as 40 years. The portion of this phase that takes the longest is the political circumstances, meaning the alignment of the problem, potential solution, and political circumstances (Baumgartner & Jones, 1993; Kingdon, 1995). This alignment is not only necessary for the actors to agree on the policy needs, but also necessary to generate the power to pursue the policy need. The power of the president cannot be overstated when developing public policy; a quick review of the Health Policy History table (Appendix) reveals that no health policies have passed the House of Representatives and Senate and been signed into law by a president that does not have some level of presidential sponsorship. This phase can also be economically characterized as sellers (policy suppliers) balanced against buyers (policy demanders), with a policy resulting when the two sides have

agreed on the value of the problem and policy solution (Longest, 2010). Once the policy has cleared the legislative chamber(s), including the appropriate committees and subcommittees, it goes to the executive, who can either sign the policy into law or veto it. If the executive signs the policy into law, it moves to the appropriate agency for the implementation process to begin. If, however, the executive vetoes the policy, it goes back to the legislature where the legislature can decide to let the policy die, rework the policy by addressing the concerns raised by the executive, or seek to override the veto.

Once the policy is signed into law, it moves to the appropriate agency(ies) for implementation. The implementation process consists of meeting with interest groups, experts, and agency officials to develop regulations delineating how the law will be implemented and managed. These proposed regulations are published for comment in the *Federal Register* for a designated period to time (30–90 days). After the comments have been collected and reviewed, a final rule is issued by the agency and the rules are entered into the *Code of Federal Regulations (CFR)*.

Once the final regulations have been developed, the appropriate agency(ies) begin the implementation and management process of providing the policy benefit to the constituency. As the agency(ies) gain experience with the policy, they often find aspects of the policy that need modification. Depending upon the nature of the modifications, they may be handled through modification to the regulations or may require additional legislative action. Regardless, these identified problems start the agenda-setting process over again as new solutions are identified and debated. The reasons for policy modification minimally include the policy not working as intended, unintended consequences of the policy, or a shift in political alignments, resulting in a shift in agreed solutions to the policy problem. Policy formulation, implementation, and modification will be discussed in more detail in Chapters 6, 7, and 8, respectively.

▶ Power

Power in policy making is an individual's or group's ability to control or allocate resources. Formal power emanates from elected or appointed office, whereas informal power emanates from influence. Both types of power may control resources, including money and people (knowledge and votes) (see **TABLE 3.4**). A classic example of power is found in the debate leading up to and the enactment of Medicare and Medicaid. Throughout the debate, the American Medical Association (AMA) put forth a vigorous rebuttal to the need for Medicare and Medicaid, marshaling the largest amount of money to date and engaging their member physicians (AMA represented 75% of U.S. physicians in 1965). Thus, through a power lens, the AMA put forth a large amount of influence by allocating a large amount of money, a large number of people (physicians), and a large amount of knowledge (physicians). President Johnson (D) exercised his power through exquisite management of policy processes by almost constant contact with legislative leaders, ensuring the policy was designed to appeal to the

TABLE 3.4 Power

■ Formal	■ Informal
• Elected or appointed office	• Influence
• Resources	• Resources
○ Money	○ Money
○ People	○ People
□ Experts	□ Knowledge
□ Votes	□ Votes

elderly, poor, and physicians, while giving credit for the policy design and success to legislators. Despite these efforts, the physicians were still pushing back against Medicare and Medicaid after they were signed into law. President Johnson exercised power by bringing the physicians to agreement with the policy through a process that later became known as Johnsonizing, where he would corner a group or individuals into agreeing for the need for a policy before TV cameras (Blumenthal & Monroe, 2009). More recently, the Democratic Senate Majority leader used the power of the legislative calendar to keep legislation from coming to vote and Tea Party conservatives have exercised power in both the House and Senate to influence policy language on issues such as the debt ceiling and immigration and resignation of the Speaker of the House.

The healthcare professions have seen a dynamic shift in market power that has also eroded the profession's political power. Over the past 50 years, physicians (and increasingly, those who manage the business and financial aspects of medical practice) have pursued consolidation of the once sacrosanct private physician practice. Progressive consolidation movements began with physicians first developing or joining group practices, followed by integration of those practices into larger organizations, such as health systems. Three drivers of this erosion are technological advancement, the demand for increased practice specialization, and graduate medical education. All have led to increased physician dependence on larger organizations (health systems) as a resource for the purchase of the advanced technological equipment and as a location to perform the associated procedures.

The fourth erosion of physician power is the decentralization of patient care, with the progressive delegation of patient care responsibilities to mid-level providers and a variety of other allied health professionals and technicians. Finally, physician power has eroded as health insurance companies, regulatory agencies, and health system administrators have provided stern direction to them on how to practice medicine. These five phenomena minimally represent the power shifts that have occurred over the past 50 years—certainly others could be added to this list. One proxy measure of this power erosion is physician resistance to major national healthcare legislation, with the ACA being the first time physicians have not put up a fight to resist such legislation. As a result of this erosion of power, physicians no longer have the influence they once had over the policy process, with the power shifting to those handling the financial and business aspects of medical care.

Another way to view power is through the lens of merger and acquisition activity. Organizations traditionally engage in merger and acquisition activity to gain economy of scale efficiencies, market share, and bargaining power. Post-ACA, an additional merger and acquisition rationale is administrative control associated with new payment models that reward high quality of care, coordination of care, and positive patient outcomes. For the years 2000–2009, there were a mean of 60 (range 38–85) health system mergers,[2] whereas the years 2010–2017 had a mean of 98 (range 74–115) mergers or an increase of 61%. While the increased number of mergers and acquisitions is significant, the numbers do not reflect the size of the mergers. A proxy measure for size is FTC review and approval, which is triggered by an increase in market concentration[3] that inhibits competition or by the value of net revenues. FTC merger review data indicates that for the years 2000–2009, there were a mean of 0.6 (range 0–2) merger reviews, whereas the years 2010–2017 had 2.75 (range 0–6) merger

---

2 Health system mergers include: hospital–hospital (horizontal integration), hospital–health system (horizontal or vertical integration), and health system–clinic (vertical integration of physician offices).

3 Measured by calculating the Herfindahl-Hirschman Index by summing the squares of the individual firm's market share: unconcentrated <1500, moderately concentrated 1500–2500, highly concentrated >2500.

reviews or an increase of 450% (Kaufman Hall, 2018). While the aforementioned data reflects hospital–health system–physician office merger activity, another arena of activity includes health insurance company mergers and acquisitions with a few odd twists such as the CVS (pharmacy and pharmacy benefit manager) acquisition of Anthem (health insurance). Both of these types of mergers are attempts to gain administrative control and increased bargaining power. One concern about increased market share of either health systems or insurance companies is price increases, with the current on this topic mixed.

▸ Cost, Quality, and Access

When building health policies and systems, researchers frequently use the cost–quality–access triangle (see **FIGURE 3.3**) as a method of organizing how the health system is built and how to measure its success. From a conceptual lens, the three sides should be equal, as in an equilateral triangle, indicating a system in balance. The U.S. health system is an example of how an unbalanced system produces lower quality and less access, despite higher costs (see **FIGURE 3.4**). The best, although not perfect, comparisons for the U.S. health system are other similar countries, such as the Organization for Economic Cooperation and Development (OECD) countries. When the United States is compared on costs to OECD countries, the U.S. costs as a percent of GDP are generally 34%–88% higher (World Bank, 2016). OECD countries all have some type of universal coverage, whereas even under ACA, the United States has an uninsured rate of 13.1% (Cohen & Martinez, 2014) and underinsured rate of 23% of adults aged 19–64 years in 2014 (Collins, Rasmussen, Beutel, & Doty, 2015).

Thus, while access to health insurance has increased due to the implementation of the ACA, access to healthcare services has yet to be directly correlated (see Figure 3.4). This lack of correlated access is due to both a shortage of primary care providers (HRSA, 2013) and high out-of-pocket costs associated with high deductible plans (Collins et al., 2015). Regarding quality, the United States has begun to focus on quality and link it to payment (McClellan, McKethan, Lewis, Roski, & Fisher, 2010; Medicare.Gov, 2015). However, we still rate lowest of all OECD countries (Davis, Stremikis, Squires, & Schoen, 2014). The United States is currently undergoing a payment transition that is attempting to link quality and cost through a variety of value-based payment methods (Medicare.Gov, 2015).

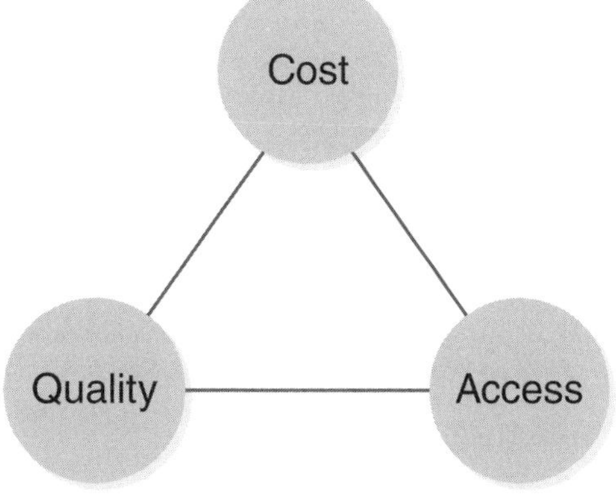

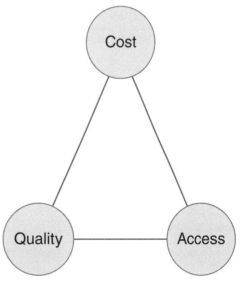

FIGURE 3.3 Cost, Quality, Access Triangle Overview

FIGURE 3.4 Cost, Quality, Access—United States

References

Baicker, K., Cutler, D., & Song, Z. (2010). Workplace wellness plans can generate savings. *Health Affairs, 29*(2), 304–311. doi:10.1377/hlthaff.2009.0626

Baumgartner, F. R., & Jones, B. D. (1993). *Agendas and instability in American politics.* Chicago, IL: The University of Chicago Press.

Baxter, S., Sanderson, K., Venn, A. J., Blizzard, L., & Palmer, A. J. (2014). The relationship between return on investment and quality of study methodology. *American Journal of Health Promotion, 28*(6), 347–363.

Blumenthal, D. (2006). Employer-sponsored health insurance in the United States—Origins and implications. *The New England Journal of Medicine, 355*(1), 82–88. doi:10.1056/NEJMhpr060703

Blumenthal, D., & Monroe, J. A. (2009). *The heart of power: Health and politics in the oval office.* University of California Press. Retrieved from https://data.worldbank.org/indicator/SH.XPD.CHEX.PC.CD

Bradley, E. H., & Taylor, L. A. (2013). *The American health care paradox: Why spending more is getting us less.* New York, NY: Public Affairs.

Carroll, A., & Ambrose, J. M. (2002). Any-willing-provider laws: Their financial effect on HMOs. *Journal of Health Politics, Policy and Law, 27*(6), 927–945. doi:10.1215/03616878-27-6-927

CDC—Social Determinants of Health—Definitions (2016). Retrieved from http://www.cdc.gov/socialdeterminants/Definitions.htm

Cohen, R. A., & Martinez, M. E. (2014, January–March). Health insurance coverage: Early release of estimates from the national health interview survey. Retrieved from http://www.cdc.gov/nchs/data/nhis/earlyrelease/insur201409.pdf

Collins, S. R., Rasmussen, P. W., Beutel, S., & Doty, M. M. (2015). *The problem of underinsurance and how rising deductibles will make it worse* (Issue Brief). The Commonwealth Fund.

Congressional Research Service. (1990). *Insurance regulation by the states* (CRS report).

Cooper, R. W. (2009). Preservation of state-based insurance regulation: An ongoing challenge in the U.S. and the European Union. *Journal of Insurance Regulation, 27*(4), 81.

Culter, D. M., & Lleras-Muney, A. (2007). *Education and health* (Policy Brief #9). National Poverty Center.

Davis, K., Schoen, C., & Stremikis, K. (2010). Mirror, mirror on the wall: How the performance of the U.S. health care system compares internationally, 2010 update. The Commonwealth Fund.

Fouse, L. G. (1904). State regulation of insurance. *The Annals of the American Academy of Political and Social Science, 24*(1), 69–83. doi:10.1177/000271620402400105

Fronstin, P., & Roebuck, M. C. (2015). *Financial incentives, workplace wellness program participation, and utilization of health care services and spending* (Issue Brief 417). Employee Benefit Research Institute.

Hellinger, F. J. (1995). Any-willing-provider and freedom-of-choice laws: An economic assessment. *Health Affairs, 14*(4), 297–302. Retrieved from http://search.proquest.com.ezproxy.gvsu.edu/docview/204609190?accountid=39473

HRSA Health Workforce Analysis. (2013, November). Projecting the supply and demand for primary care practitioners through 2020. Retrieved from https://bhw.hrsa.gov/health-workforce-analysis/primary-care-2020

KaufmanHall. (2018). 2017 in review: The year M&A shook the healthcare landscape. Retrieved from https://www.kaufmanhall.com/sites/default/files/legacy_files/2017-in-Review_The-Yearthat-Shook-Healthcare.pdf

Kingdon, J. W. (1995). *Agendas, alternatives, and public policy* (2nd ed.). New York, NY: Longman.

Longest, B. B. (2010). *Health policy making in the United States.* Chicago, IL: Health Administration Press.

McClellan, M., McKethan, A. N., Lewis, J. L., Roski, J., & Fisher, E. S. (2010). A national strategy to put accountable care into practice. *Health Affairs, 29*(5), 982–990.

McCray, S. B. (1993). Federal preemption of state regulation of insurance: End of a 200-year era? *Publius, 23*(4), 33.

Medicare.Gov. (2015). Linking quality to payment. Retrieved from http://www.medicare.gov/hospitalcompare/linking-quality-to-payment.html?AspxAutoDetectCookieSupport=1

Morrisey, M. A., & Ohsfeldt, R. L. (2003). Do "any willing provider" and "freedom of choice" laws affect HMO market share? *Inquiry, 40*(4), 362–374.

National Conference of State Legislatures. (2015). Scope of practice overview. Retrieved from http://www.ncsl.org/research/health/scope-of-practice-overview.aspx

National Conference of State Legislatures. (2016). CON-Certificate of need laws. Retrieved from http://www.ncsl.org/research/health/con-certificate-of-need-state-laws.aspx

Pickens, M. (2003). The NAIC's 2003 agenda modernizing state insurance regulation: A legacy of consistency, efficiency & trust. *Journal of Insurance Regulation, 21*(3), 117.

Squires, D., & Anderson, C. (2015). *U.S. health care from a global perspective: Spending, use of services, prices, and health in 13 countries* (pub. 1819, Vol. 15). Commonwealth Fund.

Telfair, J., & Shelton, T. L. (2012). Educational attainment as a social determinant of health. *North Carolina Medical Journal, 73*(5), 358.

WHO Social Determinants of Health. (2015). Retrieved from http://www.who.int/social_determinants/sdh _definition/en/

Wooten, J. A. (2014). A legislative and political history of ERISA preemption, Part 4: The "deemer" clause. *Journal of Pension Benefits, 22*(1), 3.

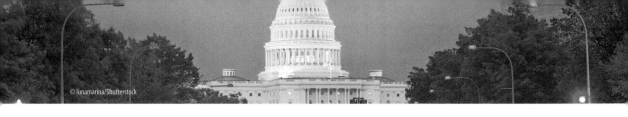
© lunamarina/Shutterstock

CHAPTER 4

Comparative National Health Systems and Health Policy

This chapter is designed to give healthcare leaders an understanding of comparative national health systems and health policy by covering the following topics:

- How healthcare measurement for the United States compares to OECD
- What different national health system models exist and what the United States can learn
- How the international differences in dynamics of cost, quality, access, and innovation affect healthcare measurements, outcomes, and policy

The need for healthcare services is common to all people of the globe and has been addressed throughout the world in ways that are sensitive to national cultures and economies. Scholars have developed four categorical models to assist researchers and policy makers in understanding the characteristics, similarities, and differences of these systems.

▶ United States Health Delivery

The United States has some of the most sophisticated, technologically advanced healthcare services in the world and is considered the hub of healthcare technological advances. Despite these great accomplishments, the United States also has one of the most fractured and fragmented systems in the world, with some measures of national health outcomes ranking among the worst. The Commonwealth Fund (2017) sponsored a study of world health systems, ranking 11 OECD countries on a variety of access, cost, and quality measures. While the United States was rated third on effective care and fourth on patient-centered care, five measures (quality care, safe care, coordinated care, patient-centered care, and timeliness of care) were rated toward the middle, and four measures (cost-related access problems, efficiency, equity, and healthy lives) were rated last, pulling the final rating to last (or 11th) out of 11 OECD countries. In addition to these poor system delivery ratings, the United States had a 2011 health expenditure per capita of $8508, roughly double that of the other ten countries in this study (see **TABLES 4.1** and **4.2**).

More current data (2015) from OECD Health Statistics and the World Health Organization yielded similar findings when the

TABLE 4.1 OECD Quality and Care Measures

Country	Primary Insurance Type	Adult Access to Care	Did Not Have Prescription Reviewed	Chronic Care Management	Primary Care Feedback	OECD Healthcare Quality Indicators	Avoidable Deaths	Prevention	Access and Quality Subtotal	Sub-rank
England	National Health System	1	5	2	1	8	7	1	25	1
New Zealand	National Health System	6	6	2	3	6	10	5	38	5
Norway	National Health System	6	8	9	7	3	3	9	45	10
Sweden	National Health System	5	11	8	2	1	4	5	36	4
Australia	National Health Insurance	6	2	2	9	2	2	5	28	2
Canada	National Health Insurance	11	2	2	11	6	6	4	42	7

Country	Type									
France	Statutory Health Insurance	9	10	6	8	9	1	11	54	11
Germany	Statutory Health Insurance	2	4	11	5	11	8	3	44	9
Netherlands	Statutory Health Insurance	3	8	7	3	9	4	1	35	3
Switzerland	Statutory Health Insurance	3	7	9	10	4	9	10	43	8
United States	Statutory Health Insurance, National Health Insurance, National Health System	10	1	1	6	4	9	8	39	6

oecd.org/els/healthsystems/healthdata.l

TABLE 4.2 OECD Quality and Care Measures

Country	Primary Insurance Type	Public View of Health System	Public View Subtotal	Sub-rank	Life Expectancy (years)	Under 5 Mortality Rate per 100,000 (Years)	Life Expectancy and Infant Mortality Subtotal	Sub-rank	Total	Rank
England	National Health System	1	26	1	8	8	16	10	42	2
New Zealand	National Health System	5	43	4	3	10	13	9	56	7
Norway	National Health System	6	51	9	3	1	4	1	55	6
Sweden	National Health System	7	43	4	3	1	4	1	47	3
Australia	National Health Insurance	4	32	2	1	3	4	1	36	1
Canada	National Health Insurance	8	50	7	3	8	11	8	61	8
France	Statutory Health Insurance	10	64	11	3	3	6	5	70	10
Germany	Statutory Health Insurance	8	52	10	8	3	11	6	63	9
Netherlands	Statutory Health Insurance	3	38	3	8	3	11	6	49	4
Switzerland	Statutory Health Insurance	2	45	6	1	3	4	1	49	4
United States	Statutory Health Insurance, National Health Insurance, National Health System	11	50	7	11	11	22	11	72	11

Oecd.org/els/healthsystems/healthdata.htm & The World Bank: The WHO.

United States was compared to 11 OECD countries. Access, quality, and safety measures were rated best for prescription review and chronic care coordination, and tenth for adult access to care, yielding an overall ranking of six. The public's view of the U.S. health system came in last at 11, moving the U.S. ranking from sixth to seventh. Life expectancy was the lowest for this set of OECD countries, as was infant mortality, yielding a category and overall rating of 11 out of 11, or last place (see Table 4.2). When the OECD and World Health Organization categories are aggregated and applied to categories (National Health System, National Health Insurance, and Statutory Health Insurance), the United States is consistently rated third or fourth in these categories as well (see **TABLE 4.3**).

Finally, it is noteworthy that the U.S. health system, coupled with medium to poor healthcare quality and access, has the highest cost as a percentage of GDP and per capita of comparative OECD countries (see **TABLE 4.4**, **FIGURES 4.1** and **4.2**). When compared to health system type, the

U.S. cost per GDP is higher by a range of 67.5%–87.5% (see **TABLE 4.5**). While the United States has experienced significant growth in healthcare expenditures since the implementation of Medicare and Medicaid in 1965, the growth in expenditures has been in line with comparative OECD countries until circa 1980 when growth began to exceed OECD growth and has continued to do so at an exponential pace since then.

The aforementioned factors of low quality, limited access, and high cost, with an increasing change among the national expenditures per GDP and cost per capita, raise the questions, "Why the difference?" "What is going on to cause these discrepancies?" and "How can the United States address these concerns" to bring them back into line with comparative OECD countries? Multiple policy attempts to bring these discrepancies under control and into line with comparative OECD countries have been ineffective. These failures have caused many healthcare and policy professionals to ask the question, "What can we learn from other OECD countries and apply to our system?"

TABLE 4.3 System Rankings

Health System Type	Access and Quality Subtotal	Sub-rank	Public View Subtotal	Sub-rank	Life Expectancy and Infant Mortality Subtotal	Sub-rank	Total	Rank
National Health System	36	2	41	1	9	3	50	2
National Health Insurance	35	1	41	1	8	1	49	1
Statutory Health Insurance	44	4	50	3	8	1	58	3
United States	39	3	50	3	22	4	72	4

Oecd.org/els/healthsystems/healthdata.htm & The World Bank: The WHO.

TABLE 4.4 Comparative Characterists and GDP

Country	Primary Insurance Type	Funding	Private Insurance	HC as % GDP 2000	HC as % GDP 2010	HC as % GDP 2015
Denmark	National Health System	Income tax	37% Complimentary	8.7	11.1	10.6
England	National Health System	General tax	11% Supplemental	6.9	9.5	9.8
Italy	National Health System	Corporate, VAT, general, and regional taxes	7% Complimentary	7.9	9.4	9.1
New Zealand	National Health System	General taxes	35% Complimentary	7.5	11.2	9.4
Norway	National Health System	General taxes	7% Complimentary	8.3	9.3	9.9
Sweden	National Health System	General taxes	5% Complimentary	8.2	9.5	11.1
Australia	National Health Insurance	General revenue and income taxes	48% Complimentary	8.1	9.0	9.3
Canada	National Health Insurance	General tax (provincial and federal)	67% Complimentary	8.7	11.2	10.1
Israel	National Health Insurance	General taxes	Several plans	7.1	7.4	7.8
Japan	Statutory Health Insurance[1]	General taxes and insurance	70% Complimentary	7.5	9.6	11.2

Country	Type	Financing	Coverage			
France	Statutory Health Insurance	Payroll and general revenue taxes	90% Complimentary (government vouchers)	9.8	11.2	11.0
Germany	Statutory Health Insurance	Payroll and general revenue taxes	11% Complimentary and cover cost-sharing	10.1	11.3	11.1
Netherlands	Statutory Health Insurance	Payroll and general revenue taxes	84% Complimentary	7.4	10.5	10.8
Singapore	Statutory Health Insurance[2]	General taxes	Several plans	2.7	4.0	4.9
Switzerland	Statutory Health Insurance	General taxes	Several plans	9.9	11.1	11.5
United States	Statutory Health Insurance, National Health Insurance, National Health Insurance	Payroll and general revenue taxes	56% Private insurance	13.7	17.0	16.9

[1]Japan is closest to the statutory health insurance (Bismarck) model; however, the fee schedule is set annually by the central government.

[2]Singapore is closest to the Swiss model except that health plans are largely derived within a "corporatist governance" system. Thus, health plans share some similarities with the "Bismarck" model.

Data from World bank data.worldbank.org/indicator/SH.XPD.TOTL.ZS The Commonwealth Wealth Fund international.commonwealthfund.org.

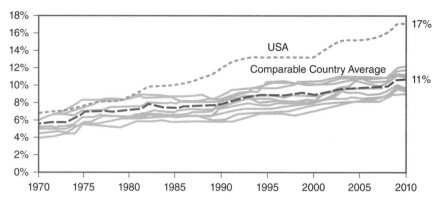

FIGURE 4.1 Comparative Expenditures per GDP

Kaiser Family Foundation analysis of 2013 OECD data "OECD Health Data: Health expenditure and financing: Health expenditure indicators," OECD Health Statistics (database). Doi: 10.1787/data-00349-en (Accessed on June 25, 2014).

Notes: Because 2012 data were unavailable, 2011 were used for Australia and the Netherlands. Data for Canada and Switzerland are estimated values.

▶ National Health Systems: Models

We open this section with a disclaimer: every national model of healthcare delivery is unique to the individual country's culture, economy, and population. Despite the uniqueness of each of these models, nations across the globe can learn from the successes and failures of other similar nations by defining broad models that reflect common components of these systems. It should also be noted that none of these systems is "pure socialism," all have some provisions through complimentary insurance to address those needs not covered by the national plan. These models will be discussed from greatest to least government intervention.

The *national health system* model, more commonly known as "socialized medicine" and sometimes referred to as the Beveridge model,[1] is the model with the greatest government intervention. In these systems, the

government owns and is the system, the infrastructure, and all associated resources. These systems are funded through either federal or joint federal and provincial government's tax revenues. All of the physical assets (buildings, land, and equipment) are owned by the government, all staff (physicians, ancillary, and administrators) are employees of the government, all citizens or residents are covered by the government, and all medical bills are paid for by the government. In systems such as this, no one is denied access to care and no one has a copay or deductible.

In contrast, no one is guaranteed same day service except for emergencies and no one is guaranteed timeliness for elective procedures. Many people in these systems like to think their care is free, and it is free in the sense that they have no out-of-pocket obligations. However, care is not free; rather, the cost is passed along to them through general, value-added, or payroll taxes. Several countries that use this model include: Denmark,

---

1 Named for William Beveridge, the British Prime Minister who, in the aftermath of World War II, oversaw the initial design and implementation of the United Kingdom's National Health System.

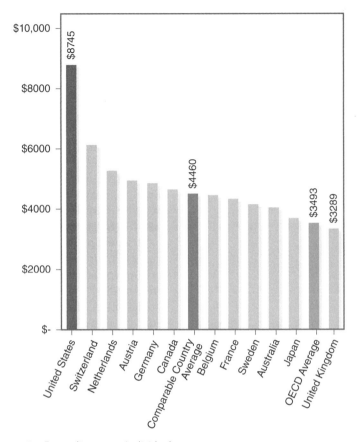

FIGURE 4.2 Comparative Expenditures per Individual

Kaiser Family Foundation analysis of 2013 OECD data "OECD Health Data: Health expenditure and financing: Health expenditure indicators," OECD Health Statistics (database). Doi: 10.1787/data-00349-en (Accessed on June 25, 2014).

Notes: Because 2012 data were unavailable, 2011 were used for Australia and the Netherlands. Data for Canada and Switzerland are estimated values.

United Kingdom, Italy, Japan, New Zealand, Norway, and Sweden. These countries generally rate high on quality and all hold their healthcare costs between 9% and 11% of GDP. In the United States, we use this system for the Military Health System,[2] Veterans Administration, and Indian Health Service, with all three systems generally getting fair to good reviews for quality and satisfaction.

Next is the *national health insurance* model, in which the government acts as the third-party payer or insurance company; this model is funded through general and income tax revenues, and services are provided by

---

2 Not to be confused with Tricare, the healthcare plan for military dependents and for servicemen on leave or detached duty away from a regular, active duty military installation.

TABLE 4.5 Percentage of GDP Difference		
Health System Type	**HC as % GDP 2015**	**% Lower than U.S. GDP**
National Health System	10.0	70.0
National Health Insurance	9.1	87.5
Statutory Health Insurance	10.1	67.5
United States	16.9	

providers through private markets. Providers within these private markets are not employees of the government; rather, they work within nonprofit and for-profit organizations. Within this system, no one is denied access to healthcare services, provided they meet a minimal requirement such as citizenship or residency. Two countries that use this model are Australia and Canada. The quality results are mixed from moderate to fair, and they hold their costs as a percentage of GDP within the 9%–11% range. In the United States, we use this system for traditional Medicare that generally gets favorable reviews for quality and satisfaction.

Third is the *Statutory Health Insurance* model, sometimes known as the Bismarck model,[3] in which the government mandates that all citizens or residents have health insurance provided through the private markets that are funded by a combination of payroll and general tax revenues. There are multiple health insurers in these markets that provide

health insurance plans based on government-mandated requirements and who also provide complementary coverage for cost-sharing or services not covered under the mandated requirements. All of the providers within this system are private and work within private, mostly nonprofit, organizations. Several countries that use this system include: France, Germany, Netherlands, Singapore, and Switzerland. Lastly, this model is a direct outcome of the corporatist models of government predominant in Western Europe and Scandinavia (exclusive of the United Kingdom, inclusive of Ireland)[4] (**TABLE 4.6**).

It should be noted that all of these countries use traditional health insurance products (except Singapore, which uses a set of three medical savings accounts, based on population-specific needs). Generally, these countries provide medium- to high-quality care and hold their costs as a percentage of GDP to 11%–12%. Medicare Advantage is the best comparison the United States has to these programs, in which seniors have the option of opting out of traditional Medicare and purchasing an "approved" plan through the private markets. A close, but not exact, comparison is our employer-based market, where 57% of our citizens get their health insurance coverage through their employer, who is given a tax credit for providing health insurance.

The final model is the *out-of-pocket* model, in which citizens and residents get whatever level of healthcare services they can afford. This is a brutal system of "haves" and "have-nots," in which you receive healthcare services based on the amount of money you have or are willing to pay. Within this system, citizens and residents often receive needed medical care by paying a physician to provide their care and, if necessary, to get them into a hospital.

---

3 Named for Otto von Bismarck, the German Chancellor, who in the latter half of the 19th century oversaw the design and implementation of the initial version of this model.

4 The primary reason the authors do not expect to see the United States adopt a statutory health insurance model is because all prior efforts to introduce a corporatist model of governance in the United States have failed.

TABLE 4.6 Case Comparison of United States with Three National Health System Model

Government Funding Across Healthcare Service Delivery and Social Support Systems

Country	Model	Health Care	Social Spending (Includes Public Health, Mental Health, and Social Insurance Programs)
Germany	Statutory Health Insurance (Bismarck)	Almost none	Almost all
Netherlands	Statutory Health Insurance (private mandate)	Almost none	Almost all
Canada	National Health Insurance (Beveridge)	Almost all	Almost all
United States (Federal Government only)	Mixed	Medicare Medicaid HRSA DHS IHS	Public health, mental health, social security, HUD

OECD, Commonwealth Fund & World Bank.

For those who cannot afford to pay a physician for care, they go without medical care and either endure the morbidity of their illness or succumb to mortality as a result of it. Often, these individuals will resort to some variation of traditional or natural medicine to meet their healthcare needs. Countries that use this system include many of the undeveloped or underdeveloped countries throughout the world. One intriguing country in this category is India, which boasts world-class hospitals and healthcare services for those who can pay and even has a thriving medical tourism sector, contrasted against members of its poorer population who do not have access to modern medical care and often resort to traditional medical practices. These countries have poor quality of health care and hold their national costs as a percentage of GDP to less than 10%. The comparison population in the United States is the uninsured, who survive on what they can get through charity care or by foregoing care.

▶ Social Determinants of Health

Within the United States, social determinants of health have been addressed at the local community and state levels. The results of these isolated interventions have been primarily positive, with income support, coordination of community services, housing support, and nutritional support, all resulting in improved health outcomes and reduced health spending (Bradley et al., 2016; Taylor et al., 2016). Current local and state-level models addressing social determinants of health use an ROI

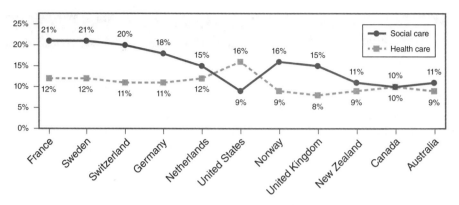

FIGURE 4.3 Health and Social Care Spending as a Percentage of GDP

Data from Bradley, E. H., & Taylor, L. A. (2013). The American Health Care Paradox: Why spending more is getting us less. *Public Affairs.*

model to justify the cost of providing these services. While ROI-focused models provide a financial justification for the provision of these services, ROI rationale is not sustainable in the long term and will eventually need to move to focus on public goods[5] for sustainability (Nichols & Taylor, 2018). Focusing on the provision of social determinants of health as public goods is how most of the OECD justify their provision at the federal level (**FIGURE 4.3**).

▶ Cost, Quality, Access, and Innovation

Comparison of national healthcare delivery models has been developing for several years with early research being more descriptive and more recent research evolving into cost, quality, and access categories, with the recent addition of innovation.

Cost comparisons frequently begin with cost per GDP and total expenditures per citizen or resident. These numbers are a good place to begin the comparison, as debates about healthcare systems frequently end up in a discussion of costs. Cost is a barrier to care for many nations, since not even wealthy nations

have unlimited resources. Cost is also a proxy for quality, because the amount of money spent is often a barometer of low quality due to too little being spent on the provision of services for them to be of any reasonable quality. Conversely, higher costs are not an indicator of high quality. Rather, higher costs could be an indicator of waste and lack of efficiency. Likewise, low costs are not an indicator of access, because the reimbursement may be too low for providers to cover their cost of care. High costs, however, can be an access barrier, with the costs so high that individuals and payers cannot afford the purchase of services. Once researchers get beyond these initial cost measures, they begin to compare wages and costs of resources, such as doctor's visits, hospital stays, pharmaceuticals, and technological innovations.

Another aspect of cost is how acquisition and provision of services are incented. From the recipient side, there is a moral hazard concern that if an individual's cost is too low or free, the resulting behavior is an excessive use of services. In contrast, if an individual's cost is too high through total out-of-pocket expenses, co-pays, or deductibles, the resulting behavior is a delay in the use of services, often resulting in more expensive care. From the provider side, if the payment method is fee-for-service,

5 See Chapter 6 for a discussion of public goods.

the resulting behavior is often overuse of services, because the amount of money received is directly correlated to the amount of services provided. In contrast, if the payment method is capitation, in which the provider is provided a set amount of money to care for a population, the incentive is to do less in order to garner more profit. The United States is currently moving to payment based on patient outcomes and is experimenting with a variety of methods, such as value-based purchasing and bundled payments. Through a national budgeting lens, many countries control their national costs through the use of global budgets, where they set a limit for national expenditures, although most of them pay their providers by a fee-for-service method. The U.S. free market system does not use global budgets that are viewed by many Americans as an infringement on their personal liberty.[6]

Quality is another topic that can be fraught with a variety of definitions and descriptions. Some of the more commonly accepted quality of care measures are length of life, maternal and infant mortality, child death before age 5, immunizations, and the percentage of a country's disease load that is communicable, as opposed to noncommunicable. These quality measures may also serve as proxy measures for access to and efficacy of healthcare services. Quality has a correlation to access, with the assumption that lack of access will result in delays or foregone access services, resulting in low-quality health results, such as increased morbidity or mortality rates.

Cost is also correlated to quality when too little is spent on healthcare services, resulting in poor health outcomes. For example, if maternal and infant mortality are high, quality concerns include access to prenatal and postnatal care, a safe delivery environment, and nutrition. Parsing quality concerns more closely, countries begin to look at individual diseases and judge

quality based on how closely treatment regimens adhere to current evidence-based practices.

Public health efficacy is another aspect of quality that is often measured by the percentage of a country's disease load that is communicable, as opposed to noncommunicable, and the nature of the communicable disease. If the communicable diseases are GI or parasitic, the missing public health action may be the need to separate the drinking water from refuse water. If the communicable diseases are infectious, the source may need to be isolated and eliminated, standard infection control practices need to be followed, and appropriate medical treatment provided.

Access is another area that looks at the efficacy of a healthcare system and how easy it is for individuals to get access to providers and receive care. The first topic associated with access is who is going to pay for the care. In countries with a national health system, the central government pays for a determined set of services, with supplemental health insurance necessary for any services not covered by the national plan. In countries with national and statutory health insurance systems, a determined set of services is covered and supplemental insurance is required for services not covered by the national requirements. In all of the countries with the aforementioned three payment models, access to routine and emergent services is relatively routine and timely; however, access to elective services can result in long wait times. In countries with an out-of-pocket model, access to healthcare services is based on one's ability to pay.

Even when payment is ensured, other barriers to access that are commonly cited are transportation, physician availability, child care, and language. Particularly for low-income families, the cost of transportation to get to a physician or provider can be a barrier if they do not have their own personal transportation

---

6 The state of Maryland is the exception to this. Retrieved from https://www.advisory.com/-/media/Advisory-com /Health-Policy/2016/Maryland-All-Payer-Model-White-Paper.pdf

and have to rely on public transportation or someone else transporting them. Second, physician availability can refer to physical location, hours of availability (office hours or scheduling), or physician to population ratio. All of these have fairly routine remedies, such as physicians having several locations that are easily accessible to the concerned populations, expanded office hours, and open scheduling. Physician to population ratio is more difficult to address and usually involves recruitment or using non-physician providers. Child care can be addressed by physicians having child-friendly offices, subsidized child care centers, and stipends for child care. Finally, language barriers are addressed by the availability of medical interpreters that can either be on-site or telephonic.

Innovation is the fourth and most recent addition to these models, and while the most common perception of innovation is scientific and technological, countries can also innovate on model delivery and payment methods. When considering scientific and technological innovation, the United States surpasses all other countries in the breadth and depth of its scientific and technological production and diffusion. The supports the United States provides for this are funding through the National Institutes of Health and Center for Disease Control, federal and private grants for applied research (Health Resources and Services Administration), and proprietary research for marketable products. Once these products have completed the developmental and regulatory review processes, they are available to any provider willing and able to pay for them, thus making their access and use relatively common. Conversely, with countries that control their costs through global budgets, the availability and use of newer technological products are limited.

References

Bradley, E. H., Canavan, M., Rogan, E., Talbert-Slagle, K., Ndumele, C., Taylor, L., & Curry, L. A. (2016). Variation in health outcomes: The role of spending on social services, public health, and health care, 2000–09. *Health Affairs (Project Hope), 35*(5), 760–768. doi:10.1377/hlthaff.2015.0814

Nichols, L. M., & Taylor, L. A. (2018). Social determinants as public goods: A new approach to financing key investments in healthy communities. *Health Affairs (Project Hope), 37*(8), 1223.

Taylor, L. A., Tan, A. X., Coyle, C. E., Ndumele, C., Rogan, E., Canavan, M., … Bradley, E. H. (2016). Leveraging the social determinants of health: What works? *PLoS One, 11*(8), e0160217. doi:10.1371/journal.pone.0160217

The Commonwealth Fund. (2017). Retrieved from http://international.commonwealthfund.org

The Organization for Economic Cooperation and Development. (2017). Retrieved from http://www.oecd.org/els/health-systems/health-data.htm

The World Bank. (2017). Retrieved from https://data.worldbank.org/indicator/SH.XPD.CHEX.PC.CD

The World Health Organization. Retrieved from https://www.google.com/search?client=safari&rls=en&q=world+health+organization&ie=UTF-8&oe=UTF-8

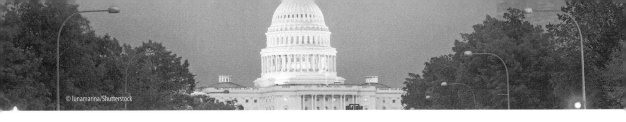

CHAPTER 5

Policy Theories

This chapter is designed to give healthcare leaders an understanding of policy theories by covering the following topics:

- How theories, frameworks, and models describe the policy process
- How innovation and diffusion affect policy
- How population groups are defined and positioned within the policy process
- How leaders can influence and position their influence in the policy process
- How to bring the theoretical models together

As you work through this chapter and the following chapter, it is our hope that you begin to see the close link between the practice of healthcare administration and the formation and implementation of health policy. Just as important, we hope you see ways in which private sector healthcare actors and their innovations may influence policy change. While it is often the case that healthcare administrators (rightly) feel powerless in the face of government regulation, these same administrators can—through state and national trade associations, each system's government affairs experts, and successful innovation—influence government regulations and policy.

Health administrators face top-down change imposed by state and federal agencies as well as from private sector payers (health plans and insurers) in the form of directives related to reimbursement. While not all changes can be classified as "social change" or even as "innovative," a surprising amount are. In response to government mandates, healthcare administrators often respond with innovation, aided and abetted by technological advances, and/or by past successful innovations. These innovations sometimes lead to changes in government policy.

In Chapter 14, we present the ways in which change agents and entrepreneurs interact to create innovations in healthcare delivery that, if successful, lead to changes in government policy. We also clarify how these two groups of actors diffuse successful innovations across regions, states, and the nation.

▶ Conceptual Frameworks, Theories, and Models

Conceptual frameworks, theories, and models are tools used to bring order and understanding to the policy-making process. They differ by the breadth and density of what they are describing and the precision associated with their final outcome. For simplicity's sake, these three phenomena will be treated as theories and divided into process and interest group categories (**TABLE 5.1**). The process category is primarily focused on how ideas are generated,

debated, and developed into legislation. The interest group category focuses on how various groups influence idea, policy, and regulatory development.

▶ Introduction to Problems and Solutions

Gaining a basic understanding of process and interest group theories will provide healthcare leaders an understanding of how policy problems are generated and defined, and how potential solutions are developed prior to entering the formal policy development

TABLE 5.1 Interest Group Frameworks, Theories, and Model Characteristics	
Process-Oriented Conceptual Frameworks, Theories, and Models	**Interest Group–Oriented Conceptual Frameworks, Theories, and Models**
Social constructivism ■ Positive associations ■ Negative associations	
Multiple streams ■ Problems ■ Policies ■ Politics ■ Policy window ■ Policy entrepreneur	Institutional rational choice ■ Behavior-based ■ Action arena ■ Values ■ Official and unofficial policies ■ Consensus ■ Punishment
	Network approach ■ Issue action group ■ Policy advocates and experts ■ Values ■ Cohesion
Punctuated equilibrium ■ Stable incrementalism ■ Shock	Advocacy coalition ■ Common belief systems ■ Education ■ Specialization ■ Resources ■ Deal with wicked and difficult problems

Modified from Sabatier, P. A., & Ebooks Corporation. (2007). *Theories of policy process*. Boulder, CO: Westview Press.

process. Public and private sector managers encounter and solve problems on a daily basis; in fact, their ability to solve problems is a basic competency of leadership. It is only when these problems rise to a level where they are having a negative impact on large portions of the population or the ability of public or private organizations to provide services to the population, that the *societal problem* becomes a *public policy problem*. All public policy solutions follow a similar process, in which they are identified, defined, and redefined by professional and trade groups. Once all parties have agreed to the definition of a problem, they begin to pose and debate potential problem solutions that align their political philosophy. Finally, when all of the circumstances are appropriately aligned, a public policy solution is presented to the appropriate legislative body and enters into a formal process that could result in the enactment of a law.

▶ Social Constructivism

Anne Schneider and Helen Ingram describe social constructivism and policy design in *Policy Design for Democracy* (1997). The theory of social constructivism and policy design begins with the establishment of three categories—individuals, power, and political environment—and then subdivides these three categories into eight elements (**TABLE 5.2**). The *individuals* category describes how individuals process information through heuristics and a bounded relativity process that reinforces previous biases and stable social constructs, while discarding information that does not conform to these previous biases or social constructs. *Power* is acknowledged to be unequally distributed and augmented by a discussion of the *faces of power* that include the aspects of influence, conflict, and control of resources and information. One noteworthy aspect of power that is counterintuitive is not its

ability to progress political ideas and solution to the agenda, but rather, it is its ability to keep ideas that do not conform to stable social constructs off the agenda. The *political environment* describes the uncertainty of the political environment, messaging to citizens affecting their orientation and participation, and a feed forward process. *Feed forward* is a process in which new policies are developed as a result of the influence of past policies and politics (Caronia & Caron, 2019), a process very similar to incrementalism, described by Almeida and Gomes (2018), Kingdon (1984, 1995), and Baumgartner and Jones (1993). For example, the Social Security Act of 1935 had 11 acts, whereas the current Act has 21 titles, with each title resulting in significant benefits to an additional target (socially constructed) population.

Next, Schneider and Ingram describe how population groups are constructed based on level of power and perception of social construction (**TABLE 5.3**). While the population groups move in a progressive continuum, the social constructs identified by the four quadrants assist in framing or understanding these socially constructed population groups. The groups include *advantaged*, which are positively constructed and high power, resulting in a high share of benefits and a low burden (Pierce et al., 2014). Next are *contenders*, which are negatively constructed and low power. While they receive a fair amount of benefit and low burden, their negative construct allows them to be easily undermined. *Dependents*, which are positively constructed and low power, receive limited benefits and hidden burden. Finally, *deviants* are negatively constructed and low power, receiving limited to no benefits and no high burden. One phenomenon associated with the continuum of movement throughout these four quadrants is that population groups are not static. Rather, they are dynamic as they move through the various quadrants due to their influence and public opinion.

TABLE 5.2 Social Construction Categories

Individual	Power	Political Environment
1. Inability to possess all information, resulting in the use of mental heuristics as filters 2. Biased mental heuristic filters, resulting in retention of confirmatory information and rejection of all other information 3. Used in a subjective, evaluative manner 4. Bounded relativity of subjective reality when stable patterns of social construction are perceived	1. Not equally distributed within a political environment Dimensions or faces of power (Luke, 1994; Bachman & Bartz, 1962) a. Observable behaviors, influence, and conflict b. What is not present and the ability to keep items off the agenda c. Ideology and potential influence of the rationale for the creation of preferences Dimensions or faces of power (Schneider & Ingram, 1993, 1997) a. Influence and the arousal of political resources (e.g., skill, voter mobilization, and votes) b. Public opinion and control policy-associated information c. In-depth case studies	1. Policy creates policies that feed forward to create new policy and politics 2. Policies send messages to citizens that affect their orientations and participation patterns 3. Policies are created in an environment of political uncertainty

Modified from Pierce, J. J., Siddiki, S., Jones, M. D., Schumacher, K., Pattison, A., & Peterson, H. (2014). Social construction and policy design: A review of past applications. *Policy Studies Journal, 42*(1), 1–29, doi:10.1111/psj.12040.

TABLE 5.3 Target Population Classifications

	Positively Constructed	Negatively Constructed
High power	Advantaged	Contenders
Low power	Dependents	Deviants

Modified from Pierce, J. J., Siddiki, S., Jones, M. D., Schumacher, K., Pattison, A., & Peterson, H. (2014). Social construction and policy design: A review of past applications. *Policy Studies Journal, 42*(1), 1–29, doi:10.1111/psj.12040.

TABLE 5.4 Policy Design Elements

Policy Design Elements (Schneider & Ingram)		
1. Target population	2. Problem or goal definition	3. Rules
4. Rationales	5. Assumptions	6. Benefitd & burdens
7. Tools	8. Implementation structure	9. Social construction

Modified from Pierce, J.J., Siddiki, S., Jones, M.D., Schumacher, K.,Pattison, A., & Peterson, H. (2014). Social construction and policy design: A review of past applications. Policy Studies Journal, 42(1), 1-29, doi:10.1111/psj.12040.

Finally, once these groups are socially constructed, the focus shifts to policy design, which includes nine elements (**TABLE 5.4**). These elements begin with the target population, progress through rationales and assumptions, and end with social construction. The process of social construction involves identifying a population, constructing how that population lives and functions based on institutional and cultural norms, and identifying problems, requiring public policy resolution based on this construct. Normally, these constructs are agreed on by society, as positively and negatively incented policies are targeted at the constructed group. Once these policy resolutions have been implemented, they are evaluated and adjusted as necessary to achieve the desired policy result (**FIGURE 5.1**).

Social construction occurs within the material world and results from the interaction of individuals and groups with the environment. Problems are a result of tension that arises when two conflicting thoughts or values are held simultaneously (Valentine, Sovacool, & Brown, 2017). Social construction is built on the structure of populations and social classes, how social groups interact within and between these societally established classes, and the resulting conflicts or problems that result from this interaction. The nature of constructed groups is based on

their power within the environment that can emanate from legitimate position, the ability to provide reward or coerce behavior, expert knowledge, or referent such as a well-known political or social figure.

An example of social construction in health care is the uninsured population (deviants). We episodically support their healthcare needs through free clinics, federally qualified health centers, and charity policies. When the uninsured are described by the data, they fall into two categories: (1) chronically uninsured individuals who are generally single minority males in low paying jobs (dependents), and (2) acutely uninsured individuals in middle and upper middle class families whose primary wage earner is in between jobs (contenders). Both of these categories need different supports to access healthcare services. The chronically uninsured (dependents) need access to regular medical care that they can currently receive through federally qualified health clinics. The acutely uninsured (contenders) need continuation of current healthcare provider relationships that are available to them through COBRA insurance provisions, which most find unaffordable. Contrary to the socially constructed impression of the uninsured (deviants) as irresponsible and unemployed, most of the uninsured are either working or looking for work. A likely policy

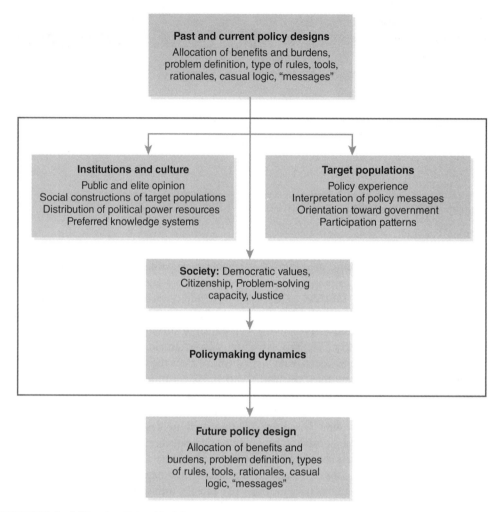

FIGURE 5.1 Social Constructivism Model

Reproduced with permission of Taylor & Francis, from Ingram, Helen, Schneider, Anne L., & Deleon, Peter. (2007). *Theories of the policy process* (2nd ed.); permission conveyed through Copyright Clearance Center, Inc.

to address the uninsured need for health insurance, resulting in access to healthcare services, could be to require them to provide evidence of work in order to receive health insurance coverage. However, a more accurate understanding of this population(s) yields the knowledge that they are either already working or in the process of gaining new employment, and that requiring work from this population to demonstrate "responsibility" on their part may actually be counterproductive

and not address their need for support in their current work situation.

▶ Innovation and Diffusion

Innovation refers to new ideas or policy approaches to address current public problems, whereas diffusion refers to using current ideas in different jurisdictions. There are few innovative ideas for national health system models and payment systems. Currently, there are four national healthcare models (national health system, national health insurance, statutory health insurance, and out-of-pocket) that vary as to the degree of governmental intervention, from complete ownership to no interaction. Innovation would result from coming up with a fifth model that is different than the previous four, although it would likely be some variation of these four models. Currently, CMS is mandated by the ACA to host an innovation center that is testing innovative models of care that are all variations of care coordination, under the premise that coordinated care is less fragmented and less expensive. They are also testing payment methods that all involve shifting risk to providers and incenting payment based on quality outcomes. When these two general concepts are compared to all other national models, they are considered innovative because no other models directly engage healthcare professionals in coordinating care. From a payment lens, all other models pay providers on a fee-for-service basis with some type of pay for performance provisions.

Diffusion is what CMS hopes will happen with the models they have tested through the innovation center. *The dissemination of tested and proven models to other jurisdictions is the heart of diffusion.* These proven models allow jurisdictions to learn what does and does not work from each other, as well as learn the nuances of implementation and management of innovative systems. There are several models of diffusion, including national and regional models, leader-laggard, isomorphism, vertical, and internal determinants models. *National models* are adopted by all states and are influenced by the level of interaction state leaders have with federal governmental officials. An example of national diffusion is expanded Medicaid that has resulted in three general approaches: (1) as designed by the ACA,

(2) variations of the ACA design that allow for private market influence and products, and (3) refusal to adopt. *Regional models* posit that states in a region will behave like each other, with these similarities rooted in both regional culture and political climate. Using the expansion of Medicaid again, regional diffusion notes three large clusters of states that either have or have not expanded Medicaid (**FIGURE 5.2**). One cluster includes Northeast and Eastern Midwest states, another large cluster includes the West Coast, and a third cluster (which has not expanded Medicaid) runs from the Southeast up through the Midwest. *Leader-laggard* models suggest that certain states are leaders in various aspects of public policy and others follow once they see how their well-regarded peers have performed. Again, Medicaid expansion (Figure 5.2) could be used as an example of this phenomenon, with the more socially liberal states on either coast leading the way and more moderate states following. Another aspect of this model that has to be considered with this example is state-level political control. The leaders in Medicaid expansion were states that had strong Democratic control of the legislature, governorship, or both. Those states with some level of Republican control that expanded Medicaid have either a long history of providing social support programs, pragmatic Republican governors, or both. Additionally, when they did expand Medicaid, many of them did so with a CMS waiver to alter the program and bring it closer to Republican values.

Isomorphism argues that states that are similar behave in similar ways, thus copying each other as they adopt and implement public policy. The regional clustering of states that either have or have not expanded Medicaid could be an example of isomorphism, with the similarity of these states' values reflected either in the political control in their state or in their history of support for social service programs. *Vertical* models argue that states emulate the federal governmental, as opposed

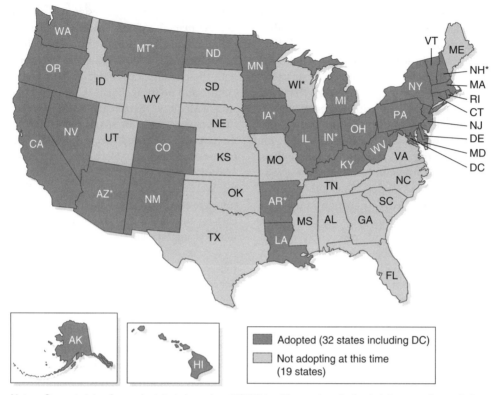

Adopted (32 states including DC)

Not adopting at this time
(19 states)

Notes: Current status for each state is based on KCMU tracking and analysis of state executive activity. *AR, AZ, IA, IN, MI, MT, and NH have approved section 1115 waivers. WI covers adults up to 100% FPL in Medicaid, but did not adopt the ACA expansion.

FIGURE 5.2 Medicaid Expansion

"Status of State Action on the Medicaid Expansion Decision," KFF State Health Facts, updated January 1, 2017. https://www.kff.org/health-reform/state-indicator /state-activity-around-expanding-medicaid-under-the-affordable-care-act/

to state, models or that higher levels of government use their coercive power to force change. Continuing with the expanded Medicaid example, in a 2012 Supreme Court decision, the Court found the expansion of Medicaid as written in the ACA, which tied all Medicaid funds to the implementation of expanded Medicaid, to be too coercive, and found that traditional Medicaid funds could not be linked to the expansion of Medicaid. Finally, *internal determinants* models argue that states consider political, economic, and social variants of the state when adopting other models. Again, this is the essential argument with the expansion of Medicaid.

Other variants on diffusion include the mechanisms of learning, economic competition, imitation, and coercion. *Learning* includes the idea that states are laboratories where we try various solutions to social and democratic problems. The idea behind this concept is that states implement different governmental and non-governmental programs based on their social and political climates and that the laggards or late adopters learn from the successes and failures of the leaders or early adopters. *Economic competition* carries the idea that states bordering each other are economically competing with each other and are not allowing their border neighbors to outcompete them economically or under compete them socially. The fear of states is that providing an economic climate that is less favorable than their border neighbor will result in loss of jobs to their neighbor, or conversely, that offering social services richer than their neighbor will result in the pull of those seeking social services from their neighbors. *Imitation* is similar to isomorphism, or the idea that states imitate successful programs implemented by other states. A nuance of this idea is that states with similar values will imitate like states. *Coercion* is either vertical or horizontal. *Vertical coercion* results when a higher level of government forces a lower level of government to perform in a manner they would not normally endorse without the associate negative incentive. *Horizontal coercion* occurs across jurisdictions of similar size, where jurisdiction forces another similar size jurisdiction to perform in a manner they would not normally endorse. Ultimately, innovation and diffusion find that there are few new ideas and that when jurisdictions do adopt the ideas of other jurisdictions, they do so based on similarity of the original jurisdiction or their leadership in a given policy area.

▶ Multiple Streams Theory

Multiple streams is the thesis of *Agendas, Alternatives, and Public Policies,* published by John Kingdon in 1984 and updated once (1995) with an additional chapter of his reflections on the theory. Since its original publication, countless scholars and researchers have used this theory to frame their research. This theory posits that all public policies begin with the identification of a problem. The problem is usually identified by leaders and advocates of a social group and is originally ambiguous, while multiple actors debate the problem and its merits,

functioning similarly to how the "garbage can" model of problem identification and solutions functions (Cohen, March, & Olsen, 1972). Throughout this process, a problem is refined and re-defined within the communities affected by the problem and in the public literature. As this debate draws near a close, groups begin to provide potential policy solutions for the problem. The potential policy solutions are modeled and debated for their merits and demerits throughout the various communities, ultimately taking on a political tone as political parties join the debate based on the groups for which they are advocating and the alignment of their political philosophy with the potential solutions. Finally, a policy window emerges that is normally prompted by an event that brings the problem, potential policy solution, and politics into alignment. These events can be exogenous, such as the 9/11 attack on the twin towers that resulted in passage of the Patriot Act and the consolidation of several existing federal agencies into the Department of Homeland Security, or endogenous, such as through a political campaign resulting in the Patient Protection and Affordable Care Act. Once this alignment occurs and the public agrees on the need to address this problem, a policy entrepreneur takes the policy and ushers it through the legislative process that results in a new public policy or law. It should be noted here that the policy solution at this stage may still be ambiguous, with the resulting policy reflecting the most politically feasible, as opposed to idealistic, policy outcome. An example of this occurred in the development of the ACA, when liberal Democrats idealistically wanted to propose a single-payer health system. However, this proposal did not have sufficient political support and the resulting legislation was far more moderate and based on Republican ideas. This process is normative and takes 20 years on average to complete (range 5–50 years), is dynamic, and is limited to the agenda-setting and legislative processes.

Positive examples of this include the enactment of Medicare, Medicaid, and the Patient Protection and Affordable Care Act. In each of these scenarios, the need for a national healthcare program had been debated (problem definition) for several years. Both political parties had their proposals for how to address the problem based on their political philosophy and constituent feedback. In each scenario, the policy window opened with the national election of a democratic congress and president, and the president acted as the policy entrepreneur, backed up by co-entrepreneurs in both chambers of congress. The opening of the policy window is normally a narrow period that needs to be acted on quickly or else the legislative opportunity is forfeited. A negative example of this is the Health Security Act proposed by President Clinton, for which the policy window closed before the policy was developed and voted on.

▶ Punctuated Equilibrium Theory

Punctuated equilibrium is a theory developed by Baumgartner and Jones (1993) about how information is processed, drawing on Herbert Simon's work on serial processing, parallel processing, and bounded rationality. Serial processing is when thoughts or ideas are processed sequentially, with the next action based on the former action. Parallel processing is when individuals and organizations process several thoughts or ideas at the same time. The modern term for parallel process is multitasking. While it sounds impressive to be able to process several ideas or tasks at the same time, both Simon's research (Simon, 1947, 1976) and current cognitive research (Duncan & Mitchell, 2015; Ophir, Nass, Wagner, & Posner, 2009; Takeuchi et al., 2014) indicate that

while parallel processing improves with practice, we still serial process ideas and tasks. Neither individuals nor organizations can parallel process. We can process several ideas or tasks over short periods of time, but we do so by concentrating on each task or idea individually. Thus, most of what we do remains in stasis or equilibrium while we work through or focus on processes or topics that have risen to the forefront and demand our attention.

Punctuated equilibrium theory states that most policy topics are either static or in a state of equilibrium and are progressively maintained incrementally until something (an event) occurs to break the topic from its parallel equilibrium to series processing. This event is associated with the phenomenon of bounded rationality and serial processing of information. Bounded rationality is the idea that we have a limit to how much information we can process at one time and that when we process information, we do so in a serial process. Thus, when policy makers focus on a topic, they do so in a serial process that often results in the development of a policy window. When this policy window or break occurs, it does so with a kerfuffle-like flurry of activity for a short time. Once the event has ceased, the equilibrium is higher than normal for a short time and then evens back to parallel processing, incremental activity. When these policy activities are graphed, they demonstrate leptokurtic, positively skewed distribution. When this process is described graphically, it demonstrates static, incremental activity, a large amount of activity leading to an acute spike in activity, followed by a larger amount of residual activity that quickly declines into static equilibrium.

The number of Congressional hearings focused on Veterans Affairs (**FIGURE 5.3**) demonstrates a classic example of static equilibrium punctuated with a leptokurtic, positively skewed curve, followed by

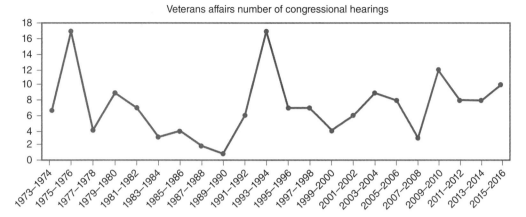

FIGURE 5.3 Leptokurtic Curve—Veterans Affairs

data source Congress.gov., graphic Higbea 2017.

a gradual decrease in activity. An intriguing variation to this theory occurs with all health laws and Congressional hearings by committees assigned health topics if graphed from 1973 to present (**FIGURE 5.4**). While the leptokurtic, positively skewed punctuations occur at least three times, the post-leptokurtic volume of activity never returns to the original baseline. Rather, a new baseline is established at approximately the median of the most recent leptokurtic curve. Thus, the activity demonstrates a continued build up or importance of health activity at the federal level.

The original work by Baumgartner and Jones (1993) was on budget authority; however, a more relative recent example is the policy process surrounding the Patient Protection and Affordable Care Act. Since the enactment of Medicare and Medicaid in 1965, there have been only a few major healthcare policy proposals, such as the Prospective Payment System (1983—passed), Health Security Act (1993—failed), Health Insurance Portability and Accountability Act (1996—passed), and the Medicare Modernization Act (2003—passed). A review of healthcare legislative activity throughout

this time period demonstrates generally at least 1000 healthcare-related bills submitted per Congress (**TABLE 5.5**), with less than 5% passed into law and most of them being updates and minor revisions. Prior to the 2008 presidential election, healthcare legislation was in a state of incremental stasis. Throughout the presidential campaign, Senator Obama made national health reform a campaign topic (creating an event) and, while he had some definite ideas, the proposal was ambiguous. Once in office for a year, President Obama brought up the need for national healthcare reform and allowed congressional leaders to draft the final bill (ambiguity of ideas). The bill was large, with over 2000 pages, and was passed along party lines. Since that time, there have been at least 50 bills to modify (most signed by the president) or repeal (none passed through both chambers of Congress) the bill, multiple district and appeals court challenges, and three Supreme Court challenges.

Baumgartner and Jones argued that when political images (created by elites and broadcast to the public through mass media) are positive, government permits, and even facilitates, industry experts to develop a

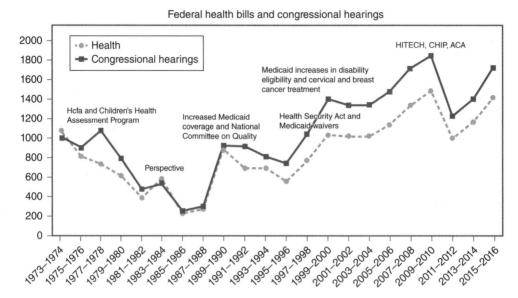

FIGURE 5.4 Leptokurtic Curve—All Health Bills and Congressional Hearings

data source Congress.gov., graphic Higbea 2017.

policy subsystem that controls policy related to that industry (e.g., the design and enactment of industry regulations). They posit that the development of the policy subsystem is an effort to insulate the industry from the influence of democratic forces. Also noteworthy is their argument that the development of a policy subsystem is more likely when the issues at hand appear to be technical and specialized in nature, requiring the turnover of control to persons trained to deal with these issues. The policy subsystem that is created controls policy activity through the limitation of the number of venues available for change, and also attempts to maintain a positive policy image.

Policy subsystems may be broken; however, they are broken by the activity of those actors outside of the policy subsystems who disagree with their outputs. The avenues for breaking these subsystems are the myriad other more receptive venues available to these actors (sometimes referred to by Baumgartner

and Jones as policy entrepreneurs). These other venues include, but are not limited to, elected officials, legislative bodies, government agencies, the mass media, other industries, the public at large, and the market. The process of breaking up a policy subsystem is marked by what they term a "succession of 'venue-access events'" (1993). These events result in the expansion of the discussion of issues related to those in the hands of the policy subsystem to venues beyond the subsystem's control. They state that "... the job of a policy entrepreneur is often that of identifying the most receptive alternative venues for the policy" (1993).

Coincident and interactive with the venue-access events is a change in policy image. The policy image becomes less positive, and the exposure of images related to the policy (positive and negative) increases. These two types of events are interactive and mutually supporting as the increase in the number of venues looking at a problem is

TABLE 5.5 Bills Submitted to Congress

Congress	Years	Enacted	Total	Got a Vote	HC Bills	HC Law
113	2013–2015	296	10,637	474	3975	92
112	2011–2013	284	12,299	390	3662	67
111	2009–2010	385	13,675	601	4616	109
110	2007–2009	460	14,042	861	4871	131
109	2005–2006	483	13,072	597	4216	149
108	2003–2004	504	10,669	694	3895	155
107	2001–2002	383	10,781	602	3685	121
106	1999–2001	604	10,840	650	3831	166
Total		3399	96,015	4869	32,751	990
Mean		424.88	12,001.88	608.63	4093.88	123.75
Percentage		3.54%		5.07%	36.65%	3.02%
Total						1.03%
Bills vote and enacted				69.81%		

Govtrack.

increasing, and journalists are drawn to the issue because of increasing elite attention. Changes that may weaken a policy subsystem occur largely outside the public eye in the early stages, with little media attention at the beginning stages of venue expansion and image change. As mentioned earlier, the possible venues for weakening the policy subsystem include state involvement, advances in research and technology, and market activity. Understanding these conditions at the local level inevitably requires close connection with the community and its contexts. This is exactly a finding of a recent study on "public" entrepreneurs by Mack, Green, and Vedlitz (2008). They found that the connection with the local community exhibited by many community-level entrepreneurs to be one of the most important attributes of successful change efforts.

▶ Agenda-Setting

Multiple streams (Kingdon, 1984) and *punctuated equilibrium* (Baumgartner & Jones, 1993) are both agenda-setting theories developed to describe and predict the agenda-setting process. The need for an agenda goes back to Simon's work on serial processing and bounded rationality, or an unlimited amount of problems competing for a limited amount of time. Or, as stated by Dearing and Rogers (1996), "The *agenda-setting process* is an ongoing competition among issue proponents to gain the attention of media professionals, the public, and policy elites." The first item of business by issue proponents is to get on the agenda by raising the public image of a problem or issue to the level requiring action. Next, issue proponents need to promote the

immanence of their issue or problem up the competing hierarchy of competing issues or problems to a place of prominence and action. The process of gaining access to and hierarchically moving up the agenda is described by Dearing and Rogers (1996) and modeled in **FIGURE 5.5**. The continued relevance of these models, with a few inter-process revisions, was developed by Almeida and Gomes (2018).

First, the concept of an agenda is general and needs to be divided into three agendas that present in a progressive fashion. These agendas are a media agenda, a public agenda, and a policy agenda. Next is the concept of the interrelationships among actors affecting the agenda(s), including experience and communication among elites; gate keepers, influential media, and media events; and public perception of an agenda item's importance.

▶ Network Approach

Interest groups are a product of political necessity and convenience that allow a group unified by a cause or concern to come together with a

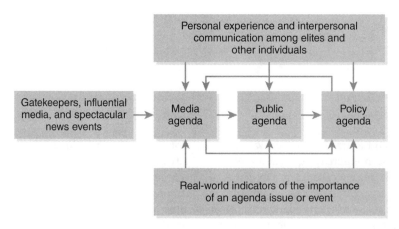

FIGURE 5.5 Components of the Agenda-Setting Process

variety of actors to speak in unison. The organization of interest groups varies from official advocacy activities associated with professional organizations, such as physicians, nurses, or administrators, to specific topical concerns, such as diabetes or heart disease. The organization of interest groups includes topical experts, legislative experts, and actors who have an interest in the group's cause or concern in general and in how the ultimate legal remedy will personally affect them. These groups function effectively when the interested actors provide resources to the expert actors, which allows them the time necessary to develop solutions to identified problems and raise the problem with their solutions to public and political attention, including getting their ideas before governmental administrators, legislators, and staffers. The ultimate goal of any interest group is to get their ideas into legislation and passed into law. Once the law has been signed, interest groups continue their advocacy work throughout the implementation, operations, and modification phases. If the interest group is satisfied with the final legal remedy, they may choose to disband; however, if they desire to focus on refinements to the legal remedy or to focus on other topics, they may desire to remain together and continue their work.

The focus of the *network approach* is how groups gather around specific issues with a common cause, knowledge, and values, and how they use these commonalities to shape the issues of their interest. One of the earliest examples of this approach is the *iron triangle*, positing that Congress, the bureaucracy, and interest groups are both synergistic and symbiotic, all requiring the support of each other to thrive and survive. A result of this required support was the development of subgovernments in which everyone involved in an issue knows each other and there seems to be a blurring of the line between public and private involvement of the actors. These network groups are self-organizing, self-governing groups of public and private actors who are unified by their desire to solve public problems. Within these networks, the actors have differing capabilities, with the distribution of these capabilities throughout the network resulting in various concentrated pockets of power. The greatest concentration of power normally goes to the state actors who have the ability to impose statutes and regulations upon society. To a lesser extent, private actors have the power to shape statutes and regulations, although they are more likely to use their power to stop unfavorable statutes or regulations.

Next, policy networks can be described by their level of cooperation with the two types of cooperation: (1) concentration, in which there is little conflict or bargaining and hierarchical cooperation, and (2) fragmentation, in which there is high conflict or competition, symmetrical bargaining, and horizontal cooperation. With those network descriptors in mind, the network approach will be further explored through the development of (1) issue action groups, (2) policy advocates and experts, (3) values, and (4) cohesion.

Issue action groups can be described as geographical international or national policy networks. The scholarly study in this realm focuses on the legislative and administrative domains and is primarily concerned with the central level of control (intervention) the government can exert to force policy change. Another way to describe issue action groups is as general or specific policy variables. The variables differ in the incentives or disincentives associated with a policy or with destabilizing shocks to the policy domain. Destabilizing shocks can result from changes in ideas, values, and knowledge that can result in the dissolution and reorganization of policy specific domains or issue action groups.

Within the healthcare arena, there are various levels and degrees of intervention, varying from the national, state, and local levels.

There is frequent tension within these groups, particularly when one level of government defines a public problem, develops a solution, and imposes that solution on a lower level of government. When this occurs between the federal and state levels, charges of federalism often come up and the legal authority to impose the policy solution is challenged in court. A recent example of this is the Supreme Court's decision in 2012 stating that the federal government expansion of Medicaid, designed as an all or nothing proposal (expand or lose all Medicaid funding), was too coercive and unconstitutional. In this case, several Republican state attorney generals self-organized, filing several suites. One state attorney general took the lead in each case and then they dissolved as a group once the Supreme Court settled their cases (concerns).

The other way issue action groups organize is based on situational variables, focusing on the stability of the environment within which the issue action group works. Disrupters that can destabilize the system include changes in ideas, values, and knowledge. Healthcare changes in ideas and knowledge often coincide with innovation (technological, model, or payment). Recent examples of this type of activity include the work currently underway through the CMS Innovation Center that is testing new models of how care is organized, coordinated, and delivered, and tied to innovative payment methods that focus on patient outcomes and the quality or value of the care delivered. These changes are causing tension and stress, as the healthcare system reorganizes to accommodate the changes coming out of the Innovation Center. There are a large variety of organizations and issue action groups in ferment as industry and professional groups join together to defend the stability of their environment, while recognizing that change is inevitable. All are seeking to influence the pace of change as much as possible.

Throughout the healthcare domain, there are issue action groups for every sector, industry, professional group, and disease. All of these groups behave as described earlier, operating on the various governmental levels, as appropriate, and within the specific arenas, as appropriate. Hospitals are one example of an industry group that has developed a rather sophisticated policy network group, frequently led by the American Hospital Association. This industry group has been in existence since 1899 and both promoted the interests of hospitals with the various levels of government and shepherded their transformation over the past 100 plus years. Hospitals changed from places for the poor to die, to technological centers of excellence, to coordinators of healthcare services. They went from stand-alone hospitals to both vertically and horizontally integrated healthcare systems. Currently, the industry is struggling to reorganize itself and reorganize how care is delivered, while payment structure transforms from fee-for-service to outcome-based and value-based payment. Throughout this journey, the AHA has worked to organize hospitals around the various issues that have surfaced and sought to influence the legislative and regulatory processes in the best interest of hospitals.

The other situational area that issue action groups form around is values that can change over time as the values of society evolve. One example of a value that has evolved over time is individual autonomy and self-determination. Some of the initial work on this topic and an example of international context came as a result of atrocities performed on individuals during World War II in the Nazi concentration camps, resulting in the Helsinki Accords: Declaration of Human Rights (1975), in which the participating countries agreed to uphold basic human rights. As a result of this accord, institutional review boards have been established that require researchers to ensure that research participants have consented to the research and are aware of any potential dangers they may encounter as a result of the research.

▶ Advocacy Coalition

The Advocacy Coalition Framework (ACF) is a framework designed ". . . to deal with 'wicked' problems—those dealing with substantial goal conflicts, important technical disputes, and multiple actors from several levels of government . . ." (Sabatier & Ebooks Corporation, 2007). Additionally, the ACF ". . . has at least four basic premises: (1) that understanding the process of policy change—and the role of policy-oriented learning therein—requires a time perspective of a decade or more; (2) that the most useful way to think about policy change over such a time span is through a focus on 'policy subsystems' . . . the interaction of actors from different institutions who follow and seek to influence governmental decisions in a policy area; (3) that those subsystems must include intergovernmental dimension . . . they must involve all levels of government (at least for domestic policy); and, (4) that public policies (or programs) can be conceptualized in the same manner as belief systems . . . as sets of value priorities and causal assumptions about how to realize

them" (Sabatier & Jenkins-Smith, 1993). The model for this framework has been essentially unchanged since its inception (see **FIGURE 5.6**) and includes (1) relatively stable parameters, (2) external (system) events, (3) degree of consensus needed for major policy changes, (4) constraints and resources of subsystem actors, and (5) policy subsystems.

The characteristic of a wicked or difficult problem that ACF groups deal with was originally environmental in nature; however, healthcare concerns certainly fall within this category as well. The wicked problem of health care includes the desire to provide healthcare access for everyone in the country while maintaining the cost at around 10% of GDP and ensuring individual choice, responsible behaviors, and quality outcomes. Within the context of this problem is a debate over the level of government interventions required to ensure the aforementioned outcome. Common belief systems within U.S. society include the belief

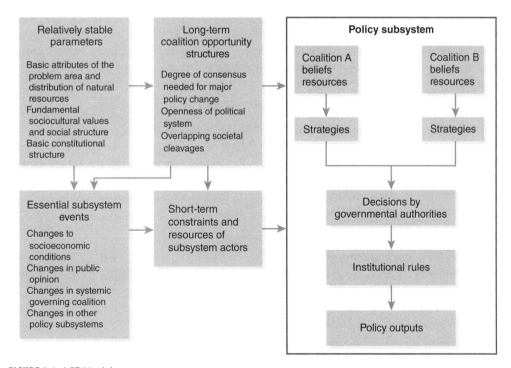

FIGURE 5.6 ACF Model

that everyone should have access to health-care services. However, the differences revolve around the level of individual responsibility and government intervention (commodity/market justice or right/social justice). The resources of the subsystems involved in the debate are rather robust; however, the resources of those ultimately providing the services and paying for them are limited. Roughly 57% of the nation has employer-based insurance that most of this group find affordable, although it is becoming less affordable as costs continue to increase. Another 20% of the nation has some type of governmentally provided healthcare services that require minimal personal outlays and most of this group find affordable. Approximately 7% of the nation purchases personal or individual health insurance policies. The affordability for this group is mixed—individuals at either end of the income levels have little problems affording their policies due to financial resources or governmental subsidies, but the middle group has difficulty affording these policies. About 10% have no health insurance and find its purchase unaffordable. Taken a different way, employers are finding it increasingly difficult to continue purchasing health insurance for their employees even with the tax credit and increased employee cost-sharing. Meanwhile, the citizenry is divided, with some expressing concerns about the increased level of government involvement while others are concerned about ensuring access to coverage.

Specialization is an area in which both sides of this debate have considerable depth in formal training and healthcare and policy experience. Additionally, a large amount of learning has occurred over the past 100 years through debates regarding governmental intervention and healthcare system structure. For example, the Democrats have learned from the Health Security Plan (Clinton in 1993) the importance of not debating the topic so long that the policy window closes on them and have learned positively by diffusing the Massachusetts plan into the ACA. This framework is used throughout the various stages of

the policy process, as the various subgroups seek to either influence the positive outcome of legislation and see it passed to become law or block from becoming law what they view as poor legislation.

The various coalitions formed by the AMA over the past century have been focused on blocking healthcare legislation (Medicare, Medicaid, Health Security Act). However, during the debate of the ACA, the AMA did not oppose the law; rather, they worked with other coalitions to see it pass with as little negative effect as possible for their membership. One posited reason for this change in tactic is that the AMA's level of influence has diminished over the past century, as membership went from representing 75% of the physicians in 1950 to 15% of physicians during the ACA debate.

▶ Institutional Rational Choice

Institutional Rational Choice (**FIGURE 5.7**) is a framework that describes how various groups interact and are self-governed. The original work on Institutional Rational Choice was conducted by Elinor Ostrom (1993) when she studied water rights in California and how the groups involved with the water rights behaved, developed their values, and were governed. The model (see Figure 5.7) is rather simple, yet elegant, and includes physical or material conditions; attributes of community; rules-in-use; action arena, including action situations and actors; patterns of interaction; evaluative criteria; and outcomes.

The physical or material conditions in the most recent healthcare debate are the cost, quality, and access of healthcare services for all U.S. citizens (residents have been excluded from this debate). The attributes of the healthcare community can be stratified by industry sector, providers versus payers, and various aspects of cost of care, including charges for services, cost of services, payment for services, cost of

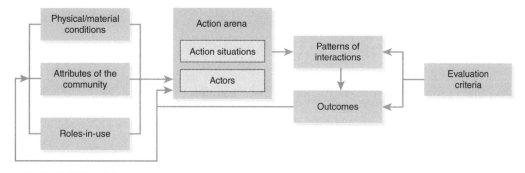

FIGURE 5.7 IRC Model

Data from Ostrom, E. (1990). *Governing the commons: The evolution of institutions for collective action.* Cambridge University Press.

technology, cost of healthcare infrastructure, cost to employers, cost to individuals, cost to the government (percent of GDP), clinical quality of care, patient perceived quality of care, access to care with health insurance, access to care without health insurance, outcomes of services provided, morbidity, mortality, the ethical values of the community, behaviors, such as no medical care, that can be prescribed without a physician order and no payment will occur without a physician order, physician centric versus patient centric model of care, and the list can go on to include the legislative and governmental arenas. Rules in use include (1) no prescribed service or payment without a physician order and (2) comprehensive service only provided to individuals with "good" health insurance. The action arena is where healthcare services take place and from a medical lens would include a physician office, outpatient clinic, hospital, or other institution, such as a long-term care facility. However, when viewed through the lens of healthcare services, the action arena includes our homes and places of work and education. When viewed through the lens of healthcare policy, the action arena is public debate driven by debate within legislative chambers. The point is that the action arena shifts based upon the actors involved in the process.

The patterns of interactions are varied as well based on the action arena. For example, in the medical arena, the interaction patterns are driven by the physician–patient relationship, with the lead in that relationship varying depending on whether the model is physician-centric or patient-centric. In the legislative arena, there are normal patterns of how legislation progresses, including through the various stages as well as through the legislative process of committees and legislative leaders. Members of either of these processes have consensus on how the process will operate. If actors violate the rules of the process, the other actors have the ability to punish that actor in order to maintain the rules of the process. Examples of this include patients firing physicians and physicians firing patients for noncompliance. In the legislative arena, this punishment often comes in the form of removal from plum committee assignments or lack of inclusion in policy development when the actor has a defined skill set.

Although policy entrepreneurs are incidentally referenced by Baumgartner and Jones (1993) in their study of policy subsystems and policy change, their theory is relevant to the issue of how local policy entrepreneurs may go about interacting in both political and market venues (components of Mintrom's milieus, introduced in Chapter 14) in order to achieve change. Baumgartner and Jones presented a theory explaining both policy stability and punctuated changes in policy within the United States. They argued that both stability and punctuated change were manifestations of a process that is "the interaction of beliefs and values concerning a particular policy . . . [the policy image] . . . with the existing set of political institutions .... [venues of policy action]" (1045).

Baumgartner and Jones argued that when political images (created by elites and broadcast to the public through mass media) are positive, government permits, and even facilitates, industry experts to develop a policy subsystem that controls policy related to that industry (e.g., the design and enactment of industry regulations). They posit that the development of the policy subsystem is an effort to insulate the industry from the influence of democratic forces. Also noteworthy is their argument that the development of a policy subsystem is more likely when the issues at hand appear to be technical and specialized in nature, requiring the turnover of control to persons trained to deal with these issues. The policy subsystem that is created controls policy activity through the limitation of the number of venues available for change, and also attempts to maintain a positive policy image.

▶ Bringing the Theoretical Models Together

After reviewing the aforementioned models, it is natural to question the meaning of the models and whether they work in isolation or in unity. We posit they work in unity (**FIGURE 5.8**), with each framework, theory, or model describing a unique aspect of a dynamically interactive process. All of the action begins in the *action arena*, with a variety of private and political *actors* responding to a *socially constructed condition* that is in the process of being identified and defining *socially constructed* as a *problem*.

As the debate regarding the *problem* begins, a variety of physical, material, and political *external forces* shape the debate. The affected communities seek to ensure that the context of

the problem and any solutions remains contextually intact. During this time, *interest groups* begin exerting their power, resources, and knowledge, as they seek to ensure their positions and solutions are considered and those of their opponents are blocked. As this debate progresses to the *solutions level*, the action arena fractures along political and philosophical lines, with the structures essentially duplicating themselves as the actors align around general political and philosophical solutions. As these fractured action arenas emerge, additional policy entrepreneurs (individual and institutional) emerge with their own nuanced policy solutions aligned with specific group(s) of the political base. All of the aforementioned activity progresses along in a stable, incremental fashion until an endogenous or exogenous shock occurs, blasting open the policy window.[1]

Once the policy window opens, the intensity of the debate dramatically increases, as all of the policy entrepreneurs seek to position their solution as the basis for legislation. After the basis for legislation is decided, the other (non-winning) policy entrepreneurs seek to at least have aspects of their solutions considered and included as part of final legislation. Needless to say, the solutions emanating from the party in power have a greater likelihood of becoming a major part of the legislation, although, depending on the nature of the debate and the political timeline, the minority party may have opportunity to have their concerns addressed and included.

Following final passage of legislation, the executive takes whatever action is deemed appropriate, either signing the bill into law or vetoing it. After this, the process starts all over again, whether working through the implementation, operations, and modification process or going back to the legislature for additional action.

---

1 Government policy in the aftermath of 9/11 provides an example of policy change after an exogenous shock. Federal funding for updating and strengthening emergency preparedness across all levels of governance swiftly followed the events of September 11, 2001. The federal policy passed through the appropriations stage equipped with ample financial resources, which is not a common occurrence.

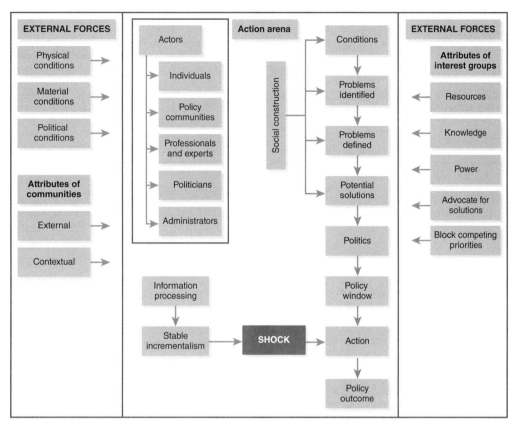

FIGURE 5.8 Bringing It All Together

Courtesy of Dr. Raymond J. Higbea, copyright 2017.

References

Almeida, L. A., & Gomes, R. C. (2018). Cadernos. *EBAPE. BR, 16*(3), 444–455. Rio de Janeiro.

Baumgartner, F. R., & Jones, B. D. (1993). *Agendas and instability in American politics.* Chicago, IL: University of Chicago Press.

Caronia, L., & Caron, A. H. (2019). Morality in scientific practice: The relevance and risks of situated scientific knowledge in application-oriented social research. *Human Studies,* (1–31). doi:10.1007/s10746-018-09491-2

Cohen, M. D., March, J. G., & Olsen, J. P. (1972). A garbage can model of organizational choice. *Administrative Sciences Quarterly, 17*(1), 1–25.

Dearing, J. W., & Rogers, E. M. (1996). *Agenda-setting.* Thousand Oaks, CA: Sage.

Duncan, J., & Mitchell, D. J. (2015). Training refines brain representations for multitasking. *Proceedings of the National Academy of Sciences, 112*(46), 14127–14128. doi:10.1073/pnas.1518636112

Kingdon, J. W. (1984). *Agendas, alternatives, and public policies.* New York, NY: Longman.

Kingdon, J. W. (1995). *Agendas, alternatives, and public policies* (2nd ed.). New York, NY: Longman.

Mack, W. R., Green, D., & Vedlitz, A. (2008). Innovation and implementation in the public sector: An examination of public entrepreneurship. *Review of Policy Research, 25*(3), 233–252. doi:10.1111/j.1541-1338.2008.00325.x

Ophir, E., Nass, C., Wagner, A. D., & Posner, M. I. (2009). Cognitive control in media multitaskers. *Proceedings of the National Academy of Sciences of the United States of America, 106*(37), 15583–15587. doi:10.1073 /pnas.0903620106

Ostrom, E., Schroeder, L., & Wynne, S. (1993). *Institutional incentives and sustainable development: Infrastructure policies in perspective.* Boulder, CO: Westview Press.

Pierce, J. J., Siddiki, S., Jones, M. D., Schumacher, K., Pattison, A., & Peterson, H. (2014). Social construction and policy design: A review of past applications: Social construction and policy design. *Policy Studies Journal, 42*(1), 1–29. doi:10.1111/psj.12040

Sabatier, P. A., & Ebooks Corporation. (2007). *Theories of policy process.* Boulder, CO: Westview Press.

Sabatier, P. A., & Jenkins-Smith, H. C. (1993). *Policy change and learning: An advocacy coalition approach.* Boulder, CO: Westview Press.

Schneider, A. L., & Ingram, H. M. (1997). *Policy design for democracy.* Lawrence, KS: University Press of Kansas.

Simon, H. A. (1947). *Administrative behavior: A study of decision-making processes in administrative organization* (1st ed.). New York, NY: Macmillan.

Simon, H. A. (1976). *Administrative behavior: A study of decision-making processes in administrative organization* (3rd ed.). New York, NY: Free Press.

Takeuchi, H., Taki, Y., Nouchi, R., Hashizume, H., Sekiguchi, A., Kotozaki, Y., . . . Kawashima, R. (2014). Effects of multitasking-training on gray matter structure and resting state neural mechanisms: MT-training affects brain structure and function. *Human Brain Mapping, 35*(8), 3646–3660. doi:10.1002/hbm.22427

Valentine, S. V., Sovacool, B. K., & Brown, M. A. (2017). Frame envy in energy policy ideology: A social constructivist framework for wicked energy problems. *Energy Policy, 109*, 623–630. doi:10.1016/j.enpol.2017.07.028

Appendix

Steps in Social Cost/Benefit Policy Design

- Problem definition
- Specification of goals/objectives
- Alternative solutions
- Search & understand
- Target groups
- C/B analysis (with discounting)
- Estimate risk
- Decision criteria
- Recommendation

▶ Researching/Analyzing Policy: Questions to Ask:

- Where did it come from?
  - Branch
  - Committee/agency/court
- When did it originate (first become policy)?
  - Time frame
  - Understand what was happening at the same time.
- What groups/individuals does it affect?
  - Industry/interest group
- What are the costs of the policy?
  - Direct and indirect: to whom
- What are the benefits of the policy?
  - Direct and indirect: to whom
- Did the policy work?
  - Who said it did and why? (What are their factual and nonfactual reasons?)
  - Who said it didn't and why? (What are their factual and nonfactual reasons?)
- If you had to measure it, how would you design a fair set of measures?
- What changes to the policy would make it more effective at doing what it was intended to do?
  - Additions/deletions/alterations

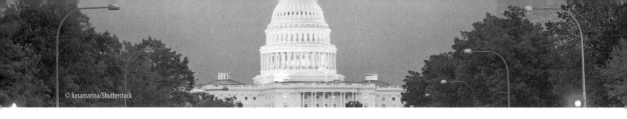

CHAPTER 6

From Theories to Application: Policy Choice and Analysis

This chapter is designed to give healthcare executives an understanding that policy analysis begins with policy design, including an understanding of how policy components are chosen to achieve intended end goals. This chapter will give healthcare leaders that understanding by covering the following topics:

- Public choice theory
- The multi-attribute problem
- Policy analysis: four models of increasing complexity
- Forecasting policy outcomes
- Monitoring policy outcomes

As you work through this chapter and the following chapter, it is our hope that you begin to see the close link between the practice of healthcare administration and the formation and implementation of health policy. Just as important, we hope you see ways in which private sector healthcare actors and their innovations may influence policy change. While it is often the case that healthcare administrators (rightly) feel powerless in the face of government regulation, these same administrators can—through state and national trade associations, each system's government affairs experts, and successful innovation—influence government regulations and policy.

Health administrators face top-down changes imposed by state and federal agencies, as well as from private sector payers (health plans and insurers), in the form of directives related to reimbursement. While not all changes can be classified as "social change" or even as "innovative," a surprising amount are. In response to these government mandates, healthcare administrators often respond with innovation, aided and abetted by technological advances, and/or by past successful innovations. These innovations sometimes lead to changes in government policy.

Continuing from Chapter 5, you will now be presented with the theory and mechanisms for how the components of government policy are chosen to effect desired, or *intended*, outcomes. We then present one expandable policy analysis model (the Basic Model) and three sets of increasingly complex expansions to the model: cost-benefit components, cost-effectiveness components, and social cost-benefit components. Next, we explain the differences between the two uses of policy analysis: forecasting the effects of future policy and monitoring existing, implemented policy.

▶ Public Choice: A Model of Policy Choice

Health leaders operate in an environment that straddles both the public and private sectors in what, at first glance, can seem an impossibly chaotic world. Private sector health systems must collaborate with local and state health agencies while also complying with federal, state, and, sometimes, local government regulations emanating from multiple agencies at each level of governance. Contracting for the delivery of health promotion, prevention, and screening programs and payment for Medicare and Medicaid recipients are the responsibility of health leaders in government agencies located at the federal, state, and/or local levels. We strongly believe that the most effective theory for understanding this complexity is *public choice*.

Public choice is a theory (others believe a set of similar theories) that combines economic theories of free markets with political theories of behavior and voter choice. Public choice attempts to explain political and policy outcomes, as well as to identify when and how government should intervene in the private sector with new or altered public policy. To understand when government should or should not act, it is best to start with an understanding of two

TABLE 6.1 Goods Matrix

	Rival	Nonrival
Excludable	Private	Club
Nonexcludable	Common	Public

Data from Samuelson, Paul A. (1954). The pure theory of public expenditure. *Review of Economics and Statistics, 36*(4), 387–389; Samuelson, Paul A. (1955). Diagrammatic exposition of a theory of public expenditure. *Review of Economics and Statistics, 37*(4), 350–356. doi:10.2307/1925849. JSTOR 1925849.

characteristics of "goods" that humans produce: excludability and rivalness. Excludability refers to the ability of producers of a good to prevent the use/consumption of a good by those who have not paid for it. Rivalness refers to goods that, when consumed by one consumer, the good is either "used up" (such as a food item) or at least cannot be simultaneously consumed by others (such as a seat at the cinema). From these two characteristics, we have the familiar 2×2 matrix of the four possible types of goods (**TABLE 6.1**).

Most policy makers in westernized democratic systems consider free markets to be the most effective mechanism for the production of excludable goods. Most would further state that government should avoid inhibiting the market for production of excludable goods, except in cases in which provision produces negative externalities (e.g., air pollution). The production of nonexcludable goods, however, is either under produced by free markets (in the case of common goods) or not produced at all (in the case of public goods). If the public wants some set of nonexcludable goods, then it should express its will for these goods through democratic voting mechanisms that send a signal to government to produce specific nonexcludable goods. The public expressing this will for the government provision of nonexcludable goods is found by voting for individual candidates that express the same in the form of campaign promises and for parties that express the same in party platforms.[1]

Health care is clearly a good that is both rival and excludable (unless government steps in and provides for either direct care or payment to those providing direct care) and thus a private good. We find William Dunn's model more effective in understanding the locus of goods wherein government should intervene to ensure the provision of goods. Dunn argues that there are three types of goods based on the same two characteristics, these being specific, quasi-collective, and collective goods. He identifies quasi-collective goods (see **FIGURES 6.1** and **6.2**) as:

> . . . specific goods whose production has significant spillover effect for society. Although elementary education can be provided by the private sector, the spillovers are considered so important that the government produces great quantities at a cost affordable to all. (Dunn, 2012, p. 204)

Although Americans do not yet agree on how much health care the government should produce (or pay for the production of), the federal government (and the states) fund the production of healthcare services beyond what would be produced if left solely to the free market.

There are multiple sets of axioms that identify the goals and limits for public choice. We prefer the five propositions presented by Stokey and Zeckhauser (1978, p. 257):

1. The purpose of public decisions is to promote the welfare of society.
2. The welfare levels of the individual members of society are the building blocks for the welfare of society.
3. Anything that affects the individual welfare therefore affects the welfare of society. Something that has no effect on individual welfare levels has no impact on the welfare of society.
4. With rare exceptions, we should accept individuals' own judgments

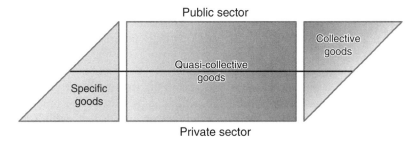

FIGURE 6.1 Three Types of Goods in the Public and Private Sectors

---

1 Regardless of the nature and/or purpose of government involvement (policy), any involvement ALWAYS produces additional costs for some of the targets of the policy. It is assumed that the intended outcomes are benefits that exceed these costs.

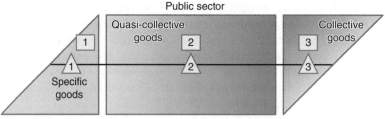

Triangles: Health systems
1. Payment: Conditions for receiving medicare/caid reimbursement
2. Prevention: BCCC&N programming
3. Promotion: Intimate partner violence surveillance system

Squares: Government agencies
1. Payment: CMS or state medicaid agency
2. Prevention: State-level childhood immunization registry
3. Promotion: Local water fluoridation

FIGURE 6.2 Health Leader Positions: Private and Public Sectors

as the appropriate indicators of their own welfare.

5. We would <u>like</u> to have an unambiguous procedure for aggregating the welfares of different individuals so that we can compare the welfare of society.

▶ The Multi-Attribute Problem

As you likely surmised, the last axiom is rarely attainable! Hence, policy makers and policy analysts all face what is known as the "multi-attribute problem." Public policies almost always have more than one goal and objective measured with more than one outcome. These outcomes have different *attributes*. With multiple goals, objectives, and outcomes, with each of the latter often possessing multiple different attributes (often a combination of positive and negative), crafting a public policy that attains the highest level on all attributes is not possible (Yan, Tieju, & Huynh, 2017). Thus, all public policy is a balance between attaining the perceived promises of elected officials—both legislators and chief executives—and the platforms of the majority political party.

Policy Perspectives

A partial solution to the multi-attribute problem is reached by examining policy goals from different perspectives. By simultaneously examining from each perspective, a balanced set of components can be proposed, assessed, and either included or excluded in the final policy. Equally useful for analysis, the four perspectives permit analysts to "break down" analysis of policy into more manageable components. The four perspectives are technical, economic, legal, and social (Dunn, 2012)[2] (see **TABLE 6.2**).

---

2 The perspectives introduced here are often referred to as "rationalities," as first articulated in rational choice theory, from which public choice theory is derived.

TABLE 6.2 Policy Perspectives	
Perspective	**Description**
Technical	Choice of components based on effectiveness in obtaining a desired outcome
Economic	Choice of components based on efficiency of obtaining a desired outcome
Legal	Choice of components based on legality of each component
Social	Choice of components based on maintaining or improving societal norms or institutions as a desired outcome
Substantive	Choice of final components regarded as "best fit" from prior four perspectives

Standard Criteria for Policy Outcomes

Flowing from the five perspectives are six standard criteria for both designing and analyzing policy: effectiveness, efficiency and adequacy, equity, responsiveness, and appropriateness. As will become clear, not all six standards are applied every time government officials design public policy. In many cases, this is because not all standards are relevant.

Effectiveness examines how close a policy component gets to attaining a desired outcome (e.g., does it attain 50%, 80%, or 100% of the desired outcome?). Efficiency examines the cost of a component in achieving a desired outcome. Adequacy examines the relationship between effectiveness and efficiency. This is represented by the four types of policy contexts that exist across effectiveness and efficiency. The four types of policy contexts present different constraints on those designing policy and aid those analyzing existing policy in understanding why the final components of a policy were chosen over other components (see **TABLE 6.3**). Equity, responsiveness, and

appropriateness will be addressed at the end of this chapter in the model for social cost-benefit analysis.

▶ Policy Analysis Models

Policy analysis models range from simple to complex, based on time available, resources available, and the analysis outputs necessary for decision-making (see **FIGURE 6.3**). At the apex of the inverted pyramid, we provide an analysis process built on one expandable framework—the Basic Model. From there, we add in three models in increasing complexity: cost-benefit analysis, cost-effectiveness analysis, and social cost-benefit analysis. The Basic Model is the simplest and quickest method for organizing and informing a decision maker on the business effects of existing or proposed law. You should note (see **TABLE 6.4**) that three of these four models can be applied across all four policy types; however, the cost-effectiveness model can only be applied to policy types I and II.

Cost-benefit analysis is when the cost of an implemented policy is subtracted from the benefit achieved through its implementation.

TABLE 6.3 Policy Contexts by Type			
Type	**Desired Effectiveness**	**Available Resources**	**Example**
I	Variable	Fixed	Community mental health
II	Fixed	Variable	Immunization policy
III	Variable	Variable	NIH funding
IV	Fixed	Fixed	Medicaid

Note: When analyzing policy, bear in mind that occasionally policy is written as one type, but upon implementation, becomes a different type.

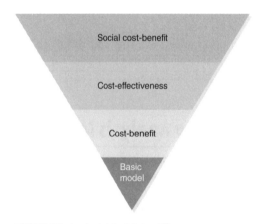

FIGURE 6.3 Analysis Models by Effort

If the resulting number is positive, the program is deemed to have a positive effect, whereas if the resulting number is negative, the program is not deemed to have a positive effect. The difficulty with this equation comes from determining the cost and the benefits achieved by the program. Particularly with social programs, determining a dollar value for the benefits can be difficult because you are often projecting the dollars that would have normally been spent elsewhere, as compared to the dollars spent on a social issue. Cost-effectiveness adds in the assessment of proportion of desired outcomes attained (i.e., does the policy attain 100% of intended outcomes or some portion less than intended?). At the base (top of the inverted pyramid), we present social cost-benefit analysis that builds on the prior three models by providing methods for incorporating the qualitative analysis of broader social costs and benefits into the final analysis.

Shared Analysis Concepts

Prior to presenting the analysis models, we present the analysis concepts shared across all four: the Fundamental Rule, pairwise comparisons, discounting, and satisficing. Phrased simply, the Fundamental Rule is, "In any choice situation select the alternative that produces the greatest net benefit" (Stokey & Zeckhauser, 1978, p. 137). The best policy choice among alternative policies is the policy delivering the greatest net benefit. This model then requires analysts to reduce all costs and benefits to a common quantitative measure—most often monetary (i.e., in dollars). This leads directly to the concept of pairwise comparison. The most effective and simple way to compare between possible policy components is to compare these components in pairs to assess

TABLE 6.4 Analysis Models by Effort and Applicability to Policy Types		
Model	**Analytical Effort**	**Applicability to Types**
Basic	Low	Types I through IV
Cost-effectiveness	Medium	Types I and II
Cost-benefit	Medium	Types I through IV
Social cost-benefit	High	Types I through IV

either efficiency (cost-benefit) and/or effectiveness (cost-effectiveness).

Discounting is the technique used to appropriately assess the value (positive or negative) of future dollars in a multiple year cost-benefit or cost-effectiveness analysis. Whenever valuing the expenditure or gain of future dollars, we must reduce the value of both; humans do not assign the value of a current dollar to the gain or loss of future dollars. Discounting for future dollars (gained or lost) in policy is identical to that applied in health care, except for the rare cases previously noted. Only in rare cases must you change your discounting methodology when applying the technique to policy analysis. The most obvious example is when individuals consider the purchase of long-term care insurance. At any one time, approximately 5% of Americans 65 years or older are using services covered under typical long-term care insurance policies. However, over the course of the average American's lifespan, from age 65 until the end of life, the probability that any one individual will use these same services is approximately 50%. Thus, when examining long-term care insurance, the appropriate "discount" applied to the dollars now spent on long-term care insurance is one-tenth the amount most Americans perceive (Campbell & Morgan, 2005).

Satisficing is the concept that when policy makers face resource constraints, sometimes they consciously choose to maximize some intended outputs from a policy over other intended policy outputs. Those outcomes that are maximized are often referred to as primary outcomes, while those that are "satisficed" are known as secondary outcomes. When analyzing any policy, keep in mind that those intended outcomes not maximized are still attained by the lowest cost components (based on pairwise comparisons) that produce some lower, yet still "satisfactory," outcome.

Policy Analysis: The Basic Model

What we describe as the "Basic Model" for policy analysis is designed to be the simplest, quickest, yet thorough, model for presenting any decision maker with the minimum information necessary to understand the effects of any existing or proposed law on healthcare operations. Before describing the format, we will explain how best to complete the information gathering for the accomplishment of the analysis.

Get the full text of law and then read it. Odd as this may sound, the quickest way to understand a law is not to read what others think about it. Rather, you should first obtain the full text of the law and read it. As you read the law, use the format of the Basic Model provided to fill in (first in bulleted form) the components. This is best accomplished in one sitting.

After reading the law and filling in the components of the Basic Model, identify sources of research you will need to access regarding the effects of the law. In addition to the governmental agencies identified earlier in this chapter, search online databases of peer-reviewed journals and independent research studies for valid research findings or clearly stated facts (always ensuring the facts are referenced). Be aware that you face the "fact/value" dichotomy as you look for evidence to ascertain if the policy was successful or not. This dichotomy is based on the idea that facts can be measured, whereas value (moral and ethical values, not currency) cannot. A scientific understanding of health policy needs to be based first on facts, but not to the extent that moral/ethical values are removed from consideration.

Keep foremost in your mind that this analysis may be cited by a decision maker in the course of advocating for policy change or making business decisions. Always provide evidence for any claims you include regarding need, effectiveness, costs, savings, etc. You support a claim by correctly referencing valid research studies or statements of fact based on accepted data sources. These findings may come from journal articles, but many are also found in research studies published by foundations, trade associations, advocacy organizations, and government agencies. Next, we describe the most basic format for a thorough, yet quick, analysis of any government policy.

Introduction

A description of the policy you are assessing. Depending on the complexity of the policy, this could be as short as one paragraph or as long a page (or slightly longer).

Policy Beneficiaries

Detail the beneficiaries. Policies are designed to benefit some group that is deemed to need some benefit that is best provided by government based on either rational one or two. This group (or these groups) are identified in this organizational framework as beneficiaries. Do not assume that targets are beneficiaries! It is often the case that the beneficiaries are hardly mentioned in the language of the law. Often beneficiaries of a law are not required to do anything at all.

Policy Targets

Detail the target(s). Policies apply instruments to clearly identified targets. Targets are a group or groups that are identified in the law as being subject to new (or changed) instruments in order to achieve some benefit. Targets are sometimes, but often are not, the intended beneficiaries of the law.

Policy Instruments

Present and explain the policy instrument(s) and how these are expected to affect changed behavior. Instruments are any of the following:

- New or altered rules/regulations (or new rules/regulations)
- New or altered incentives/disincentives to encourage/discourage behavior
- New or altered penalties/sanctions for breaking rules/regulations
- New or altered processes for interfacing with others (individuals/organizations/government)
- Any adjudication procedures specific to the policy

Describe each instrument in enough detail to ensure a reader would know which of the groups it falls into. Example: if some breaking of a rule results in a fine, you would have first clearly identified the workings of the rule, and then noted that breaking the rule results in a fine.

Policy Outcomes

Describe the policy's intended outcome(s). These are the stated end goals of the policy as contained in the law. These are the easiest to find because laws must include the intended end goals (outcomes) of the law. Outcomes of a policy not stated in the law are known as unintended outcomes.

Describe the policy's unintended outcome(s). These require more effort, but both supporters and detractors of policy offer up unintended outcomes that are both positive and negative. You can best start by identifying the beneficiaries and the targets and then identifying what trade associations and/or advocacy organizations are concerned with these. The relevant trade associations and/or advocacy organizations will have inevitably either conducted studies or commissioned studies to prove these unintended outcomes are occurring or will occur.

Recommendation for Advocacy

Explain how you would change the policy to be more effective and or equitable. Here, you may recommend altering any or all of the analyzed components: beneficiaries, targets, instruments, or outcomes.

Cost-Benefit Analysis Component: Outcomes Section

When adding the cost-benefit component to your analysis, the additional analysis should be added to your outcomes section.

1. Go through your list of intended outcomes and identify what portion of each can be quantitatively measured, and note the unit of quantitative measurement for each. Identify which of these quantitative measures can be "monetized"—converted into dollars. For any remaining intended outcomes, identify common quantitative measurements (e.g., births, deaths, quality of life years lost or gained).[3]

2. Do the same with your list of unintended outcomes.

3. Sum all monetized costs (being sure to discount future costs) across all targets.

4. Sum all monetized benefits (being sure to discount future benefits) across all beneficiaries.

5. Report the balance (positive or negative) in the Outcomes section.

6. Report your cost-benefit findings in the Recommendations for Advocacy section.

7. Sum all common quantitative measures not in dollars in the same manner as Steps 1–4, then report the balance in the Outcomes section. (You can do no more with these computations unless you include the cost-effectiveness component.)

Cost-Effectiveness Analysis Component: Outcomes Section

Cost-effectiveness should be added to the outcomes section following step 7 of the cost-benefit component. Referring back to the policies in Table 6.3, you will notice that cost-effectiveness analysis can be considered

---

3 Quality of Life Years—QALYs—is a concept from managerial epidemiology for quantifying and comparing the life added/lost across different clinical choices or different population-based programs. When paired with cost data, this permits rigorous pairwise comparison of healthcare policy components.

an "end stage" analysis for any policy that fits either Type I or Type II—there will not be a substantive social component "left over" for analysis. You will have to choose from three calculations for this component, based on the text of the policy.

Analysis choices based on Types I or II:

1. Fixed effectiveness: Which approach has the lowest cost?
2. Fixed resources: Which approach delivers the most total effectiveness?
    a. Maximum effectiveness total: Which approach produces maximum effectiveness at the lowest cost?
    b. Satisficing effectiveness total: Which approach produces satisficing level of effectiveness at the lowest cost?
    c. Combination of maximizing and satisficing effectiveness

If you are analyzing an existing policy that you categorize as 2b or 2c, you need to both estimate (and assess) the intended level of satisficing and assess if another approach would attain a higher level or more numbers at the same overall cost.

Social Cost-Benefit Analysis Model

Social cost-benefit analysis incorporates the remaining three of the six standards (equity, responsiveness, and appropriateness) into the analysis framework. The analysis findings for each standard should be reported in the Outcomes section, with relevant discussion of proposed changes based on the findings contained in the Recommendations section.

Equity is a standard that, when applied, seeks to distribute existing or new government benefits or services in a "fair" and/or legal manner. Both Medicare and Medicaid are federal government policies that have an equity standard governing the applicability to the intended beneficiaries. Responsiveness is the standard criterion for assessing whether all of the intended beneficiaries of a policy fully receive the intended benefits of the policy. Appropriateness refers to the overall "balance" of the policy across the prior five criteria.

Equity is drawn from the legal and social perspectives (refer to Table 6.2). Analyzing (either for choice in constructing a new policy or for assessing a policy in place) for equity requires assessing a policy using one or more of the following objectives:

1. Maximize individual welfare: Maximize all affected individuals' welfare at the same time.
2. Protect minimum individual welfare: Increase some individuals' welfare while holding all others' constant.
3. Maximize net societal welfare: Social benefits for the group outweigh the costs. This is identical to the concept in the Fundamental Rule.
4. Maximize redistributive welfare: Maximize specific benefits to specific groups. Medicare (for the elderly) and Medicaid (for the poor) are both policies designed to maximize (or at least increase) redistributive welfare with respect to access to healthcare services.

When analyzing a policy on this standard, you should ask yourself which of these four objectives the policy seeks to fulfill, keeping in mind that these objectives are not mutually exclusive. You then report your findings of which of these four objectives are intended outcomes of the policy and assess (using quantitative measures wherever possible) the extent of success toward these intended outcomes made on the matching equity objectives.

Responsiveness refers to the extent to which a policy delivers the intended outcomes to all beneficiaries as intended. This standard is best explained through a common example. While most of the intended beneficiaries of a state's Medicaid program may be successfully enrolled in the program, access to Medicaid-covered services may vary a great deal across enrollees due to differences such as availability of healthcare providers, distances necessary to travel, and presence of co-pays.

Lastly, appropriateness refers to how a policy "measures up" across all five prior standards. Assessing this process is primarily quantitative for the first three (efficiency, effectiveness, and adequacy) and some combination of qualitative and quantitative for the last two (equity and responsiveness).

Forecasting Policy Outcomes

As mentioned at the outset of this chapter, forecasting is the use of policy analysis to estimate the effects of future policy change. Forecasting may fit into one of three types, based on the quantitative information at hand for analysis. These are, in decreasing levels of scientific rigor, projection, prediction, and conjecture.

> **Projection** is forecasting based on extending trends in quantitative data into the future, often using pairwise assessments from similar policies to project effects of different components into the future.

> **Prediction** is forecasting based on causal arguments based on commonly accepted understanding of cause and effect. An example would be, "An increase in Medicaid reimbursement levels would lead to an increase in the number of providers that accept patients on Medicaid."

> **Conjecture** is forecasting based on expert opinion of future states. Conjecture is similar to the arguments used at the beginning of the agenda-setting stage for a proposed

new, or large change in existing, policy. An example would be, "Medicaid reimbursement levels do not require raising as there will always be enough providers willing to accept existing levels as an expected part of serving within a community."

Monitoring Policy Outcomes

As noted in the introduction to this chapter, monitoring is policy analysis applied to existing policy. Easier than forecasting, the collection of actual outcomes data is the most obvious difference between monitoring and forecasting. However, monitoring of policy outcomes may have one or more of four separate purposes: compliance, auditing, accounting, and explanation. Any one or combination of the four may be a part of monitoring a policy. The distinctions between the purposes are easily identifiable and clear.

> **Compliance**: Monitoring to ensure that a policy is implemented as defined in law.

> **Auditing**: Assessing that the intended benefits of the policy reach the intended beneficiaries as intended. (Useful for assessing equity and responsiveness.)

> **Accounting**: Collection of quantitative data on the intended outcomes (and as unintended outcomes occur, these as well).

> **Explanation**: Use of the information from compliance, auditing, and accounting purposes to produce a causal explanation for the actual outcomes of the policy. "Causal" meaning, did the policy cause the observed outcomes (intended and unintended) or were they caused by something else?

References

Campbell, A., & Morgan, K. (2005). Federalism and the politics of old-age care in Germany and the United States. *Comparative Political Studies, 38*(8), 887–914.

Dunn, W. (2012). *Public policy analysis: An introduction* (5th ed.). New York, NY: Routledge Press.

Stokey, E., & Zeckhauser, R. (1978). *A primer for policy analysis.* New York, NY: W.W. Norton.

Yan, H., Tieju, M., & Huynh, V. (2017). On qualitative multi-attribute group decision making and its consensus measure: A probability based perspective. *Omega, 70*, 94–117.

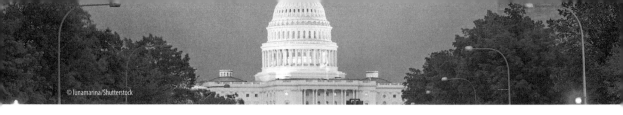

CHAPTER 7

Policy Formulation and Economic Scoring

This chapter is designed to give healthcare leaders an understanding of policy formulation and scoring by covering the following topics:

- Sources of policy, theory, and philosophy
- The agenda-setting process and how bills develop
- Congress 101: senators, representatives, and staff (oh my!)
- How policies are formulated
- How bills are economically scored
- Roles of various levels of government in the development of legislation and how legislation becomes law
- Case study of agenda-setting: controlling vote outcomes

▶ Policy Sources

Within the United States, there are two basic sources of policies: the laws, statutes, and ordinances drafted and passed by the legislative body, and the rules, rulings, orders, and memorandum of administrative and judicial bodies interpreting and implementing the laws, statutes, and ordinances. The U.S. Constitution, Article I, Section 1 states, "All legislative powers herein granted shall be vested in a Congress of the United States, which shall consist of a Senate and House of Representatives." Article I, Section 8 of the U.S. Constitution details how once the legislative body agrees to and passes a law, it moves to the executive who has the option of signing the legislation into law or vetoing the law and sending it back to the legislature.[1]

The U.S. Constitution is silent on what happens to a law signed by the executive other than stating in Article II, Section 3 that the president

---

1 State and local jurisdictions within the United States follow a similar pattern of vesting their legislative powers to the state or local version of "Congress" and similar law affirming the power of enactment (signing) to the corresponding executive.

"… shall take Care that the Laws be faithfully executed …." During the first 150 years of our country, this "… faithful execution …" of the law was rather irregular and unpredictable (Carey, 2013, p. 5). When coupled with the weight of uncertainty of the enlarged administrative state stemming from the New Deal, Congress acted in 1946 by passing the Administrative Procedures Act that was subsequently signed into law. Multiple laws and presidential direction have given additional structure to the rulemaking process that includes rules, regulations, executive orders, and presidential memorandum all having the force of law.

In addition to the sources of policy, there are various foci of policy rationale. Longest (2010) describes the policy rationale focus as *allocative* if it provides a net benefit to one group at the expense of another and as *regulatory* if it influences actions by administrative direction. Weissert (2012) describes types of policy rationale as *substantive*, changing what is done; *procedural*, changing how things are done; *distributive*, providing benefits to a group; *redistributive*, taking from one group to the benefit of another; and *regulatory*, restricting the behavior of actors.

▶ Theory and Philosophy

Before launching into a discussion about policy formulation, it is worth the time to briefly review the theories and political philosophies associated with policy formulation. All of the theories discussed in Chapter 4 are pertinent to the topic of policy formulation. First, a condition has to become raised to the level of a problem that cannot be addressed by the private sector. The target and beneficiary groups associated with the problem have to be socially constructed (Schneider & Ingram, 1997) as they are defined (Baumgartner & Jones, 1993; Kingdon, 1993) through the intervention of interest groups (Sabatier & Jenkins-Smith, 1993) and progress through the stable equilibrium phase (Schneider & Ingram, 2016). Once the problem has been defined, the political

parties craft solutions in line with their political philosophies, with the Democrats aligning with big policy solutions crafted from a social justice lens, and the Republicans aligning with incremental changes that respect established institutions crafted from a market justice lens.

▶ Agenda-Setting

The processes of agenda-setting and policy formulation can span a time of 10–50 years. Agenda-setting is undoubtedly the longer of these two processes, with policy problems, potential solutions, and potential legislation debated over 10–50 years. Once the political alignment has occurred and the policy window has opened, the process is relatively quick and cannot exceed 2 years (the length of each Congress).

The model developed by Higbea (**FIGURE 7.1**) will be used to frame this discussion. This model (Figure 7.1) combines the stages (phases) heuristic and multiple streams theories in a dynamic format. The dynamism of this model is that it recognizes that policies move in dynamic directions, going back and forth through the stages heuristic, and that they seldom sit idly within any stage of this process. How advocacy or attempting to influence is conducted depends on where the policy is in this process.

Throughout the agenda-setting phase, interest groups, professional associations, and political leaders gain an understanding of the issue, define the issue, and understand how it will affect constituents and the public in general. This process takes place in a variety of arenas, such as newscasts and news sites reporting on both the facts of and opinions on the topic by various leaders, community meetings, professional publications and meetings, and conversing directly with political representatives and leaders.

Once the problem has been defined and agreed to by the actors, the process moves to identifying potential solutions. As these potential solutions are debated, they become

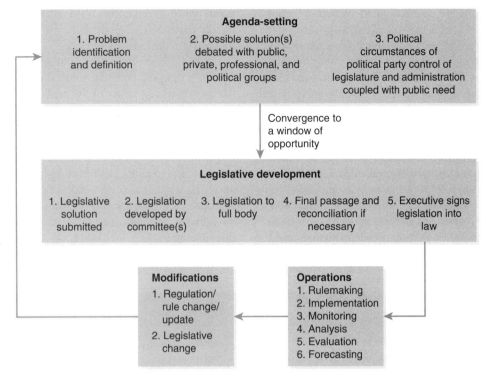

FIGURE 7.1 The Policy Process Model
Courtesy of Dr. Raymond J. Higbea, copyright 2017.

aligned with the actor's political philosophy and interests (personal, professional, political, and business). Normally, these potential solutions will align with political philosophies, with the Republicans aligning themselves with incrementalism and market justice solutions and the Democrats aligning themselves with dynamism and social justice solutions. These potential solutions are debated in the same forums as the problem definition was debated, with the potential addition of legislative committee and subcommittee hearings. Throughout this phase of the process, opinion leaders and policy entrepreneurs begin to emerge as various community, professional, and political groups refine potential solutions and coalesce around them. Ultimately, the political leaders from this group will become the policy entrepreneurs that usher any defined policy through the legislative process.

Within these debates about potential solutions, the healthcare leader may become conflicted when professional or business solutions do not align with his/her personal or political philosophies. In these situations, the healthcare executive needs to clearly identify for whom he/she is speaking when discussing the policy problem and solutions with public and political officials. How the executive responds to this conflict depends upon the severity of the conflict and the degree of personal introspection. If the conflict is not severe, the executive may agree to disagree, yet go along with the professional or business group. However, if the conflict is strong, the executive may need to continue the debate within the professional or business group or, depending upon the level of support, begin another group. The influence trend throughout the policy process is going to move more strongly toward the interest groups and away from individuals.

As the potential solutions become refined over time (at least 10 years), as posited by the Advocacy Coalition Framework (Sabatier & Jenkins-Smith, 1993), the process enters into stasis or equilibrium, as described by Kingdon (1995), with both sides waiting for the event or political circumstances that will punctuate the equilibrium and open the policy window of opportunity. The event that punctuates the equilibrium (Baumgartner & Jones, 1993) can be natural, such as a crisis, or manufactured, such as a political promise. Almeida and Gomes (2018) reaffirm the necessity of the aforementioned policy approaches and add the importance of understanding the dynamics of the situation and its key concepts. Regardless of the nature of the event, policy entrepreneurs need to be ready to rapidly move on the opportunity and get their solution into the legislative process.

While multiple actors participate in agenda-setting and potential political solutions, the agenda-setting power of the president cannot be understated. The U. S. Constitution does not vest the president with any legislative powers; however, without the president's agreement, legislation passed by Congress will not become law. A review of major healthcare legislation or proposed legislation since 1900 indicates that without the president's sponsorship, 100% of the bills fail, and with the president's sponsorship, 33% of the bills fail (**TABLE 7.1**). Thus, the power of the president is imperative to getting

TABLE 7.1 Bills Sponsored by President

Years	Number of Bills	Sponsored by President	Not Sponsored by President	Became Law	Did Not Become Law
1910–1999	1	1	0	0	1
1920–1929	1	1	0	1	0
1930–1939	3	3	0	1	2
1940–1949	6	5	1	3	3
1950–1959	3	2	1	1	2
1960–1969	6	6	0	4	2
1970–1979	15	11	4	5	10
1980–1989	10	10	0	10	0
1990–1999	10	10	0	6	4
2000–2009	10	10	0	8	2
2010–2019	2	2	0	2	0

Congress.gov.

legislation on the agenda. However, even the president's power to set the agenda does not guarantee passage of proposed legislation.

▶ Congress 101: Senators, Representatives, and Staff (Oh My!)

The differences in the electoral context faced by representatives and senators lead to differences in the two chambers that affect the legislative process. Because senators are elected to 6-year terms, and these terms are staggered, only one-third of the seats in the Senate are up for reelection in our 2-year Congressional elections. Thus, senators spend less time in "campaign mode" and more time on policy making, hence the common reference to the Senate as the "deliberative" body. Because there are only 100 senators who face lessened electoral pressure, each senator is more powerful than the average representative in the 435-seat House. Differences in Senate rules and the increased possibilities for service on important committees add to the potential power of individual senators.

All 435 members of the House of Representatives face re-election every 2 years. This is because the authors of the Constitution intended it to be the "representative body" and to be more responsive to public pressure. As such, it must face more frequent elections to ensure members receive input from the voting public on performance (as measured by votes). In the modern era of political campaigns, this responsive design and 2-year term length have placed representatives into permanent "campaign mode." With more members in competition, individual House members must

devote more time and effort to obtaining desirable committee seats, resulting in longer time frames to obtain leadership roles.

Congressional staff fall into two distinct groups: those who staff the committees and subcommittees and those who staff the Washington offices. Committee staffers—responsible to the committee chair and members—tend to be older, more experienced issue area experts and often policy entrepreneurs. In general, committee staff are more powerful, which is in part based on the importance of the committee and in part based on the power of the chair of the committee.

The office staff are responsible to the individual member and his/her constituents. Office staff are more focused (especially in the House) on the reelection of the member. In most cases, office staff are younger and less experienced than committee staff. Additionally, the power of the office staff varies directly with the power of the member of Congress for whom they work.

▶ Legislative Process

The legislative process begins with the introduction of a bill to one of the legislative chambers (see **TABLE 7.2**).[2] Of course, a bill must be developed prior to its introduction, with the work of developing the bill normally the responsibility of staffers assigned to individual legislators and committees. Staffers are an extremely valuable group of individuals who have a variety of constituency and policy-development skills and knowledge that are necessary for any legislator to succeed. As staffers develop bills, they keep in mind the political philosophy each legislator represents and input, including policy language, from major interest groups.

Once a bill has been introduced, it is assigned to a committee for review and markup.

---

2 The U.S. Congress will be used for this discussion. State and local legislative bodies use similar, although often not as robust, processes.

TABLE 7.2 Health-Related Committees of the U.S. House of Representatives and Senate

U.S. House of Representatives

Committee	Subcommittee	Jurisdiction
Appropriations	Labor, Health and Human Services, Education, and Related Agencies	Department of Health and Human Services
Education and The Workforce	Health, Education, Labor, and Pensions	… employment related health security … health … ERISA
Energy and Commerce	Health	Multiple health programs … Medicare, Medicaid, HHS, CDC, Indian Health Service, NIH
Small Businesses	Health and Technology	Implementation of PPACA … availability and affordability of healthcare coverage for small businesses
Veterans Affairs		Veteran health
Ways and Means	Health	Payments for health and health services, health research, Medicare, Medicaid, tax credits and deductions (IRS)
U.S. Senate		
Agriculture, Nutrition, and Forestry		Food stamps and human nutrition
Appropriations	Labor, Health and Human Services, Education, and Related Agencies	HHS (except FDA, HIS, and Construction), AHRQ, CMS, CDC, HRSA, NIH, and multiple other agencies and programs

Committee	Subcommittee	Topic
Banking, Housing, and Urban Affairs		Nursing home contractors
Environment and Public Works		Clean air and water
Finance		Medicare, Medicaid, CHIP, HHS
Health, Education, Labor, and Pensions	Employment and Workplace Safety	Worker health and safety
	Primary Health and Retirement Security	HRSA, SAMSA, ERISA, Oral Health
Homeland Security and Government Affairs		Emergency Management
Veterans Affairs		Veteran health

However, there are instances when the speaker of the House or majority leader of the Senate will hold the bill indefinitely, essentially killing the bill before it gets to committee. Depending upon the complexity of the bill, it may be divided up and sent to several committees based on the committee's jurisdiction. Neither the U.S. House of Representatives nor the U.S. Senate has a designated health committee; rather, they have health-related topics, programs, and agencies divided up among several subcommittees (see Table 7.2). In the U.S. House of Representatives, there are 26 committees and multiple subcommittees. Of these subcommittees, six are assigned health-related topics, programs, and agencies. In the U.S. Senate, there are 20 committees and multiple subcommittees. Of these subcommittees, seven are assigned health-related topics, programs, and agencies. Once the bill is assigned to a committee, the committee chair is responsible for assigning the bill to a committee meeting agenda, discussing the bill with the minority leader on the committee,[3] calling witnesses for testimony and professional opinion, and scheduling hearings, markup, and votes on the policy.

Bills can languish in committees for weeks as legislators conduct hearings to make certain that interest groups advocating either for or against the bill have an opportunity to make a statement regarding the bill and answer questions of committee members. The bill also goes through the markup process in which the committee reads every line of the bill and marks it up, either agreeing with it or making changes to it that must be voted on, thus clearly stating how each committee member stands on a given topic.

Once the committee gets a bill that they can agree on and that can get a majority vote, the bill is moved back to the chamber leader, who goes through the process of whipping up votes and, when enough support is ensured, schedules the bill for debate and vote by the full chamber. Depending on the rules the chamber is working under, the bill may be open for amendments, and, if so, the amendments must be voted on. If the bill passes, it is moved to the other chamber for consideration.

The other chamber can respond by (1) preparing a bill in parallel that they vote on, (2) waiting for the bill to come from the other chamber, or (3) ignoring the bill from the other chamber. Once a bill has passed and been referred to the other chamber, they can (1) vote on the bill and agree with it, (2) develop amendments that will cause the opposing bills to align, or (3) send the bill to conference committee, where the two sides reconcile differences and produce a bill that meets the concerns of both chambers and then must be voted on and approved by both chambers. If both sides cannot agree on how to reconcile the bill, it dies and new legislation must be developed. However, if the bill passes both chambers, it moves to the executive (president) who has four options: sign the bill into law, not sign the bill within 10 days—if Congress is in session, it becomes law; if Congress is not is session, it does not become law—or veto the bill. If the president vetoes the bill, two-thirds of both chambers are necessary to override the veto (U.S. Constitution Article I, Section 7).

Since the 106th Congress (1999–2001), Congress has had on average 12,000 bills (**TABLE 7.3**) submitted per session, 5.3% got a vote and 3.3% were implemented as law. During that same time period, Congress submitted on average 3917 healthcare-related bills, or 37.9% of all bills submitted, per session, and 1.5% of total healthcare bills submitted were implemented as law. As noted by the aforementioned figures, approximately 95% of the bills submitted to Congress in a given year did not get a vote and likely did not get out of committee. However, when a bill did get a vote, its likelihood of passing was rather high, with approximately 70% of the bills that got a

---

3 A collaborative action that is normally followed, although based on the topic and relationship between the leaders, may not be followed.

TABLE 7.3 Health-Related Committees

Health-Related Committees of the U.S. House of Representatives and Senate

U.S. House of Representatives

Committee	Subcommittee	Jurisdiction
Appropriations	Labor, Health and Human Services, Education, and Related Agencies	Department of Health and Human Services
Education and the Workforce	Health, Education, Labor, and Pensions	… employment related health security … health … ERISA
Energy and Commerce	Health	Multiple health programs … Medicare, Medicaid, HHS, CDC, Indian Health Service, NIH
Small Businesses	Health and Technology	Implementation of PPACA … availability and affordability of healthcare coverage for small businesses
Veterans Affairs		Veteran health
Ways and Means	Health	Payments for health and health services, health research, Medicare, Medicaid, tax credits and deductions (IRS)

(continues)

TABLE 7.3 Health-Related Committees   *(continued)*

Health-Related Committees of the U.S. House of Representatives and Senate

U.S. House of Representatives

Committee	Subcommittee	Jurisdiction
U.S. Senate		
Agriculture, Nutrition, and Forestry		Food stamps and human nutrition
Appropriations	Labor, Health and Human Services, Education, and Related Agencies	HHS (except FDA, HIS, and Construction), AHRO, CMS, CDC, HRSA, NIH, and multiple other agencies and programs
Banking, Housing, and Urban Affairs		Nursing home contractors
Environment and Public Weeks		Clean air and water
Finance		Medicare, Medicaid, CHIP, HHS
Health, Education, Labor, and Pensions	Employment and Workplace Safety	Worker health and safety
	Primary Health and Retirement Security	HRSA, SAMSA, ERISA, Oral Health
Homeland Security and Government Affairs		Emergency Management

vote passing. Thus, through the agenda-setting lens, bills have to be submitted often and regularly to be available for consideration and possible enactment in a moment when equilibrium is punctuated. It is noteworthy that once a bill is seriously considered through the committee hearing and markup process, it has a high likelihood of getting passed. This enactment rate has a lot to do with how Congressional leaders work with their caucuses and refuse to bring up legislation that has a slim margin of support (see **TABLE 7.4**).

TABLE 7.4 Total Bills, Votes, and Enactments								
Congress	**Years**	**Enacted**	**Total**	**Got a Vote**	**HC Policy**	**Health in Bill**	**Committee**	**HC Law**
115	2017–2018	232	12,021	791	1267	4225	122	11
114	2016–2071	329	12,063	661	1418	4466	110	21
113	2013–2015	296	10,637	474	1161	3738	48	22
112	2011–2013	284	12,299	390	997	3426	23	5
111	2009–2010	385	13,675	601	1483	4286	67	15
110	2007–2009	460	14,042	861	1332	4562	83	30
109	2005–2006	483	13,072	597	1131	4022	51	21
108	2003–2004	504	10,669	694	1011	3667	61	23
107	2001–2002	383	10,781	602	1013	3543	70	16
106	1999–2001	604	10,840	650	1017	3631	49	9
Total		3960	120,099	6321	11,830	39,566	684	173
Mean		396	12,010	632	1183	3957	68	17
Percentage		3.3		5.3	9.9	32.9		1.5
Bills Voted and Enacted				62.6%				

Economic Scoring

Since 1974, all major legislation has been required to have an economic score before being considered by Congress. Stated otherwise, Congress needs to understand the economic cost and impact of every major piece of legislation as part of its consideration. The Congressional Budget Office (CBO) was established as a non-partisan neutral office to provide Congress with economic information regarding government operations and potential legislation. This office has traditionally used static scoring methods when providing economic scores for legislation. Throughout the years, several scholars and politicians have stated that this method is inaccurate and that the economic cost and impact of a policy are under predicted, and have argued for the use of dynamic scoring.[4] Both sides of this debate have scholarly evidence to which they can point in support of their position; thus, the results are mixed and uncertain at present. One of the policy issues that the 114th Congress has passed into law is the requirement that CBO use dynamic scoring for all major legislation. The final results are yet to be seen; thus, any pronouncement of victory by the dynamic scoring side needs to be delayed until the results surface over the next few years, when we can then judge whether dynamic scoring provides more accurate results. The Joint Committee on Taxation (JCT) is a joint committee of House and Senate appropriations committees that works collaboratively with the CBO on scoring any legislation that has tax implications.

Congressional Research Service

The Congressional Research Service was established in 1914 as a branch of the Library of Congress to provide legal and policy analytic support for both chambers of Congress. Its members participate in every phase of the legislative process, from policy drafting to enactment. They are known for the high quality of their work and are considered by legislators to be a trusted analytic source. While they provide a variety of legal and policy analytic products, they are best known for the policy summaries they prepare for every major piece of legislation.

In summary, once a public problem makes it through the agenda-setting process and is considered for development as a piece of legislation, Congress has a high level of support in the forms of economic, legal, and policy analytic support for policy development and analysis. Legislators also call upon their own expertise and enhance their understanding of a bill through the markup process. The area of policy development and enactment that is more challenging is the political aspect that requires making certain everyone has been heard and their concerns considered and addressed if possible. When all of this works as designed, the country ends up with a well-designed piece of legislation that can be enacted into law and become a benefit to the citizens of our country.

Authorizations, Appropriations, and Conference Committees

Less obvious to those unfamiliar with Congress and the legislative process is the distinction between authorization and appropriation. Authorizations are laws that create new (or alter existing) agencies and create new (or alter existing) programs for these agencies. Appropriations are separate laws that determine the funding levels for authorizations. Generally, authorizations are passed first, followed by appropriations. It is not unusual for components of passed authorizations to receive more funding than expected, less funding than expected, or even no funding at all.

---

4   An economic scoring model that includes the macroeconomic costs and impact of a policy.

Conference committees are ad hoc groups of legislators formed to resolve differences in bills passed by both the Senate and the House. These committees are made up of members from both chambers, appointed by senior leaders from the same. Conference committees determine how to "reconcile" language across both bills, creating a single bill that is subject to an "up or down vote" (no discussion) in both chambers.[5] Once passed in both chambers, the bill is then sent to the president for signing into law.

Bills sent to conference committees are distinct in several ways. First, this represents a "second chance" lobbying opportunity for groups unhappy with the content of the bill but who "lost." Similarly, it is a common time for the president to step in and push for his preferences that were not placed in the bill. Although noted earlier that reaching conference increases probability of passage, bills do "die" there. Most common are highly controversial components of bills too important to an influential subgroup within one chamber to be left out. Once in conference—subject to the discussion and decision of a selected committee from both chambers—these components are easier to remove. The normal budgetary process is supposed to be complete before October 1st each year, with a formally approved budget complete prior to that date. However, from 1995, the budget process has been conducted with a series of continuing resolutions (funds flow at prior authorized levels for some specified time period) followed by a conference committee that produces an "omnibus" budget bill. Once legislation is finally agreed upon and passed by both chambers of Congress and signed

🔍 *CASE STUDY*

Agenda-Setting: Controlling Vote Outcomes

When following news reports on the process of a proposed law (bill) in either chamber of Congress, you may run across a reference to vote counting (prior to an actual vote) and to a person in a role named "majority whip." What is being referred to is a process of identifying each voting member's preferences prior to holding a final vote on legislation. Both parties have a formal role filled by a senior member who leads this process for this purpose—the Whip. Why?

When three or more persons with different preference sets vote, the person leading the vote process may be (and often is) able to manipulate the outcome. This is true when the following assumptions are true:

1. Individuals all have preferences regarding any set of options.
2. Preferences are ranked. ("Choice A is better than Choice B.")
3. Preferences are transitive (a > b, and b > c. Thus, a > c).

The following case consists of three senior administrators who have to make a decision on use of capital in a fiscal year. The choices for use of the capital have been narrowed to three: invest in a "Big Bore" MRI, construct a new surgical wing, or invest the capital for 1 year (status quo). Figure One shows these preferences and each administrator's preference ordering. Note that each administrator has a different preference ordering (**TABLE 7.5**).

---

5 Hence, the common reference to bills that come out of conference committees as "reconciliation bills."

TABLE 7.5 Current Fiscal Year Capital Use Preference Ordering

Senior Administrator	Preferred	Second Preferred	Third Preferred
Bill	Big Bore MRI	New Surgical Wing	Status Quo
Jane	New Surgical Wing	Status Quo	Big Bore MRI
Another Guy Named Bill	Status Quo	Big Bore MRI	New Surgical Wing

TABLE 7.6 Current Fiscal Year Capital Use Preference Ordering. First Binary Vote: Big Bore MRI versus New Surgical Wing

Senior Administrator	Preferred	Second Preferred	Third Preferred
Bill	Big Bore MRI	New Surgical Wing	Status Quo
Jane	New Surgical Wing	Status Quo	Big Bore MRI
Another Guy Named Bill	Status Quo	Big Bore MRI	New Surgical Wing

TABLE 7.7 Current Fiscal Year Capital Use Preference Ordering. Second Binary Vote: Big Bore MRI versus Status Quo

Senior Administrator	Preferred	Second Preferred	Third Preferred
Bill	Big Bore Wil		Status Quo
Jane		Status Quo	Big Bore MRI
Another Guy Named Bill	Status Quo	Big Bore MRI	

into law by the president, it continues on its journey through implementation (discussed in Chapter 8) and modification (discussed in Chapter 9).

With these preference orderings known, the person leading the voting process can assure that the preferred outcome is chosen by scheduling two sequential binary votes. Figure Two shows the process when controlled by the third administrator (Another Guy Named Bill). The first binary vote is between investing in the Big Bore MRI and the New Surgical Wing. Note that the first choice of each is noted. Big Bore MRI wins this binary vote (**TABLE 7.6**).

The second binary vote is then conducted. This is between the remaining two choices, Big Bore MRI and Status Quo. Figure Three presents the remaining preferences and the vote outcome—Status Quo wins (**TABLE 7.7**).

References

Almeida, L. A., & Gomes, R. C. (2018). The process of public policy: Literature review, theoretical reflections and suggestions for future research. *EBAPE.BR, 16*(3), 444–455. Rio de Janeiro. Retrieved from http://www.scielo.br/pdf/cebape/v16n3/en_1679-3951-cebape-16-03-444.pdf

Baumgartner, F. R., & Jones, B. D. (1993). *Agendas and instability in American politics.* Chicago, IL: University of Chicago Press.

Carey, M. P. (2013). *The federal rulemaking process: An overview.* Washington, DC: Congressional Research Service.

Kingdon, J. W. (1995). *Agendas, alternatives, and public policies* (2nd ed.). New York, NY: Longman.

Longest, B. B. (2010). *Health policymaking in the United States* (5th ed.). Chicago, IL: Health Administration Press.

Schneider, A. L., & Ingram, H. M. (1997). *Policy design for democracy.* Lawrence, KS: University Press of Kansas.

Schneider, A. L., & Ingram, H. M. (2016). *Deserving and entitled: Social constructions and public policy.* New York, NY: SUNY Press.

Sabatier, P., & Jenkins-Smith, H. C. (1993). *Policy change and learning: An advocacy coalition approach.* Boulder, CO: Westwood Press.

Weissert, W. G., & Weissert, C. S. (2012). *Governing health: The politics of health policy* (4th ed.). Baltimore, MD: John Hopkins University Press.

Appendix

Presidents and Bills

Year	President	Health Policy	Sponsored by President	Not Sponsored by President	Became Law	Did Not Become Law
1912	Theodore Roosevelt	National health care on party platform	X			X
1921	Woodrow Wilson	Sheppard-Townes Act provides matching funds for prenatal and child care centers	X		X	
1933	Franklin Roosevelt	Healthcare provisions as part of Social Security legislation	X			X
1935	Franklin Roosevelt	Maternal and Child Health Provision included in Social Security Act	X		X	
1938	Franklin Roosevelt	National Health Bill (Wagner)	X			X
1943	Franklin Roosevelt	Wagner-Murray-Dingell bill for universal comprehensive health insurance		X		X
1945	Harry Truman	McCarran-Ferguson Act (PL 15) exempts insurance from most federal regulations	X		X	
1946	Harry Truman	Mental Health Act	X		X	
1946	Harry Truman	Hospital Survey and Construction Act (Hill-Burton Act) and provision of a reasonable amount of charitable care	X		X	

(continues)

Year	President	Health Policy	Sponsored by President	Not Sponsored by President	Became Law	Did Not Become Law
1946	Harry Truman	Revised Wagner-Murray-Dingell bill and Taft-Smith-Ball bill for grants to states for medical care of the poor	X			X
1949	Harry Truman	Fair Deal	X			X
1954	Dwight Eisenhower	Federal reinsurance fund proposed	X			X
1954	Dwight Eisenhower	Revenue Act provides employer tax exemption for health insurance premiums	X		X	
1956	Dwight Eisenhower	Forand Bill to provide health insurance benefits to Social Security beneficiaries		X		X
1960	Dwight Eisenhower	Kerr Mills Bill to provide funds to state programs providing medical care to the poor and elderly	X		X	
1962	John Kennedy	Medicare	X			X
1963	John Kennedy	King-Anderson Bill reintroduced	X			X
1965	Lyndon Johnson	Medicare and Medicaid	X		X	
1965	Lyndon Johnson	Neighborhood Health Centers established (currently Federally Qualified Health Centers)	X		X	
1967	Lyndon Johnson	Medicaid revised to include categories for individuals not receiving cash assistance × Early and Periodic testing and Screening benefits	X		X	
1970	Richard Nixon	Kennedy-Griffiths national compulsory health insurance bill		X		X

Year	President	Health Policy	Sponsored by President	Not Sponsored by President	Became Law	Did Not Become Law
1971	Richard Nixon	Employer Mandate	X			X
1971	Richard Nixon	Private Health Insurance Employer Mandate and Federalization of Medicaid	X			X
1972	Richard Nixon	Social Security Amendments of 1972 (Disability and End Stage Renal Disease)	X		X	
1972	Richard Nixon	Supplemental Security Income provides cash assistance to physicians and hospitals	X		X	
1973	Richard Nixon	Long-Ribicoff bill to cover catastrophic costs, replace Medicaid with program covering cost of all poor, and standardization of catastrophic coverage by private insurers		X		X
1973	Richard Nixon	HMO Act requires employers to offer an HOM option	X		X	
1974	Richard Nixon	Kennedy-Mills Bill for universal coverage		X		X
1974	Richard Nixon	Employer Mandate and Replacement of Medicaid by state-run plans	X			X
1974	Richard Nixon	Employee Retirement Income Security Act exempts self-insured employers from state health insurance regulations	X		X	
1974	Richard Nixon	Health Planning Resources Act to mandate health planning and development of Certificate of Need programs	X		X	
1977	Jimmy Carter	Bill to limit the revenue increases of all hospitals	X			X

(continues)

Year	President	Health Policy	Sponsored by President	Not Sponsored by President	Became Law	Did Not Become Law
1977	Jimmy Carter	Children's Health Assessment Program established (Medicaid expansion)	X			X
1979	Jimmy Carter	Employer mandate, federalization of Medicaid, and Medicare catastrophic coverage	X			X
1979	Jimmy Carter	Universal Coverage Plan through private insurers (Kennedy)		X		X
1981	Jimmy Carter	Federal Budget Reconciliation Act requires Medicaid to make additional payments to hospitals who serve a disappointed share of Medicaid patients, repeals requirements that Medicaid pay at Medicare rates, and requires nursing homes to be paid at "reasonable and adequate" rates	X		X	
1981	Jimmy Carter	Medicaid waivers allowing states to mandate managed care enrollment, and cover home and community based long-term care	X		X	
1982	Jimmy Carter	Allow states to expand Medicaid to children with disabilities requiring long-term care	X		X	
1983	Ronald Reagan	Social Security Amendments of 1983 (Prospective Payment System)	X		X	
1986	Ronald Reagan	Emergency Medical Treatment and Labor Act (EMTALA) requiring medical screenings	X		X	
1986	Ronald Reagan	COBRA allowing employees who lose their job to purchase health insurance for 18 months	X		X	

Year	President	Health Policy	Sponsored by President	Not Sponsored by President	Became Law	Did Not Become Law
1986	Ronald Reagan	Federal Budget Reconciliation Act allowed states to cover infants, children, and pregnant women up to 100% of the poverty level and allow Medicaid to pay Medicare premiums and cost-sharing for qualified Medicare beneficiaries	X		X	
1988	Ronald Reagan	Medicare Catastrophic Coverage Act covered prescription drugs and capped out-of-pocket expenses (repealed 1 year later)	X		X	
1988	Ronald Reagan	Family Support Act provides 12 months of extended Medicaid coverage to families leaving welfare	X		X	
1989	George H.W. Bush	Federal Budget Reconciliation Act mandates coverage for pregnant women and children under age 6 at 133% of the federal poverty level	X		X	
1990	George H.W. Bush	Federal Budget Reconciliation Act mandates coverage of children age 6–18 years under the federal poverty level	X		X	
1993	Bill Clinton	Health Security Plan	X			X
1993	Bill Clinton	McDermott-Wellstone single payer insurance bill	X			X
1993	Bill Clinton	Cooper managed competition bill	X			X
1994	Bill Clinton	Bipartisan bill to expand health insurance coverage without comprehensive reform	X			X
1996	Bill Clinton	Health Insurance Portability and Accountability Act (HIPAA)	X		X	

(continues)

Year	President	Health Policy	Sponsored by President	Not Sponsored by President	Became Law	Did Not Become Law
1996	Bill Clinton	Personal Responsibility and Work Opportunity Act delinks Medicaid and cash assistance eligibility and bans Medicaid for illegal immigrants	X		X	
1996	Bill Clinton	Mental Health Parity Act prohibits lower lifetime limits	X		X	
1997	Bill Clinton	Balanced Budget Act changes provider payments to slow growth, establishes Medicare+Choice program, and established State Children's Health Insurance (SCHIP) program	X		X	
1999	Bill Clinton	Ticket to Work and Work Incentives Improvement Act allows states to cover working disabled up to 250% of the federal poverty level	X		X	
2000	Bill Clinton	Breast and Cervical Cancer Treatment Act allows states to provide Medicaid coverage for uninsured women for the treatment of breast and cervical cancer	X		X	
2003	George W. Bush	Medicare Drug Improvement, and Modernization Act subdues prescription drug benefit	X		X	
2003	George W. Bush	Medicare creates Health Savings Account to be used with high-deductible plans	X		X	
2005	George W. Bush	Deficit Reduction Act significantly changes Medicaid-related premiums and cost-sharing	X		X	
2007	George W. Bush	Health American's Act (Wyden-Bennett) requires individuals to obtain health insurance coverage through state health insurance pools	X			X

Year	President	Health Policy	Sponsored by President	Not Sponsored by President	Became Law	Did Not Become Law
2007	George W. Bush	SCHIP reauthorization passed but vetoed—temporary extension passed	X		X	
2007	George W. Bush	Proposed plan to replace tax preference for employer-sponsored insurance with a standard healthcare deduction	X			X
2008	George W. Bush	Mental Health Parity Act amended to require full parity	X		X	
2009	Barack Obama	American Recovery and Reinvestment Act invests in health information technology (HITECH), provisions to expand primary care workforce, and finds comparative effectiveness research	X		X	
2009	Barack Obama	Children's Health Insurance Plan (CHIP) reauthorized	X		X	
2010	Barack Obama	Patient Protection and Affordable Care Act	X		X	
2010	Barack Obama	Health Care and Education Reconciliation Act of 2010	X		X	

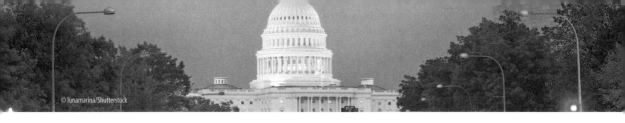

CHAPTER 8

Policy Implementation

This chapter is designed to give healthcare leaders an understanding of policy implementation by covering the following topics:

- Operations
- Rulemaking process
- Implementation
- First-, second-, and third-generation implementation theories

The contents of this chapter may seem unnecessary to those not familiar with how policy is implemented after the enactment of law. For most of us, we assume that once Congress passes a law, whatever is in the law "gets done." As future healthcare leaders, it is important to understand that implementation—and the private sector's potential for influence on implementation—does not end with the passage of a law. Understanding how public policies are implemented will assist healthcare leaders in gaining a general understanding of how federal statutes are turned into regulations and rules, how these regulations and rules are developed, and how healthcare leaders can influence the regulatory and rulemaking process.

▶ Operations

Once a policy has been signed into law, the primary responsibility for the law shifts from the legislative to the executive branch. The executive agency functions aligned with this responsibility all fall under the general heading of operations and include rulemaking, implementation, monitoring recommendations, analysis, evaluation, and forecasting recommendations. Rulemaking and implementation will be covered in this chapter, monitoring in Chapter 9, and analysis, evaluation, and forecasting were covered in Chapter 6.

▶ Rulemaking Process

Once legislation is signed into law, implementation of the law becomes the responsibility of the executive branch. While the legislative and judicial branches can have significant input into how a law is implemented, the implementation process belongs to the executive branch (**FIGURE 8.1**). When the executive branch receives a law to implement, it forwards the law to the appropriate agency(ies) based on agency jurisdictions. Prior to 1935, when a law was passed by Congress and

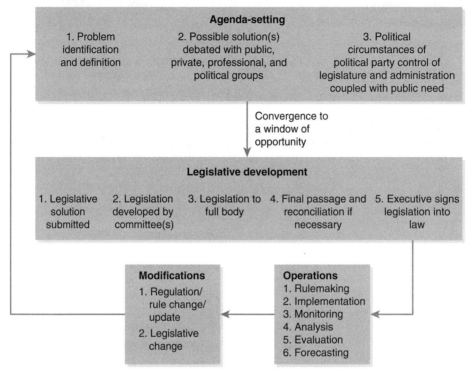

FIGURE 8.1 The Policy Process
Courtesy of Dr. Raymond J. Higbea, copyright 2017.

signed by the president, there was substantial unpredictability and lack of transparency in the process of writing final rules and regulations by executive branch agencies. This led to the Federal Register Act (44 U.S.C. Chapter 15) requiring agencies to submit for publication all proposed and final rules and regulations to laws enacted by Congress and signed into law by the president in the *Federal Register*. Since 1935, the types of documents printed in the *Federal Register* have grown to include rules, regulations, executive order, and presidential memorandum.

The type of action required by the agency depends on the intent of the law. The Administrative Procedures Act (APA) of 1946 (5 U.S.C.

§551(4)) promulgated the use of *formal rules* for legislative actions, such as rate setting. The annual Medicare rate adjustment, when the legislature sets the percentage for the rate increase and the agency (CMS) makes the adjustment and publishes the new rate, is an example of formal rules. The APA also provides guidance for *informal rulemaking*, when the agency (1) publishes proposed rules in the *Federal Register*, (2) provides for a comment period, and (3) gives consideration to all comments, prior to publishing a final rule in the *Federal Register* (see **APPENDIX TABLE 8.3**).[1]

After the agency receives the law (**FIGURE 8.2**), it convenes a group of appropriate

---

1 The Federal Register changes daily. On any given day you can connect online (https://www.federalregister.gov) and review open rules.

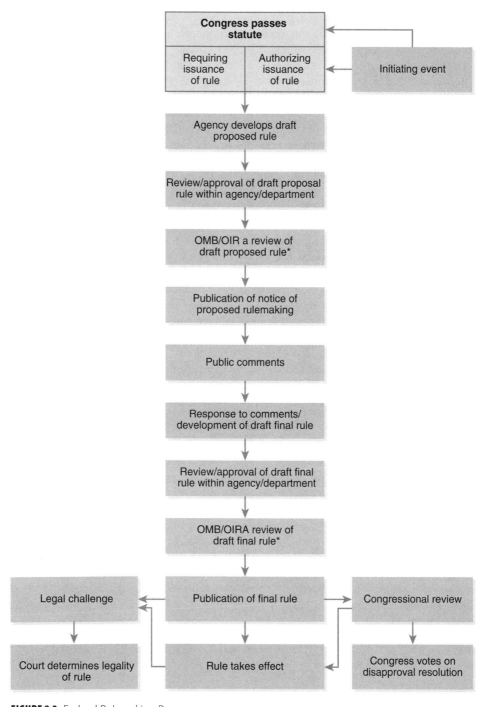

FIGURE 8.2 Federal Rulemaking Process

Carey, M. P. (2013). The federal rulemaking process: An overview. Congressional Research Service.

agency personnel who review the law to gain an understanding of its goals, objectives, and special provisions. Since laws are often not written in implementable language, agencies have the responsibility of transforming the law into implementable regulations and rules. When an agency begins the work of implementing a law, the approaches to implementation include textualism or purposivism (**TABLE 8.1**). If the agency chooses to use a *textual* approach, the text of the statute becomes the focus of the law's interpretation, with the agency looking for textual meaning and semantic context for its interpretation (Stack, 2015). If the agency chooses a *purposive* approach, the text of the statute is used as the best evidence of the purpose of the statute, providing a constraint or outer boundary for interpretation (Stack, 2015). The textual approach aligns with the APA's formal rulemaking process, whereas the purposive approach aligns with APA's informal approach.

When Congress delegates lawmaking authority to an agency, it must include use of the *intelligible principle* to be constitutionally distinctive allowing the agency to (1) develop an understanding of the purpose of the statute, (2) evaluate alternatives for action, (3) develop actions that best further the statute's purposes and principles, and (4) adopt interpretations permitted by the statute's text (Stack, 2015, pp. 875 and 876). Congress delegates rulemaking authority to the executive and executive agencies due to their administrative capacity and topical expertise. In turn, the agency assumes implementation of the statute and furtherance of the principles of the statute (Stack, 2015, p. 895).[2] This regulatory development process is painstakingly detailed and can take a significantly long time. For example, the 1996 HIPAA legislation took 15 years to fully implement and the 2010 ACA was originally scheduled to take 7 years.

Once the agency has assembled its rulemaking group, gained an understanding of the goals and objectives of the law, and determined the need for regulations, they begin the work of drafting regulations. The drafting of regulations can take extensive amounts of time as the agency seeks to

TABLE 8.1 Textualism v. Purposivism	
Textualism	**Purposivism**
Understand the meaning of text as the sole object of interpretation (p. 881).	Treats text as the best evidence of statutory purpose and a source of constraint … understand interpretation as a process of implementing statutory purposes, not merely adhering to statutory text (p. 882).
… resolves interpretative issues by seeking to discern the best interpretation of the text within its semantic context … (p. 915)	… looks to statutory text instrumentality … the text is the best evidence of statutory purpose as well as a constraint on the scope of possible interpretations … (p. 915)
… has an intrinsic interest in statutory text in the sense that it is the exclusive subject and source for interpretation … (p. 915)	The text … informs and establishes outer boundaries, but the text is neither the exclusive source nor exclusive subject of interpretation (p. 915).

Data from Stack, K. M. (2015). Purposivism in the executive branch: How agencies interpret statutes. *Northwestern University Law Review, 109*(4), 871.

---

2 It is important to note that regulations take on the authority of law and are the "hows" for the enforcement of the law.

reconcile the intent of the law with the goals of the leader and the public. "The Administrative Procedure Act (APA) of 1946 defines a rule as 'the whole or part of an agency statement of general or particular applicability and future effect designed to implement, interpret, or prescribe law or policy'" (5 U.S.C. §551(4) & Carey, 2013).

Since 1935, with the implementation of the Federal Register Act (44 U.S.C. Chapter 15), Congress and the executive branches of government have provided agencies with multiple statutes, executive orders, and memoranda to provide agencies with guidance and direction in the interpretation and implementation of statutes. While the original statutes were promulgated to give structure to the rulemaking process, later guidance was promulgated to refine and increase rulemaking efficiency (**APPENDIX TABLE 8.3**).

After a regulation has been developed and agreed to by the agency, it is posted in the *Federal Register* (44 U.S.C. Chapter 15). Formally developed regulations, such as rates, are posted as final and without comment. Informally developed regulations are posted as a proposed rule open for public comment for 30–60 days, depending on the regulation's significance, and can be open for up to 180 days. As part of the announcement of a proposed rule, the agency always clearly lists how long the comment period is open and to whom or where to submit comments. The *Federal Register* is the federal government's official written source for government documents that include notices, proposed rules, final rules, presidential documents, and other significant documents. The importance of commenting cannot be understated; unfortunately, regulations frequently receive few, if any, comments unless the proposed regulation is on a controversial and sensitive topic that may generate thousands of comments (E-Government Act of 2002, 44 U.S.C.A. §3601 note & **FIGURE 8.3**). The 1996 HIPAA Privacy regulations received 60,000 comments, and in 2014, HHS received more than 650,000 comments on proposed regulations. Once the commenting period has ended, the implementing

agency reviews and analyzes all comments and makes adjustments to the proposed regulation that are reflective of the comments, but still keep with the goals, objectives, and intent of the law.

The final rule is then filed with the *Federal Register* with an implementation date for

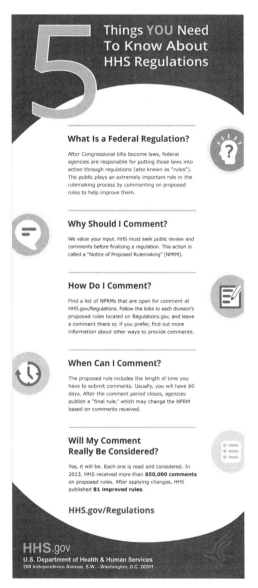

FIGURE 8.3 HHS Five Things You Need to Know About Regulations

U.S. Department of Health & Human Services.

the law to become effective. Normally, the law's effective date is several months out, in order to provide the government, public, and private agencies time to prepare for implementation by allocating or reallocating resources and revising operations and operational policies and procedures. The agency can pull back the proposed or final regulation at any time during this process if they encounter significant resistance over the regulation from legislators, other governmental officials, or the public. The judiciary does not get involved in this process unless it is petitioned to order a stay on the implementation or when a suit has been filed. Congress can also get involved in this process through their oversight function; however, they only exercise this option if the regulation is controversial or if they do not agree that the regulation is reflective of the law.

Once the rule has been promulgated, it can be challenged by judicial review through the administrative law process. The original Supreme Court's decision allowing judicial review was *Marbury v. Madison* (1803), which sought to balance presidential and political concerns against ministerial duties. *Marbury* was preempted in 1984 with *Chevron USA, Inc. v. National Resources Defense Council, Inc.* resulting in the Supreme Court's *Chevron* doctrine.[3] The Chevron decision has been credited with strengthening our form of government by (1) enhancing the separation of powers, (2) forming the basis for administrative law principles, and (3) detailing a purposive approach to rulemaking. Chevron decision is a two-step process for approaching the writing of administrative rules for newly enacted laws. Step one of the Chevron process seeks clear congressional intent by asking, "Did Congress have a specific intent with respect to the issue?" If the answer is "yes," the matter is settled. Progression to step two occurs when Congress provides an ambiguous intent by asking two questions. First, "Did Congress intend a particular result but was not clear about it?" or,

second, "Did Congress have no particular intent on the subject but mean to leave the resolution to the agency?" (Cruden & Oakes, 2016).

▶ Implementation

The judicial branch considers interpretation and implementation synonymous terms, and while this lack of distinction can be appreciated through a legal lens, these two terms carry clearly distinct and different definitions through an administrative lens. Administrators define interpretation as the "what" and "why" of a statute, and define implementation as the "how" of a statute. While public managers have implemented laws for as long as we have had governments, the formal study of implementation began with a flurry of papers published in the 1960s and Pressman and Wildavsky's publication of *Implementation* (1973).

Three "generations" of implementation theory are found in the literature, each building on the gains of the prior.[4] Mazmanian and Sabatier (1983) define program implementation as, "Those events and activities that occur after the issuing of authoritative public policy directives, which include both the efforts to administer and the substantive impacts on individuals and events." Sabatier (1986) further breaks down research on implementation of public policy into two generations: case studies (first-generation) and analytical and comparative studies (second-generation). Second-generation implementation is then further broken down into top-down (hierarchical) and bottom-up (street level bureaucrats and local officials) approaches. Third-generation implementation builds on the work of previous scholars and takes on research design approach that includes: (1) clearly defined key variables, (2) hypothesis testing based on theoretical constructs, (3) quantitative and

---

3   As discussed in Chapter 6, most of the work of public health—inclusive of environmental health—falls within either the provision of pure public goods or collective goods. Regulations for the prevention of air pollution are often used as examples of government provision of these goods.

4   This section is an adaption from Higbea, R. J. (2006). *Nongovernmental program replication and implementation: What can community-based programs to support the uninsured learn from other communities?* Dissertation, Kalamazoo, MI.

qualitative data analysis, (4) comparative analysis across jurisdictional units and policy sectors, and (5) longitudinal research times of 5–10 years (Paudel, 2009; Saetran, 2014).

Pressman and Wildavsky's case study (Implementation, 1973) of the federal Economic Development Administration's (EDA) failed efforts in Oakland, California, is a classic example of first-generation implementation. The case study goes into great detail describing economic and social conditions, as well as the actions (or lack of actions) by federal, state, and local governmental and private sector actors. They clearly describe how the complexity of implementations, such as the Oakland EDA, quickly increases with the addition of private and public actors all having some jurisdictional stake in a successful implementation and all agreeing to the overall goal, with each jurisdiction judging success based on their own jurisdiction's needs. The multitude of these measures of success that were focused on self-interest, rather than on the project, ultimately sank the project. In spite of the detailed description, Pressman and Wildavsky provide no causal evidence, theoretical analysis, or heuristic for managers to follow. Rather this case study, typical of first-generation implementation case studies, was "… pioneering but largely atheoretical, case-specific, and non-cumulative …" (Paudel, 2009).

Second-generation studies debated whether a top-down or bottom-up method of policy implementation was more effective, with scholars ultimately concluding that a synthesis or adaptive approach is most effective. This approach combines the authority held by legislators and senior administrative officials with the normative approach of street-level bureaucrats. Whether an implementing agency or organization use a top-down or bottom-up approach depends upon the organization's administrative structure, with tall hierarchical structures functioning better under the top-down approach and flat hierarchical structures functioning better under the bottom-up approach (Manzmanian & Sabatier, 1983; Palumbo & Calista, 1990; Paudel, 2009; Sabatier, 1986). Matland (1995) describes the differences between a top-down and bottom-up approach by how each approach measures success. Top-down organizations seek to measure success by quantitative measures directly tied to the program objectives. In contrast, the bottom-up organizations measure success through broader qualitative measures, such as positive impacts or effects upon the targeted population.

Several scholars described the need for the policy formulation and implementation to be conceptually clear and emphasized the importance of the implementing administrator's managerial and political skills (Palumbo & Calista, 1990). Mazmanian and Sabatier (1983) developed six conditions of effective implementation:

1. Clear and concise policy objectives
2. Sound theory, understanding principal factors and causal links, and sufficient jurisdiction
3. Structured to ensure the target agency and populations will perform as desired
4. Leaders committed to the statutory goals and possessing sufficient managerial and political skill
5. Active program supported by legislators and leaders, and supported with court neutrality
6. Statutory objectives not undermined by conflicting public policies or changes in socioeconomic conditions

Mazmanian and Sabatier (1983) also discuss four types of implementation scenarios: (1) effective implementation scenario, (2) gradual erosion scenario, (3) cumulative incrementalism scenario, and (4) rejuvenation scenario.

Effective implementation is characterized by limited and well-defined problems, modest behavioral change, strong public and private support, and high target group adherence. An example of effective implementation is how President Johnson worked with AMA leaders and Southern Democratic governors to address their concerns during the implementation of Medicare and Medicaid, resulting in smooth implementation of these programs that continue with wide public support today.

Gradual erosion is characterized by significant and well-defined problems, significant behavioral change, strong agency reliant on public and private providers of necessary implementation technology and skills, varied support ranging from strong enthusiasm to administrative vetoes, and ultimate loss of enthusiasm and program death. A current example of gradual erosion is insurance company behavior in the ACA health exchanges. The problem was well defined as an increased need for individuals to gain access to the individual insurance market. Insurance companies were quick to develop individual insurance products, despite limited actuarial data and rigid ACA requirements. After a few years of experience with business losses greater than anticipated and dwindling federal governmental reinsurance support, many insurance companies lost their enthusiasm and are cutting back participation in this market.

Cumulative incrementalism is characterized by goal-specified continuous improvement, constituency development, enhanced administrative capacity, low statutory and implementation threshold, program adherence due to monitoring, and strong central control. A recent example of cumulative incrementalism is the function of the health insurance exchange portal. The health insurance exchanges were launched with great fanfare; unfortunately, this great fanfare was undermined by an underdeveloped and poorly functioning computer portal. Once the failures were known, the federal government made immediate changes, including the hiring of new contractors and CMS leaders to supervise its development. Annually, the portal's function has improved to the point of its function becoming a non-issue.

Rejuvenation is the final implementation scenario and is characterized by poor statutory base and start up implementation, unclear legislation resulting in unclear implementation, and a long-time horizon resulting in renewed program interest. An example of rejuvenation is the implementation of Medicaid. While Medicare and Medicaid were signed into law at the same time, Medicaid's implementation has been bumpier, with states gradually agreeing to

implement the program followed by long lulls of activity. Recently, the Medicaid program has been rejuvenated through its ACA expansion that essentially removed many of the qualifiers and provided states with additional time-limited and shared financial support.

Pressman and Wildavsky's second edition of *Implementation* (1979) includes a discussion of the evolutionary nature of implementation. Their discussion considers the connection of implementation with planning and progresses from considering implementation as control (teleological–rational action–efficacy), to interaction (goals–plans–incremental discovery), to dispositions (objectives–resources–evolving and emerging constraints), and finally, to how implementation shapes policy (resources and objectives altered by actions) or as they state succinctly, "It is not policy design but redesign that occurs most of the time" (p. 172). This discussion then flips and finishes with an intuitive discussion of how policy affects implementation:

> Policy content shapes implementation by defining the arena in which the process takes place, the identity and role of the principal actors, the range of permissible tools for action, and of course supplying resources. The underlying theory provides not only the data, information, and hypotheses on which subsequent debate and action will rely, but also, and most importantly, a conceptualization of the policy problem. (p. 174)

This discussion finishes with a description of how policy learns from implementation, or into a parallel discussion of a learning organization that learns as it evolves. In the third edition of *Implementation* (1983), Pressman and Wildavsky continue describing the evolution of implementation theory, with an attempt to delineate the differences among policy analysis, implementation, and evaluation. Policy analysis is described as necessary to understand what policy makers intended to be implemented, while concomitantly implementation informs policy design. Likewise, the descriptive ways implementation informs policy design are very similar to how formative evaluation informs an ongoing policy implementation and how summative evaluation informs if policy goals and objectives were met. In conclusion, these scholars work through a discussion of the various types of evaluation models and find that evaluation's uses move along a continuum, from concrete attribution of accountability for actions, goals, and objectives on one end to abstract policy design learning on the opposite end.

Third-generation policy implementation has been described as process analysis (Sabatier, 1986), hypothesis testing, comparative and longitudinal analysis of operationalized variables (Paulmbo & Calista, 1990), and intraorganizational relations (Sinclair, 2001). Paudel (2009) finds third-generation research to differ from the previous two generations by introducing more research design and rigor through the use of testable hypotheses and analysis of qualitative and quantitative data with appropriate techniques. Finally, Saetren (2014) finds third-generation characteristics to include

"(1) key variables ... clearly defined, (2) hypotheses derived from theoretical constructs should guide empirical analysis, (3) ... use of statistical analysis using quantitative data to supplement qualitative analysis, (4) ... comparison across different units of analysis within and across policy sectors, and (5) ... longitudinal research design (i.e., research time frame of at least 5–10 years)."

Third-generation scholars focus their various analytic techniques upon describing and analyzing the implementation process or describing and analyzing the behaviors necessary for individuals and organizations to undergo change. Peters (2014) describes how three *organizational types* differ in their approaches to implementation due to their endogenous values and the type of institutionalism most closely associated with their organizational type (**TABLE 8.2**). The organizational types are (1) public sector, (2) New Public Management (public sector and private market organizations), and (3) governance (public sector and public social organizations). These organizational types differ in basic approaches due to values inherent to the organization's basic identity. The organizational values of public organizations are rooted in public service, whereas market organizations possess a

TABLE 8.2 Agencies, Institutionalism, and Implementation Structures

Agency	Public	Public and Private Market	Public and Private Social
Basic mechanism	Appropriateness	Rationality	Argumentation
Implementation structures	Normative patterns	Principal–agent relationships	Communication patterns
Implementation complexity	Least	Moderate	Most
Institutional structures	Normative	Rationality and utility	Argumentative and political

Modified from Peters, B. G. (2014). Implementation structures as institutions. *Public Policy and Administration, 29*(2), 131–144. doi:10.1177/09520767713517733.

financial, utilitarian focus, and social organizations are focused on addressing the needs of their constituents often through a network approach that introduces an inherent political nature due to similar, yet competing, values. *Institutional types* most closely associated with the aforementioned organizational types include normative, rational choice, and discussive. Normative is most closely associated with public sector organizations due to shared public service values and understanding of appropriate public sector organizational behavior. Rational choice is most closely associated with the private market sector due to the desire of these organizations to maximize their utility measured in terms of financial benefit. Finally, discussive fits private social organizations best due to a lack of shared values of the network members, resulting in a significant amount of political activity to gain implementation consensus. The value of understanding these differences for public managers responsible for implementing public policy is (1) knowing how to organize their approach to implementation based on the type of organization(s) they are working with and (2) knowing the amount and type of resources needed to ensure an effective implementation.

Another example of third-generation research is Zittoun's (2015) analysis and discussion of policy failure and how policy makers use failure to reformulate or repackage policy ideas. The first reason for policy failure occurs when a policy fails to meet its stated objectives and goals. The second reason occurs when an alternative policy objective is substituted for a clearly defined objective. This alternative objective frequently resulted in unexpected consequences that ultimately undermined an original clear set of objectives. The third reason for policy failure is associated with neither policy implementation nor measurement, rather it is a result of policy being blocked at the agenda-setting stage. Finally, proponents of failed policies turn failure of a policy proposal into a stigmatization of society as dysfunctional and in need of reform. These proponents of failed policies then call upon legislators to become standard bearers of reform, seeking through passage and implementation of their policy(ies) as reform focused on a societal good.

In summary, policy implementation tests the mettle and managerial competence of public managers who are tasked with transforming a law into operational regulations, while ensuring the goals and objectives of the law are met (see **FIGURE 8.4**). Public managers are wise to develop an understanding of organizational values and institutional types when implementing policies to help them better understand the strategies and goals associated with these organizations and the amount and type of managerial effort necessary (monitoring and politics) for successful implementation. Additionally, they should conduct the policy implementation in a conciliatory atmosphere as they develop and implement the regulations assigned to their agency. Spending time with and listening to public and private sector interest groups and organizational leaders affected by the new regulations will make the implementation process smoother.

The implementation process continues to be an important aspect of advocacy, as professionals and interest groups seek to influence the final regulations that they will become responsible for implementing in their organizations. In many ways, advocacy during the regulatory development process takes on an agenda-setting tone as groups seek to influence the regulations to their benefit. If the final regulations are not in line with their organizational goals and directions, the agenda-setting process certainly starts over again for them as they seek to influence future versions of the law, once it makes it through the operations phase and passes into the modification phase.

This chapter has covered the first of two areas wherein policy change regularly occur, often without being noticed by anyone not directly affected by the changes. This is identified as the yellow bounded area in the flowchart presented in Figure 8.4. The next chapter covers policy change that occurs predominantly in the area beyond the yellow border in Figure 8.4.

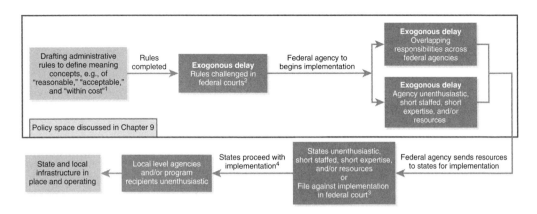

FIGURE 8.4 What Can Happen …

References

Bruhl, A. P. (2013). Hierarchically variable deference to agency interpretations. *Notre Dame Law Review, 89*(2), 727.

Congressional Budget Office. Introduction to CBO. Retrieved from www.cbo.gov/about/overview

Congressional Research Service. Retrieved from www.loc.gov/crsinfo/history.html

Cruden, J. C., & Oakes, M. R. (2016). The enduring nature of the chevron doctrine. *Harvard Environmental, 40*(2): 189–209.

Fischman, R. L., & Ruhl, J. B. (2016). Judging adaptive management practices of U.S. agencies. *Conservation Biology, 30*(2), 268–275. doi:10.1111/cobi.12616

General Accounting Office. Retrieved from www.gao.gov/about/index.html

Gluck, A. R. (2011). Intrastatutory federalism and statutory interpretation: State implementation of federal law in health reform and beyond. *The Yale Law Journal, 121*(3), 534–622.

Hiriart, Y., & Martimort, D. (2012). How much discretion for risk regulators? *The RAND Journal of Economics, 43*(2), 283–314. doi:10.1111/j.1756-2171.2012.00166.x

Joint Committee on Taxation. Retrieved from www.jct.gov/about-us/overview.html

Medicare Prescription Drug, Improvement, & Modernization Act of 2004.

Patient Protection and Affordable Care Act of 2010. Community Living Assistance Services and Support Act (CLASS).

Peters, B. G. (2014). Implementation structures as institutions. *Public Policy and Administration, 29*(2), 131–144. doi:10.1177/0952076713517733

Rice, T., Desmond, K., & Gabel, J. (1990). The Medicare Catastrophic Coverage Act: A post-mortem. *Health Affairs, 9*(3), 75–87. doi:10.1377/hlthaff.9.3.75

Stack, K. M. (2015). Purposivism in the executive branch: How agencies interpret statutes. *Northwestern University Law Review, 109*(4), 871.

The White House. Retrieved from www.whitehouse.gov/omb/organization_mission/

Zittoun, P. (2015). Analysing policy failure as an argumentative strategy in the policymaking process: A pragmatist perspective. *Public Policy and Administration, 30*(3–4), 243–260. doi:10.1177/0952076715581634

Appendix

APPENDIX TABLE 8.3 Rulemaking

Year	Law	Name	Summary
1935	44 U.S.C. Chapter 15	Federal Register Act	The act established a uniform system for handling agency regulations by requiring (1) the filing of documents with the Office of the Federal Register, (2) the placement of documents on public inspection, (3) the publication of the documents in the Federal Register, and (4) (after a 1937 amendment) the permanent codification of rules in the Code of Federal Regulations. Publication of a rule in the Federal Register provides official notice of its existence and contents.
1946	5 U.S.C. § 551 *et seq.*	Administrative Procedure Act	Written to bring regularity and predictability to agency decision-making, it provides for both *formal rulemaking*, used when rules are required by statute to be made on the record, and *informal rulemaking*, used when agencies publish proposed rules in the *Federal Register*, provides for a comment period of up to 30 days, and subsequently publishes a final rule in the *Federal Register*.
1969	42 U.S.C. §§ 4321-4347	National Environmental Policy	Requires agencies to determine whether the proposed rules will result in a significant impact on the environment. If the potential for a significant impact is determined, the agency is required to delineate the direct, indirect, and cumulative impact on the environment.
1972	5 U.S.C. App. II	Federal Advisory Committee Act	Established requirements to ensure that agencies using advisory committees receive impartial and relevant expertise and that the advice provided by advisory committees be objective and accessible to the public.
1979	19 U.S.C. §§ 2531-2533	Trade Agreements Act of 1979	Prohibits agencies from setting regulatory standards that create "unnecessary obstacles to foreign commerce" of the United States; specifically states that legitimate domestic objectives, such as safety or health, are not considered unnecessary obstacles.

(continues)

APPENDIX TABLE 8.3 Rulemaking *(continued)*

Year	Law	Name	Summary
1980	4 U.S.C. §§ 3501-3520	Paperwork Reduction Act	Requires agencies to justify any collection of information from the public by establishing the need and intended use of the information, estimating the burden that the collection will impose on respondents, and showing that the collection is the least burdensome way to gather the information.
1980	5 U.S.C. §§ 601-612	Regulatory Flexibility Act	Requires federal agencies to assess the impact of their forthcoming regulations on small entities.
1981	Executive Order 12291	Rulemaking Requirements	Establishes a set of general requirements for rulemaking: (1) requires federal agencies (other than independent regulatory agencies) to send a copy of each draft proposed and final rule to OMB before publication in the Federal Register, and (2) requires covered agencies to prepare a regulatory impact analysis for each "major" rule (e.g., those with a $100 million impact on the economy).
1985	Executive Order 12498	Regulatory Plan	Requires covered agencies (all except independent regulatory agencies) to submit a regulatory plan, which covers all of their significant regulatory actions, underway or planned, to OMB for review each year.
1988	Executive Order 12630	Constitutionally Protected Property Rights	Requires each agency to be guided by certain principles when formulating or implementing policies that have "takings" implications. Requires that private property should be taken only for real and substantial threats and be no greater than is necessary.
1990	5 U.S.C. §§ 561-570a	Negotiated Rulemaking Act of 1990	As amended and permanently authorized in 1996 (110 Stat. 3870), seeks to overcome what some observers describe as an adversarial relationship between agencies and affected interest groups that often accompanies agency rulemaking.
1993	Executive Order 12866	Rules Review	Revoked Executive Orders 12291 and 12498 and established a new process for OIRA review of rules. Limited reviews of proposed and final rules to that imposing significant regulatory impact and implemented other efficiency and transparency guidelines, including cost-benefit analysis.
1993	Executive Order 12889	NAFTA Comment Period	Requires agencies to provide at least a 75-day comment period for any "proposed Federal technical regulation or any Federal sanitary or phytosanitary measure of general application."

1994	Executive Order 12898	Environmental Justice	Each agency must develop a strategy that identifies and addresses disproportionately high and adverse human health or environmental effects of its programs, policies, and activities on minority populations and low-income populations.
1995	2 U.S.C. §§ 1501-1538	Unfunded Mandates Reform Act	Title I established new procedures designed to ensure that Congress fully considers the potential effects of unfunded federal mandates before imposing them in legislation. Title II contains requirements imposed on covered federal agencies during the rulemaking process including (1) preparation of a written statement containing specific descriptions and estimates for any proposed rule or any final rule that includes any federal mandate that may result in the expenditure of $100 million or more in any year, (2) identification and consideration of a reasonable number of regulatory alternatives and selection of the least costly, most cost-effective, or least burdensome alternative, (3) development of a plan in which agencies provide notice of regulatory requirements to potentially affected small governments, and (4) development of an effective process to permit elected officers of state, local, and tribal governments (or their designees) to provide input in the development of regulatory proposals containing significant intergovernmental mandates.
1995	Presidential Memorandum	Results-Oriented Rulemaking	Directs federal agencies to focus their regulatory programs on results, not process, and to expand their use of negotiated rulemaking.
1995	Presidential Memorandum	Public Reports and Penalties	Directed agencies to waive or reduce penalties in certain circumstances, and to reduce the frequency of reports the public is required to provide to the government.
1996	110 Stat. 857, 5 U.S.C. § 601 note	Small Business Regulatory Enforcement Fairness Act (SBREFA)	Amended the Regulatory Flexibility Act to permit judicial review and to permit small entities to participate in EPA and OSHA rulemaking before a proposed rule with a significant impact on small entities is published.
1996	5 U.S.C. §§ 801-808	Congressional Review Act	Included as part of SBREFA, requires all final rules be filed with each chamber of Congress and the GAO. Established expedited procedures by which Congress may disapprove agencies' rules by enacting a joint resolution of disapproval.

(continues)

APPENDIX TABLE 8.3 Rulemaking   *(continued)*

Year	Law	Name	Summary
1996	15 U.S.C. § 272 note	Section 12(d) of the National Technology Transfer and Advancement	Requires federal agencies to "use technical standards that are developed or adopted by voluntary consensus standards bodies" to carry out policy objectives unless doing so is inconsistent with applicable law or otherwise impractical" and to consult with and participate with voluntary, private sector, consensus bodies.
1996	Executive Order 12988	Civil Justice	Requires agencies reviewing existing and new regulations to ensure that they comply with specific requirements to improve regulatory drafting in order to minimize litigation.
1997	Executive Order 13045	Protection of Children from Environmental Health Risks and Safety Risks	For any substantive rulemaking action that is likely to result in an economically significant rule that concerns an environmental health risk or safety risk that may disproportionately affect children, the agency must provide OIRA with (1) an evaluation of the environmental or safety effects on children and (2) an explanation of why the planned regulation is preferable to other potentially effective and reasonably feasible alternatives.
1998	44 U.S.C. § 3504 note	Government Paperwork Elimination Act	Requires federal agencies provide the public, when practicable, with the option of submitting, maintaining, and disclosing information electronically, instead of on paper.
1998	Presidential Memorandum	Plain Language Rulemaking	Directive requires agencies to use plain language in proposed and final rulemaking documents.
1999	Executive Order 13132	Federalism	Requires covered federal agencies to have an accountable process to ensure meaningful and timely input by state and local officials in the development of regulatory policies that have federalism implications.
2000	Executive Order 13175	Consultation and Coordination with Indian Tribal Governments	Prohibits agencies from promulgating any regulation not required by law that has tribal implications and imposes substantial direct costs on tribal governments, unless the necessary funds are provided or the agency consults with tribal officials and provides a "tribal summary impact statement" describing those consultations.

2001	P.L. 106-554 §§ 515	Data or Information Quality Act	Amended the Paperwork Reduction Act and directed OMB to issue government-wide guidelines that "provide policy and procedural guidance to federal agencies for ensuring and maximizing the quality, objectivity, utility, and integrity of information (including statistical information) disseminated by federal agencies."
2001	31 U.S.C. § 1105 note	Section 624 of the Treasury and General Government Appropriations Act	Requires OMB to prepare and submit with the budget an "accounting statement and associated report" containing an estimate of the total costs and benefits (including quantifiable and unquantifiable effects) of federal rules and paperwork, to the extent feasible, in the aggregate, by agency and agency program, and by major rule, and an analysis of impacts of federal regulation on state, local, and tribal governments, small businesses, wages, and economic growth.
2001	Executive Order 13211	Energy Impacts	Requires agencies to prepare and submit to OMB a "statement of energy effects" for significant energy actions.
2002	44 U.S.C.A. § 3601 note	E-Government Act of 2002	Designed to enhance the management and promotion of electronic government services and processes, and contains requirements affecting the rulemaking process.
2002	P.L. 107-198	Small Business Paperwork Relief Act of 2002	The act amends the Paperwork Reduction Act, requiring each agency establish a single point of contact to act as a liaison for small business concerns with regard to information collection and paperwork issues. Direct agencies to make a special effort to reduce information collection burden for small businesses with fewer than 25 employees.
2002	Executive Order 13272	Small Entities and Rulemaking	Requires federal agencies to (1) issue written procedures and policies, to ensure proper consideration during the rulemaking process of the impacts of their draft rules on small entities, (2) to notify the SBA Chief Counsel for Advocacy of any draft rules that may have a significant economic impact on a substantial number of small entities, and (3) to give "every appropriate consideration" to any comments the Chief Counsel provides.
2003	OMB Bulletin	Peer Review and Information Quality	Required federal agencies to (1) peer review all significant regulatory actions, to (2) peer review all especially significant regulatory actions, and to (3) provide OMB annually with a report on upcoming regulatory disseminations and anticipated peer-review actions.

(continues)

APPENDIX TABLE 8.3 Rulemaking *(continued)*

Year	Law	Name	Summary
2007	Executive Order 13422		Made significant amendments to Executive Order 12866 including (1) a requirement that agencies identify in writing the specific market failure or problem that warrants a new regulation, (2) a requirement that each agency head designate a presidential appointee within the agency as a "regulatory policy officer" who can control upcoming rulemaking activity in that agency, (3) a requirement that agencies provide their best estimates of the cumulative regulatory costs and benefits of rules they expect to publish in the coming year, (4) an expansion of OIRA review to include significant guidance documents, and (5) a provision permitting agencies to consider whether to use more formal rulemaking procedures in certain cases.
2009	Executive Order 13497		Revoked Executive Order 13422, reinstating Executive Order 12866 to its original form as issued in September 1993.
2011	Executive Order 13563	Improving Regulation and Regulatory Review	Reaffirms and supplements Executive Order 12866, including (1) timely online access to the rulemaking docket, (2) an opportunity for public comment on all pertinent parts of the rulemaking docket, and (3) a requirement for agencies to initiate retrospective reviews of their existing rules.
2012	Executive Order 13609	International Regulatory Cooperation	Requires agencies to consider the issue of international regulatory cooperation and how to eliminate differences in regulations between the United States and its major trading partners.
2012	Executive Order 13610	Institutionalizing Regular Reviews	Instructs agencies to institutionalize regular reviews of their previously issued significant regulations, and to take additional steps to increase public participation in retrospective reviews of regulations.

Modified from Cruden, J. C., & Oakes, M. R. (2016). The enduring nature of the chevron doctrine. *Harvard Environmental Law Review, 40*(2), 189.

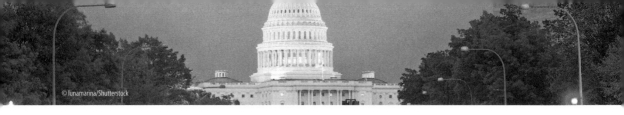

CHAPTER 9

Policy Monitoring and Modification

This chapter is designed to give healthcare leaders an understanding of policy modification and analysis by covering the following topics:

- Constituent and interest group feedback
- Federal government policy analysis and monitoring organizations
- Mechanics (federal, state, and, sometimes, local government interfaces)
- Modifications by branch
- Locus of leadership, administrative rules, implementation complexity, and dominant administrative structures
- State government initiation of modifications: a case of Medicaid policy modification

Understanding how public policies are modified is perhaps the "messiest" of skills to master of any skills covered in this text. In order to present the material for understanding monitoring and modification for effective learning, we rely on a different proportion of standard narrative explanation, case study illustration, tables, and figures than found elsewhere in this text. This will assist current and future healthcare leaders in gaining a general understanding of how and why federal statutes (and state statutes) are changed and revised. There are multiple reasons for policy changes that include, but are not limited to, political and societal environment changes, scientific changes, policy analysis and

evaluation results, interest group influence, and operational inefficiencies.

It is also important to note that modifications can be triggered at multiple places in the policy process after enactment. Furthermore, modifications may start the policy process all over again, beginning at agenda-setting and ending in the rulemaking and operations phases. Longest (2010) refers to the feedback loop that occurs among these stages and states, "[T]his cyclical relationship means that experience gained with operations of policies can influence the modification of rules or regulations subsequently used in their operation" (p. 156). In keeping with the agenda-setting theories of Kingdon (1995), Baumgartner and Jones

(1993), most modifications are incremental. Some of these modifications can have meaningless policy implications, such as when the Health Care Financing Administration changed its name to the Center for Medicare and Medicaid Services. Other modifications, such as annual Medicare payment updates, can seem small in isolation, yet large when their cumulative effect is considered over long lengths of time. For example, over the 50-year life of Medicare, 264 modifications have been enacted, yet, of those modifications, only four are major legislation, resulting in three model changes and one payment change (see **TABLES 9.1** and **9.2**).

▶ Constituent and Interest Group Feedback

Constituent and interest group feedback on implemented laws is fundamental to a functioning democracy and one of the rationales of policy modifications. It is through this feedback loop that agencies and legislators learn if a policy is meeting its desired goals and,

accordingly, if the results are positive or negative. It is also through this process that governmental actors learn if operational procedures[1] are inhibiting or enhancing policy goals. What is important for citizens to understand is that this feedback loop is two way and iterative, by nature. Multiple iterations may occur before a policy's stated goals are met. The importance of feedback cannot be overstated, for without it the agency will assume all is going well and continue operations as normal.

One of the more well-published legislative changes resulting from constituent and interest group feedback was the repeal of the Medicare Catastrophic Coverage Act of 1988 (PL 100-360).[2] This legislation was developed to provide catastrophic medical and prescription drug coverage to all Medicare beneficiaries. The bill unraveled when Medicare beneficiaries realized that the catastrophic coverage was duplicative of what many of them already had through supplemental policies, that it would result in additional costs, and that the long-term care provisions were not included. As a result of the negative feedback from Medicare beneficiaries to administrative and legislative actors, Congress repealed the Act 18 months after enacting it (Rice, Desmond, & Gabel, 1990).

TABLE 9.1 Proposed and Enacted Modifications for Medicare, Medicaid, and HIPAA

Bill	Bills Referred to Committee	Bills Reported by Committee	Bills Enacted
Medicare	7664	281	264
Medicaid	4961	264	245
HIPAA	189	18	6

1 These may be either written in the original legislation or administrative rules written after passage, or both.
2 While all changes to a policy or associated regulations have to be published in the *Federal Register*, most of these changes go unnoticed by the public unless they are directly affected by a change.

TABLE 9.2 Major Medicare Legislation	
Major Medicare Legislation	
1965	Parts A & B Enacted
1972	Disabled and ESRD added
1983	Prospective Payment
1997	Medicare+Choice
2004	Medicare Prescription Drug, Improvement, and Modernization Act

Congress.gov.

Additional consequences of this policy repeal were that prescription drug coverage was not addressed for another 16 years in the Medicare Prescription Drug, Improvement, and Modernization Act of 2004 (PL 108-173) and that long-term care coverage was not addressed for another 22 years in the Patient Protection and Affordable Care Act of 2010 (PL 111-148) (which also was then repealed).

▶ Federal Government Policy Analysis & Monitoring Organizations

Policy analysis can take several formats, ranging from content analysis—questioning whether the rules and regulations actually reflect the policy intent—to evaluative analysis. Monitoring—how well the regulations and rules are meeting the goals of the policy—includes compliance, auditing, accounting, and explanation of actual outcomes. The federal government has at least five general agencies/bodies that focus on policy analysis and/or monitoring: the Congressional Budget Office (CBO), the Joint Committee

on Taxation (JCI), the Congressional Research Service (CRS), the General Accountability Office (GAO), and the Office of Management and Budget (OMB). In additional to these offices, all of the agencies have an Office of Inspector General and other agency-level analysis capacity.

The *Congressional Budget Office* was born out of a dispute with President Nixon in 1974 over his threats to use impoundment in order to stop the flow of funds to programs that he disagreed with. Congress attempted to remedy this and other similar executive disputes by providing additional congressional capacity to control the budgetary process through passage of the Congressional Budget and Impoundment Control Act of 1974 (PL 83-344). Since its founding, the CBO has provided regular economic forecasts of how major policy initiatives will affect the budget, as well as regular updates on how the current budget projections are tracking. The CBO states their mission is to "… produce independent analysis of budgetary and economic issues to support the Congressional budget process" (CBO, n.d.). One controversy that has clouded the CBO's forecasts has been the use of static budgetary scoring methodology that provides a micro-economic forecast and has been criticized for not taking a broad enough view of the economy. Congress has directed the CBO to begin using dynamic economic scoring for major legislation, beginning in 2015, that is supposed to include the broader economic effects of budgetary changes.

The *Joint Committee on Taxation* (JCT) was established through the Revenue Act of 1926 as a nonpartisan committee to assist Congress with the development of tax policy. The JCT works closely with the CBO to project the budgetary effect of tax policy and provides assistance to Congress by:

■ Assisting Congressional tax-writing committees and members of Congress with development and analysis of legislative proposals;

■ Preparing official revenue estimates of all tax legislation considered by Congress;

■ Drafting legislative histories for tax-related bills; and

■ Investigating various aspects of the Federal tax system (JCT, n.d.).

The current composition and direction for the JCT was established by the Internal Revenue Code of 1986 and specifies the House of Representatives and Senate members of the committee and the committee's investigative duties. In addition, the Congressional Budget Act of 1974 (PL 93-344) requires the JCT to provide revenue estimates on all tax legislation (JCT, n.d.).

The *Congressional Research Service* was established in 1914 within the Library of Congress as the Legislative Reference Service with the mission of serving the legislative needs of Congress. Under the Legislative Reorganization Act of 1970 (PL 91-510), the agency was renamed the Congressional Research Service and had its statutory obligations expanded. The CRS mission is to "… serve the Congress throughout the legislative process by providing comprehensive and reliable legislative research and analysis that are timely, objective, authoritative and confidential, thereby contributing to an informed national legislature" (Library of

Congress, n.d.). The CRS is a highly respected nonpartisan professional agency that provides research analysis to Congress in multiple formats. One of the well-regarded documents the CRS provides is the policy summary of proposed legislation.

The *General Accountability Office* was established in 1921 and is a nonpartisan office that provides Congress with investigative information on how the government is spending its money. The GAO mission "… is to support Congress in meeting its constitutional responsibilities and to help improve the performance and ensure the accountability of the federal government for the benefit of the American people … provid[ing] Congress with timely information that is objective, fact-based, nonpartisan, non-ideological, fair, and balanced." Their work is performed by auditing agency operations, investigating illegal activities, evaluating how well government programs are meeting objectives, providing analysis for proposed legislation, and issuing legal decisions and opinions (General Accounting Office, n.d.).

The *Office of Management and Budget* was developed through the Budget and Accounting Act of 1921 (PL 67-13) and has a mission "… to serve the President … in implementing his vision across the Executive Branch." The OMB reports to the president and carries out its mission through the (1) development and execution of the federal budget, (2) oversight of agency performance, (3) coordination and review of regulations, (4) legislative clearance and coordination, and (5) direction of governmental actions through executive orders and memoranda. The budget development and execution aspect of the OMB is a central part of its function and vital to the smooth administration of the federal budget. The management functions are carried out through five offices that ensure that the president's management plan is developed and followed and that appropriate management policies are developed and enforced (Office of Management and Budget, n.d.).

These five federal agencies are central to the operations, analysis, and evaluation of federal policies and are a major source for policy modification. Additional governmental agencies are sources for policy modification through their internal analysis, evaluation, and constituency feedback loops. Other nongovernmental sources include the affected agencies, professional groups, and interest groups.

In summary, there are multiple sources for policy modification ideas that come from multiple governmental and nongovernmental agencies. These agencies produce sophisticated analysis and evaluation through data collection, survey, and modeling. Despite the sophistication of the aforementioned analytic techniques, often times the best source for policy modification ideas comes from end users who state that, through experience, the policy is not working. These same constituents can frequently tell you why the policy is not working and provide recommendations for how to either make the policy workable or the necessity for its repeal.

▶ Mechanics (Federal, State, and, Sometimes, Local Government Interfaces)

The mechanics of policy implementation and monitoring offer different opportunities for modification and can occur at any stage of the policy process after enactment. These opportunities "look different" for each phase of the process. As an operational history begins to develop with a policy, recommendations for modifications also begin to accrue. These recommendations begin to make their way through the policy process through agenda-setting; political actors pick up on these problems and work with their interest groups to craft remedies that are in alignment with their political philosophy. Throughout this process, political leaders, interest groups, and even private sector businesses known for their interest

in the area under discussion will take up the role of policy entrepreneur. The process will move forward or will wait for the correct political alignment and phase of policy implementation after enactment for proposing change.

When the modifications come up for debate, the tenor of the debate will depend on the severity of the need and the differences in the remedies by the two political parties, as well as groups representing the policy beneficiaries and targets. Modifications may be minor adjustments or completely different approaches, similar to the multiple options proposed by Republicans as to how they would "repair" or "replace" the ACA. The modified policy then moves its way through the legislative phase, either as a new policy or as an amendment to an existing policy. If the policy is signed into law, it is enacted through the implementation phases again, with interest group and political actors seeking to craft a final remedy to align with their political philosophy and the concerns of the constituents they represent. Then, the feedback loop or process continues and cyclically repeats itself again and again as interest group and political actors seek more modifications and continued refinement of the policy.

▶ Modifications by Branch

Each branch of government plays a part in how policies are modified, depending on the jurisdiction provided them. The executive branch has the greatest latitude in making modifications, due to their role as implementers of policies. If the recommended modifications are minor, they have the ability to make these changes without the need to seek legislative approval through the issuance of updated administrative rules. If, however, the recommended changes substantially change the focus or goals of the policy, they will need to make their way through the legislative process in which they are debated and further studied by legislators prior to developing changes to the legislation.

The executive branch can (and often does) provide recommended legislative language and assist in drafting final legislation. However, the final legislation language and passage of the legislation is the prerogative of the legislative branch. A recent example of this was the repeal of the Community Living Assistance Services and Supports Act (CLASS; PL 111-148, Sec. 8001) when, during the regulatory phase, the HHS actuaries found it impossible to price long-term care insurance and recommended repeal of the Act, which Congress acted on as recommended (PL 112-240, Sec. 642).

The legislature can take up policy modification based on constituent, interest group, or legislative recommendations for modification. Again, these changes may be minor, yet need legislative action or they may be substantive program changes. Minor modifications often result in minimal debate, whereas major changes may evoke lengthy and substantive analysis and debate. Ultimately, the legislation will either get passed into law or die due to lack of substantial support. The executive branch again enters with the president either signing the legislation and moving it on to the administration to implement or vetoing the legislation.

Finally, the judiciary may become involved if an actor challenges the constitutionality of the law (see case study "*CRC v VDH*"). They can issue stays of implementation while they consider the challenge and pend final judgment (see **FIGURE 9.1**, location 2). Ultimately, challenges to a law will result in a judicial judgment either affirming or denying the constitutionality of the law. Depending on the level of disagreement, challenges may go through multiple appeals and end up before the Supreme Court for final judgment. The Affordable Care Act has undergone several judicial challenges in its short life, with the Supreme Court affirming the constitutionality of the law (2012), yet deciding for the defendants in several other decisions. The range of potential challenges are vast; for example, the decision about how the Medicaid expansion was too coercive (2012) was based on the language of the law, whereas the decision about closely held firms (2014) not having to provide contraceptive coverage was based on a rule about how the law was implemented.

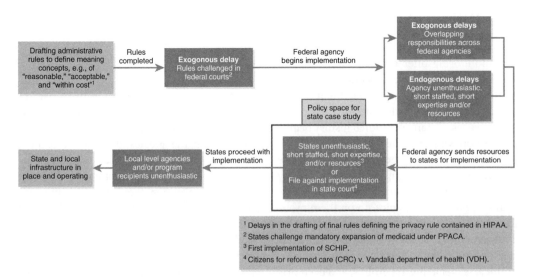

FIGURE 9.1 After the Law Has Passed …

In summary, the one factual statement that can be made about any law is that it will, at some time, go through the modification process. The modification may be minor, resulting in changes that are barely noticed, or result in major changes that are hotly debated. Furthermore, the changes can emanate in any stage of the policy process and from any branch of government, any level of governance (state or local), or the private sector.

▶ Locus of Leadership, Administrative Rules, Implementation Complexity, and Dominant Administrative Structures

Policy making in the United States is generally predicated on the presumption that government action does not require government leadership in the implementation, monitoring, and/ or modification roles. Rather, two alternatives may be employed: government agency leadership in implementation and private sector leadership in implementation. This yields two loci for leadership in the implementation, monitoring, and possible modification of policy (see **TABLE 9.3**). Note that this discussion describes the most common, expected outcomes across the intersections of dimensions. Flexibilities in U.S. government policy design result in (rare) exceptions for any of these dimensional intersections. One federal program, Medicaid, squats in between the two leadership loci. It starts at the federal level, then moves to the state government agency level, which then implements through the private sector.

Three separate dimensions interact with these two loci (the dimensions are partially interdependent) to produce a more nuanced understanding of how policy implementation, monitoring, and modification may differ. The *administrative rules dimension* refers to the expectation of the amount of writing of rules to be necessary prior to implementation. The *implementation complexity dimension* refers to the expected range of complexity with regard to beneficiaries, targets, instruments, and intended outcomes to anticipate within each locus. The *dominant administrative structure dimension* refers to the most common administrative structure associated with each locus.

When the locus of leadership remains firmly within government agencies, we find the least potential for variation in the other two dimensions. This should feel intuitive— the default for policy in the United States is to keep direct government involvement to a minimum. Thus, if the policy problem addressed is perceived as a pure collective good, government must lead implementation (see Chapter 5). When the policy problem addressed is the provision of a quasi-collective good, we should expect that implementation will be led by private sector entities.

Within the government leadership locus, both administrative rules-writing and implementation complexity should be expected to be "high" and the relationship will be quite close. The expected administrative structure is hierarchical—leadership of implementation through a chain of government agencies from the federal level to the state, and sometimes then to local government agencies. The best examples for this come from public health policy, almost all of which address the provision of pure collective goods. We ask that you recall the discussion in Chapter 1 of the Clean Water Act. The complex, detailed administrative rules for this act receive regular, painstaking review and revision, based on analysis of empirical data from monitoring activities, as well as political pressure from organizations representing both policy beneficiaries and targets of the Act. The implementation of the Act is complex, including among many other tasks, such as regular

TABLE 9.3 Policy Modification Complexities: Leadership Locus for Implementation, Administrative Rules, Policy Complexity, and Dominant Administrative Structure

Locus of Leadership for Implementation		
Government (Most common in public health policy)	Private sector (Most common in healthcare delivery policy)	
High *High = Clean Water Act*	Low to high *High = Privacy Rule* *Low = Hospital Readmissions*	Role of administrative rules
High *High = Clean Water Act*	Low to high *High = ACOs* *Low = Medicare FFS claims*	Complexity of implementation
Hierarchical (Federal agency–state agencies; sometimes then to local agencies)	Contractual	Dominant Administrative structure

measurements involving the collection of air, soil, and water samples for laboratory testing, and inspection of manufacturing firms, water treatment facilities (both private and government), agricultural waste disposal sites, etc. The persons implementing and monitoring are most often employed within federal, state, or local government agencies.

When the locus of leadership is the private sector, we anticipate more variation in the amount of rules-writing necessary prior to implementation. We expect these to range from low through high, although we should also anticipate more policies will fit in the "low" rather than in the "high" categories. This is because policy written for such leadership is more likely to cover the provision of quasi-collective goods (see Chapter 6). The administrative structure will likely be flat, consisting of contracts with private sector firms for implementation, monitoring, and feedback regarding modifications. Variation in the contractual complexity is related to implementation complexity. "Low" implementation

complexity results in administrative structures consisting of relatively straightforward contracts for payment of services rendered, for example, Medicare FFS payments to healthcare providers. "High" implementation complexity consists of complex webs of contracts amongst private sector organizations to meet the complex implementation outcomes (e.g., Medicare ACOs).

Note that in the private sector leadership locus, complexity in the writing of administrative rules does not necessarily relate to implementation complexity. As identified in Table 9.3, the administrative rules-writing for the Hospital Readmission Reduction Program was small—due to the details contained in the authorizing legislation (see the case study in Chapter 12, "Who saves? The Medicare quality and cost conundrum"). The detail in the legislation was possible as the program was the result of several successive CMS waiver demonstrations that provided the CMS sufficient experience and expertise to place implementation detail into law. However, implementing the changes to meet the program's goals is quite complex—the opposite of the administrative rules dimension.

How does this discussion help the healthcare administrator? Two ways. One, by identifying where to look for variation in administrative rules-writing, implementation complexity, and administrative structures. Two, by identifying points where modification of a policy is possible. Where levels in the first two dimensions are low, the opportunities for policy modification after passage into law are also low. Where these levels are high, the possibilities for policy modification increase.

▶ State Government Initiation of Modifications: A Case of Modification to Medicaid

Although the challenge to the Medicaid expansion component of ACA from multiple state attorney generals is a well-known and suitably illustrative example of how federal policy might be modified by state government action after enactment, this is not the only manner in which states have achieved modifications to federal Medicaid policy. The following case study, anonymized yet reflective of historical events, can be found as **point 4 in Figure 9.1**.

▶ CRC v. VDH

In the late 1990s, after more than a decade of successive 1115 waiver applications (used to propose and implement demonstrations within a Medicaid program) to enable demonstrations of programming targeted toward dual-eligible recipients. The demonstrations sought, successfully, to support dual eligibilities in their communities via provision of home-based services. The state of Vandalia's[3] Department of Health (VDH) was denied the opportunity to expand its successful PACE model (Program of All-inclusive Care for the Elderly) to the entire eligible population in the state. In frustration, the Director of the VDH, after receiving confidential prior approval from the governor, approached the statewide advocacy organization Citizens for Reformed Care (CRC) with a plan. The CRC was asked to file a lawsuit against the VDH for violating the state constitution by not providing access to PACE model benefits to all eligible residents. If this was done, the VDH would "challenge" the action up to the state Supreme Court of Vandalia, where both sides were certain the CRC would win. After the decision, the VDH would contact the CMS and note that it was now "trapped" into violating the current 1115 waiver. The CMS capitulated and did not challenge the expansion of PACE programming statewide. It is believed that the CMS Director was advised that a challenge in federal court to the state of Vandalia's expansion would eventually lead to a similar outcome at the Supreme Court of the United States.

References

Baumgartner, F. R., & Jones, B. D. (1993). *Agendas and instability in American politics.* Chicago, IL: University of Chicago Press.

Congressional Budget Office. (n.d.). Introduction to CBO. Retrieved from www.cbo.gov/about/overview

General Accounting Office. (n.d.). Retrieved from www.gao.gov/about/index.html

Joint Committee on Taxation. (n.d.). Retrieved from www.jct.gov/about-us/overview.html

---

3 Vandalia was a proposed colony that did not receive final approval from the British crown. During the American Revolution, a petition for statehood was rejected by the Continental Congress.

Kingdon, J. W. (1995). *Agendas, alternatives, and public policies* (2nd ed.). New York, NY: Longman.

Library of Congress. (n.d.). Retrieved from www.loc.gov /crsinfo/history.html

Longest, B. B. (2010). *Health policy making in the United States*. Chicago, IL: Health Administration Press.

Office of Management and Budget. (n.d.). Retrieved from www.whitehouse.gov/omb/organization_mission/

Rice, T., Desmond, K., & Gabel, J. (1990). The Medicare Catastrophic Coverage Act: A post-mortem. *Health Affairs, 9*(3), 75–87. doi:10.1377/hlthaff.9.3.75

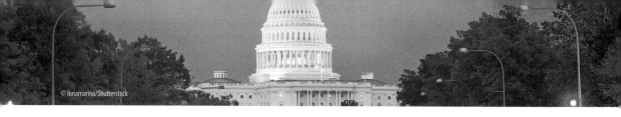

CHAPTER 10

Healthcare Payment, Cost Drivers, and Behavioral Economics

This chapter is designed to give healthcare leaders an understanding of how economics affects health policy by covering the following topics:

- Brief history of healthcare payment and long-term cost drivers
- Insurance concepts and effects on cost drivers
- Current drivers of healthcare costs
- How cost drivers in the United States compare to OECD countries
- Barriers to market entry
- Behavioral economics and health care

▶ The Market for Health Care in the United States

It is useful when thinking of the mixed methods by which health care is purchased (and delivered) to imagine that we are talking about a nested market system (see **FIGURE 10.1**).

The term "nested" reflects the variability in healthcare markets across the country at both the state and the local levels, while allowing for the role of the federal and state purchasing that cuts across local market boundaries. We can determine the geographic boundaries of these different markets, defined either by service delivery areas or politically, along state, county, or municipal lines.[1] Each market has a permeable membrane, because each market is

---

1 See the *Dartmouth Atlas* (http://www.dartmouthatlas.org/) for a description and examples of defining healthcare boundaries by delivery of service. The two most commonly used boundaries are hospital referral regions and hospital services areas.

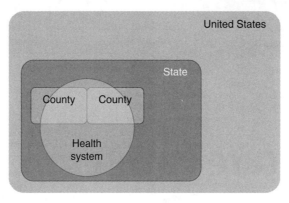

FIGURE 10.1 Nested Market Diagram
Dissertation for PhD at Michigan State University. May 2001. Courtesy of Greg Cline.

able to control, to some extent, the way in which the market operates within its own boundaries. However, each market is also increasingly affected by what is occurring in nearby markets, and in the larger state and national markets within which they are nested (through Medicaid and Medicare expenditures, which are largely beyond these local market actors' control). Also, although some healthcare coverage/services tend to still be primarily local (e.g., primary care or outpatient surgery), other services and products, such as pharmaceuticals and laboratory tests, generally operate within markets that are regional (multi-county, multi-state, and national). Thus, they increase the permeability of the smaller markets for healthcare services.

It is also useful to keep in mind that healthcare markets are far from free markets. These markets have long been dominated by two guild-like organizations (the American Medical Association [AMA] and the American Hospital Association [AHA]) that have controlled the market entry of new suppliers, as well as the way in which supply is structured and who has access to all forms of market information (Starr, 1982). The AMA and the AHA have maintained, until the late 20th century, a stranglehold on the supply side of the

market, the effects of which have been argued to materially affect most of the demand within the market. These two groups (each of which has well-organized sub-organizations at the state and regional levels, and for the AMA, at the county—and sometimes even municipal—level) have the ability to manipulate legislation that affects their professions and the markets within which they operate. They also affect the ability of purchasers to understand their options for health care, retarding demands for competition amongst providers, retarding access to quality and cost information, and slowing purchaser demands for changes in legislation and regulation. Only with the fast-paced increases in healthcare costs of the 1970s and 1980s, as well as the introduction of prospective payment by Medicare and Medicaid, have we witnessed these markets becoming more "free." With this, came efforts by various purchasers and payers to shift the costs of providing health care to their populations onto others, purchasers demanding and, in some cases, creating competition, an increase in the availability of quality and cost information to very large purchasers, and an increase in permeability of the membranes of the many smaller local markets (Rice & Unruh, 2015).[2]

---

2   This discussion should remind you of the cost pressures and responses by federal and state governments discussed in Chapter 3.

One can still argue that, in many communities, all health care is local, and that there is no dominant larger market for health care beyond the community level. This captures the facts that healthcare providers live in or near the communities in which they practice or operate hospitals and health systems, and that, for the most part, all of their patients are local. However, health systems also contract for access to patients with large health plans, whose catchment areas extend beyond the scope of any single community, including large cities, as well as sometimes crossing state borders.[3] As well, the federal government and the states, acting sometimes as payers and sometimes as purchasers, cut across local markets in their supply of services through Medicare and Medicaid.

These same health plans are then contracted by a multitude of firms (purchasers), and are increasingly contracting with state agencies (purchasers) for the right to provide care to the Medicaid population. Some firms are small, with employees who reside only locally and tend to represent a small proportion of a health plan's enrollees. Other firms may be large, and also may represent a significant proportion of a health plan's enrollees. Lastly, states are large market actors, who by entering this market with Medicaid enrollees being bid out to health plans at the lowest price (instead of acting merely as payers of Medicaid claims) have enormous market share that translates into the power to affect substantial change in the structure of local markets for health care.

Classical economics defines a perfect market as one where consumers are knowledgeable of the product or service they are purchasing and understand the cost associated with their purchase. In that sense, healthcare services existed in a perfect or near-perfect market until around the middle of the 20th century. Prior to the late 19th century and early 20th century, medical care was relatively crude, having little to offer other than attentive watching.

Developments such as understanding germ theory, the advent of anesthesia, and the development of antibiotics, vaccinations, and X-rays revolutionized medical treatment and were the advent to the development of modern medical treatment and technology. However, as medical knowledge grew, knowledge asymmetry began to develop between the medical knowledge of the physician and the patient. This knowledge asymmetry grew exponentially in the latter half of the 20th century and into the 21st century, in close correlation with the exponential growth in medical and technological knowledge. The first component of a perfect market became seriously compromised, causing the near-perfect market of the early 20th century to become an imperfect market by the mid-to-late 20th century. The growth in medical and technological advancements also correlates with an increase in the cost of care, from a nominal cost to an amount large enough to require an insurance policy to hedge against the risk of a major financial loss.

Cost of and payment for medical care were relatively transparent until approximately the mid-20th century. Prior to the advent of medical insurance, physicians frequently adjusted the cost of their services to what they deemed was appropriate for the income level of their patients. It was also not unusual for physicians and hospitals to discuss the price for medical treatment with patients and not proceed with treatment until they had possession of or were assured of payment for treatment. These practices of adjusting payment or not moving forward with treatment provided patients with an understanding of the cost of treatment and met the second condition of a perfect or near-perfect market. Following the advent of medical insurance in the early-to-mid 20th century, both the physician and the patient began to lose their direct connection, and thus, their understanding of the cost of care.

As the 20th century progressed, insurance contracting became more complex and costs were shifted from one payer to another,

---

3 A catchment area is the geographic area within which a health plan operates. It is defined by both the location of providers and enrollees.

resulting in a blurred understanding of cost by hospitals and all other providers. This lack of cost transparency has progressively been addressed, beginning in the last decades of the 20th century and continuing into the 21st century. Unfortunately, despite the work on cost transparency done thus far, cost transparency for the general public is still lacking, leaving consumers little understanding of cost. This continues to compromise the second component of near-perfect market conditions, yielding an imperfect market. In conclusion, healthcare services in the 21st century are an imperfect market.

▶ Payment

History. Prior to the Industrial Revolution, there existed no organization in the delivery of medical care or in the payment for its services. The advent of the Industrial Revolution witnessed the development of the first prepaid plans, as industries such as logging, mining, and railroads hired physicians to care for their employees. As industries continued to develop in the late 19th century, sickness funds developed to provide a disability-like payment to employees while they recovered from illness or injury. Sickness funds were sponsored by employers and unions, costing employees 1% of wages or 50 cents per month. An employee had to be certified as ill after 1 week of illness and, once certified, received a portion of wages for the 4–6 weeks of the average recovery time. In the United States, sickness funds did not pay for medical care; rather, they covered lost wages and they were only for employees. In Germany, sickness funds covered medical care and were paid for jointly by employees and employers.

Throughout this period, there was minimal government involvement in the payment for, or provision of, medical care, other than in the provision of medical care for the military. Early federal legislative action included the Bill for the Benefit of the Indigent Insane in 1854, vetoed by President Franklin Pierce (D), who deemed social services such as this should be provided by the states (**APPENDIX TABLE 10.7**). There were a number of committee actions, including the 1912 National Convention of Insurance Commissioners, that developed the first model of state laws regulating health insurance and labor actions seeking compulsory insurance, as well as a number of progressive actions seeking universal coverage that all failed secondary to the efficacy of sickness funds. The one legislative action that was passed during this period was the 1921 Sheppard–Towner Act that provided matching funds for prenatal and child care centers and was signed into law by President Woodrow Wilson (D).

Hospital insurance began at Baylor University in 1929 as an attempt to save the hospital from bankruptcy. As a creative solution to avoid bankruptcy, Baylor Hospital devised a plan where Baylor University professors could make a payment to the hospital of 50 cents per month. The hospital, in exchange for the payment, agreed to provide for the university professors' hospital care. This plan very quickly became popular with municipal employees and, ultimately, was chartered by the state of Texas as the first Blue Cross plan.[4] Physicians were not fond of insurance, claiming to be against anything that entered between the physician–patient relationship. Despite their vigorous opposition to insurance, in 1939, the first physician insurance plan was chartered in California and eventually became the first Blue Shield plan.

Over the next 20 years, federal and state activities relating to insurance and payment included a three-step process, resulting in the tax exemption for employers purchasing medical

---

4 Insurance at this time was only for the workers or employees. It was not until later in the century, when unions began negotiating benefits as part of the pay package, that family plans were included.

insurance on behalf of their employees. This process started in 1943 with the War Labor Board, which froze wages and prices but allowed the provision of non-cash wages in the form of medical insurance. Next, in 1949, the Supreme Court upheld a National Labor Board ruling that benefits could be included in labor negotiations. Finally, in 1951, employer-provided health insurance premiums were deemed a tax deduction by Congress. Other significant legislative actions include passage of the Hospital Survey and Construction Act of 1946 that provided significant financial incentives for hospital construction with the condition that the hospital provide charity care. The Fair Deal in 1949 was attempt to provide universal health insurance through the federal government but failed. In 1960, the Kerr-Mills Act provided funds to state programs providing medical care to the poor and elderly. Finally, from the provider side, in 1948, physicians launched a national campaign against health insurance, claiming that insurers were intruding between the physician–patient relationship.

The remaining 40 years of the century witnessed a marked increase in federal involvement in payment for health services, beginning in 1965 with the passage of Medicare and Medicaid. This landmark legislation marked a change in strategy, from seeking passage of a universal health plan to a more nuanced and incremental approach of providing health coverage and access to the elderly and the poor. Once this legislation passed, two sets of health-related actions consumed the remainder of the century. First was a series of bills and amendments that were successful at increasing access for "vulnerable" populations to health services through expansion of eligibility for Medicare and Medicaid. Second was a series of legislative and regulatory actions addressing the rapidly increasing (**FIGURE 10.2**) national healthcare expenditures. While the majority of these bills passed and the regulations went into effect, they were feckless, if not unsuccessful, in bringing increasing healthcare costs under control.

The 2000s have witnessed two major legislative actions focused on increasing access

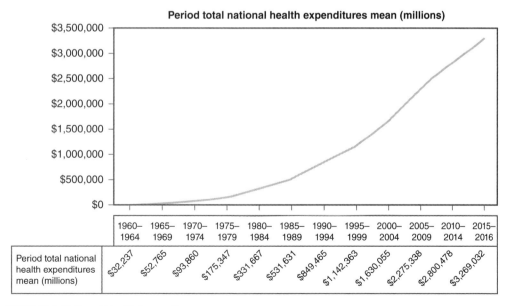

FIGURE 10.2 National Health Expenditures
Office of Actuary, at www.CMS.gov

while controlling costs. The first legislative action, in 2003, was the Medicare Prescription Drug, Improvement, and Modernization Act that subsidized the purchase of prescription drugs. Next, in 2010, the Patient Protection and Affordable Care Act (PPACA) sought to increase access and quality while "bending" the cost curve downward. Not apparent to the casual observer, a large amount of regulatory action addressing innovative payment methods began during the George W. Bush (R) administration and culminated in the Centers for Medicare and Medicaid Service (CMS) Innovation Center that was codified into law through the PPACA.

Types. The two basic methods of paying for health services are either payment prior to receiving service or payment after receiving services. Payment prior to receiving services, commonly known as prepaid plans is best known as capitation or payment to providers on a *per member per month* basis. These types of plans, also known as managed care plans, pay providers in advance to provide for the medical care of their members as the need arises. The underlying premise of these plans is to keep members healthy and avoid the cost of expensive care that comes as a result of neglecting preventive health actions. Unfortunately, since providers are allowed to keep the money they do not spend as profit, these types of plans also carry an incentive to do as little as possible to avoid incurring costs. Another type of plan similar to managed care plans is concierge plans, in which physicians contract with patients for a set dollar amount and in turn provide services 24 hours per day, 7 days per week.

The other type of payment system that pays providers after receiving services is known as fee-for-service. This payment method is commonly used in business transactions and is a central premise of the free enterprise system that rewards work based on each activity and/or resource input with additional payments. Unfortunately, this system incents volume over value and often results in over treatment and over prescribing (Brosig-Koch, Hennig-Schmidt, Kairies-Schwarz, & Wiesen, 2016; Grytten, 2017). At the extreme, this is a system ripe for fraud, as noted by the CMS's recovery of $3.3 billion in 2014 and $27.8 billion since the inception of the Health Care Fraud and Abuse Control (HCFAC) program.[5] There have been multiple attempts to control abuses of the fee-for-service payment system, which primarily include some level of bundling and range from the Prospective Payment System (1983) bundling of diagnostic-related groups to current CMS Innovation Center 30-day and 90-day readmission bundling. As stated earlier, most cost control attempts have been minimally effective.

The threat of significant financial loss is the primary reason people agree to pool their resources and purchase insurance. In prepaid plans, a significant amount of risk is held by the provider, whereas in fee-for-service plans, a significant amount of risk is held by the insurer. Most significantly, the patient (or consumer) encounters little to no risk with either of these types of payment systems. All payment reform efforts involve the shifting of risk from the payer to either the provider or patient (consumer). Payer payment reforms include bundling, quality incentives, such as pay-for-performance programs and value-based purchasing, and risk-based programs, such as Accountable Care Organizations that include fee-for-service payments with and without risk incentives based on quality and outcome measures.[6]

---

5 Retrieved from https://www.cms.gov/Newsroom/MediaReleaseDatabase/Fact-sheets/2017-Fact-Sheet-items/2017-01-18-2.html

6 This has been changing in the last few years to include quality and outcome measures for weighting by facility of those DRGs where CMS penalizes for "early" readmissions.

Patient (consumer) payment reforms include the requirements of copayments and deductibles and the establishment of health savings accounts premised on the idea that patients will avoid frivolous or expensive treatment if they bear some of the financial burden. While it seems obvious, the patient (consumer) who has no health insurance individually bears the full risk associated with payment. These individuals can be successful in reducing their financial exposure by negotiating prices with providers and, if they qualify, taking advantage of charity care programs.[7]

▶ Insurance

Insurance is a risk hedging instrument used by individuals and organizations to protect themselves from financial loss. At the heart of insurance is the concept of *indemnification*, defined as securing protection against hurt, loss, or damage. For insurance to become a profitable business, a company has to attract enough individuals not needing to file claims to offset those who do file to still make a profit. When an insurance company does not strike this balance, and has more claimants filing than resources available, they experience the phenomenon known as *adverse selection. Moral hazard* occurs when, due to lack of financial exposure or risk, an insured takes more risks than a prudent individual would. All other insurance concepts (**TABLE 10.1**) define risks or results of financial exposure associated with the insurance contract. Modern health insurance policies that provide for an array of preventive services at little to no cost to the consumer are prepaid plans and not indemnity.[8] Thus, most modern policies are hybrids

that include elements of prepaid plans (preventive care), indemnification (hospital and rehabilitation care), and patient responsibility (copays and deductibles). Insurance companies protect themselves against major loss through reinsurance policies held by reinsurance companies or insurance companies for insurance companies.

The primary cost effect of insurance is increased national cost linked to increased access to services by individuals who have minimal reason to concern themselves with the cost of care when their care is covered by a third party or insurer (moral hazard). New health insurance enrollees normally ramp up their use of services for a limited period of time before getting themselves into a state of equilibrium. Once equilibrium is reached, individuals' access to and costs of care becomes relatively flat. The National Association of Health Underwriters (2015) chronicles a number of causes associated with high cost of care and the use of insurance where individuals are essentially ignorant of the cost they are incurring (moral hazard). These causes include:

- Aging population—the link between increasing age and increasing use of health services is fairly well documented (**TABLE 10.2**)
- Pharmaceutical costs—pharmaceutical costs increased by 13.1% in 2014, accounting for a 12.2% increase in spending
- Biologicals and new technologies—imaging, biologicals, gene therapy, and precision medicine, with estimates of technological advances being responsible for 27%–48% of the increase in healthcare costs from 1960 to present
- Behavioral and lifestyle choices—up to 70% of healthcare costs are attributed to

---

7 Note that some religious groups negotiate annual prepaid plans with fixed per member per month costs and stop-loss insurance for low-frequency, high-cost acute events. These are most common in Amish and Mennonite communities.

8 Using the analogy of automobile insurance, drivers purchase collision coverage for protection or indemnification from major loss due to unanticipated damage to the car's structure. However, they do not purchase coverage for preventive maintenance (services), such as oil changes and parts replacement due to wear and age.

TABLE 10.1 Health Insurance Concepts and Consumer Protections	
Moral hazard	When an insured individual ignores risk or takes more risk due to the insurer bearing the risk liability
Adverse selection	When an insurer bears more claims from individuals than financially able to bear
Rescission	Cancellation of insurance due to unanticipated high use
Guaranteed issue	Requires insurers to underwrite a plan for anyone wishing to purchase. Depending on the state, there may be no cost limits on these plans. Goal is to prevent residents from being "uninsurable"
Guaranteed renewal	Prevents insurers from dropping individual from coverage due to recent high costs. If insurance was employer based, also protects employer if community rating laws are also in place
Community rating	State-level insurance law requiring health plans to develop plan costs for employers based on cost of insuring a representative sample of a community, rather than the insurance experience of each firm. Generally lowers costs for all, although some firms experience high costs
Exclusions for pre-existing conditions	Eliminates clauses opting insurers out from covering any or all pre-existing conditions
Coverage for specific conditions	States have passed laws mandating coverage of costs for emerging conditions, the best known being Florida's 2008 mandate requiring reimbursement for healthcare services to persons living with autism
Risk pools	The concept that a large pool of individuals will spread the risk of costly health events across the group, making it financially viable to insure all at a high level and low cost. States have tried building these, offering subsidies. To date, no state-level risk pool plan has succeeded

behavioral and lifestyle choices, with the primary negative behaviors including obesity, smoking, and illegal drug use

- System inefficiencies—these inefficiencies include:
  - Duplication of procedures and overuse of high-end procedures
  - Preventable mistakes by providers
  - Unnecessary medical treatments and prescriptions
  - Technological inefficiencies (implementation of EMRs)
  - Inconsistent focus on quality outcomes
- Medical malpractice—accounting for 7.2%–12.7% of increased costs
- Cost shifting—transferring losses from low payers to high payers
- Increased utilization—high utilization is responsible for 43% of the increase

in services directly linked to consumer demand

- Government regulations—compliance with regulations is linked to the increased administrative burden of providing health services
- Other market factors—provider and physician integration results in an additional layer of administration and, contrary to popular belief, results in an increase of 20%–40%

Through another lens, the 2015 National Healthcare Expenditures chronicles a breakdown of the 5.8% increase in healthcare expenditures, which includes the:

- *Greatest* percentage of share as
  - Private health insurance (33%),
  - Hospitals (32%),
  - Federal government (29%), and
  - Households (28%),
- *Lowest* percentage of share as
  - Other professional services (3%),
  - Home health care (3%),
  - Durable medical equipment (2%), and
  - Other nondurable medical equipment (2%),
- *Greatest* growth attributed to
  - Medicaid (9.7%) and
  - Prescription drugs (9%) and
- *Lowest* growth attributed to
  - Nursing care facilities (2.7%) and
  - Out-of-pocket (2.6%).

A final view of the high cost of health services in the United States is provided by Peterson and Burton (2007) who compared U.S. healthcare spending with that of Organization for Economic Co-operation and Development (OECD) countries and found prices correlated to the intensity of service as the primary causal factor. Squires and Anderson (2015) also compared the United States to other OECD countries and found the United States demonstrated a significantly higher use of medical technologies and had significantly higher prices. Smith, Newhouse, and Freeland (2009) estimated that since 1960, use of technology has increased healthcare expenditures from 27% to 48%. Another intriguing finding in this study is that OECD countries (including the United States) have combined health and social support spending ranging from 25% to 32% of total GDP. In all OECD countries except the United States, social support and health spending range from matching to 50% more social support than health spending, whereas in the United States health spending is 50% more than social support spending (**FIGURE 10.3**). In summary, this report demonstrates how the United States spends approximately 50% more as a percentage of GDP than the average OECD country and spends more on high-end care, with higher prices and high quality scores for complex care such as cancer care, while spending up to 50% less than other OECD countries on social support, primary care, and other less complex health services.

The United States faces a number of challenges going into the 21th century with regard to how to continue to provide some of the best care in the world, increase social support services, increase primary care access, and bring cost into line with similar countries. Gaining success in these areas will be at the heart of health policy debates as the two major political parties representing opposing political philosophies seek to reconcile differences and agree to a comprehensive national health policy that ensures access for all while protecting individual rights and freedoms.

▶ Healthcare Workforce

The healthcare workforce consists of three categories of workers: providers, such as physicians or surgeons who diagnose and establish treatment plans or provide high level technical treatment, such as surgery; allied health professionals, such as nurses, therapists, and technicians who carry out and support treatment plans; and nonclinical support staff, such as managers and leaders, finance, and human

TABLE 10.2 Personal Healthcare Expenditures by Age and Gender

Total Personal Health care Spending by Gender and Age Group, Calendar Years 2002, 2004, 2006, 2008, 2010, 201?

Level (in millions), Distribution (percent), and Average Annual Growth (percent)

| Age Group | Levels | | | | | |
	2002	2004	2006	2008	2010	2012
Total	1,367,612	1,588,153	1,805,056	2,013,936	2,194,077	2,371,800
0–18	156,125	186,052	214,559	238,569	259,094	276,833
19–44	299,383	344,534	384,824	420,420	450,250	489,229
45–64	434,621	513,205	597,186	666,656	735,032	787,562
65–84	375,141	425,859	470,870	528,985	573,099	627,978
Males	587,848	684,779	781,898	877,799	962,089	1,047,156
0–18	82,715	98,895	113,509	126,207	137,296	147,344
19–44	113,824	130,111	144,747	157,435	169,828	185,203
45–64	200,721	236,512	277,027	311,301	343,505	371,529
65–84	163,241	186,885	208,092	236,102	258,596	284,326
85+	27,347	32,376	38,523	46,754	52,864	58,755
Females	779,764	903,374	1,023,157	1,136,136	1,231,989	1,324,644
0–18	73,410	87,157	101,049	112,362	121,798	129,490
19–44	185,559	214,423	240,077	262,985	280,422	304,026
45–64	233,899	276,693	320,159	355,356	391,526	416,033
65–84	211,900	238,974	262,777	292,882	314,503	343,653
85+	74,996	86,126	99,095	112,551	123,740	131,443

Distribution (%)						Average Annual Growth (%)					
2002	2004	2006	2008	2010	2012	2002–2004	2004–2006	2006–2008	2008–2010	2010–2012	2002–2012
100.0	100.0	100.0	100.0	100.0	100.0	7.8	6.6	5.6	4.4	4.0	5.7
11.4	11.7	11.9	11.8	11.8	11.7	9.2	7.4	5.4	4.2	3.4	5.9
21.9	21.7	21.3	20.9	20.5	20.6	7.3	5.7	4.5	3.5	4.2	5.0
31.8	32.3	33.1	33.1	33.5	33.2	8.7	7.9	5.7	5.0	3.5	6.1
27.4	26.8	26.1	26.3	26.1	26.5	6.5	5.2	6.0	4.1	4.7	5.3
43.0	43.1	43.3	43.6	43.8	44.2	7.9	6.9	6.0	4.7	4.3	5.9
6.0	6.2	6.3	6.3	6.3	6.2	9.3	7.1	5.4	4.3	3.6	5.9
8.3	8.2	8.0	7.8	7.7	7.8	6.9	5.5	4.3	3.9	4.4	5.0
14.7	14.9	15.3	15.5	15.7	15.7	8.5	8.2	6.0	5.0	4.0	6.4
11.9	11.8	11.5	11.7	11.8	12.0	7.0	5.5	6.5	4.7	4.9	5.7
2.0	2.0	2.1	2.3	2.4	2.5	8.8	9.1	10.2	6.3	5.4	7.9
57.0	56.9	56.7	56.4	56.2	55.8	7.6	6.4	5.4	4.1	3.7	5.4
5.4	5.5	5.6	5.6	5.6	5.5	9.0	7.7	5.4	4.1	3.1	5.8
13.6	13.5	13.3	13.1	12.8	12.8	7.5	5.8	4.7	3.3	4.1	5.1
17.1	17.4	17.7	17.6	17.8	17.5	8.8	7.6	5.4	5.0	3.1	5.9
15.5	15.0	14.6	14.5	14.3	14.5	6.2	4.9	5.6	3.6	4.5	5.0
5.5	5.4	5.5	5.6	5.6	5.5	7.2	7.3	6.6	4.9	3.1	5.8

Centers for Medicare and Medicaid Services, Office of the Actuary, National health Statistics Group.

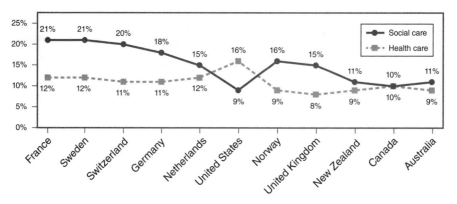

FIGURE 10.3 Health and Social Care Spending as a Percentage of GDP

Data from Bradley, E. H., & Taylor, L. A. (2013). The American health care paradox: Why spending more is getting us less. *Public Affairs*.

resources. Historically, physicians and surgeons have been around since the beginning of civilization, with their training ranging from unstructured apprenticeships to organized formal training. Nursing has followed a similar path, first with untrained families providing nursing care for ill family members, then progressing to a more organized process through religious orders, and finally becoming organized, as originally modeled by Florence Nightingale. Physician and nursing training currently is very organized, professional, and delivered through universities. Administrative support for care delivery was initially provided by religious orders and other groups organizing care, such as early hospitals. The education for nonclinical workers supporting care delivery ranges from high school for entry-level workers to graduate and professional training for leaders. The variety of workers necessary to provide care in the current era is broad, expanding, and considered a growth area in the current economy. A listing of healthcare careers is maintained by the U.S. Bureau of Labor Statistics (BLS) (**FIGURE 10.4**) and includes career description, entry level education, and median

pay (see https://www.bls.gov/ooh/healthcare/home.htm for the most current information).

▶ Physicians[9]

Agency

The need for agency arises when one individual holds information or knowledge that another individual needs or seeks. In health care, physicians act as *agents* for their patients (*principals*) who seek their knowledge and information. Physicians become agents due to their medical school and postgraduate training where they gain an inordinate amount of medical knowledge, even far surpassing the medical knowledge of allied health professionals. It is this inordinate, asymmetrical amount of knowledge that causes patients (principals) to seek advice and skills when encountering medical problems. One unique aspect of physician agency is the physician's role as both producer and provider of medical services. As a result of a physician's position as a holder of asymmetric knowledge, producer, and provider of medical services, the physician can respond as

9 Limited license physicians include any professional who can be addressed "physician" and is not an MD or DO such as podiatrists and dentists. These professionals face similar agency, payment, business models, barriers, and licensure phenomenon as MDs and DOs.

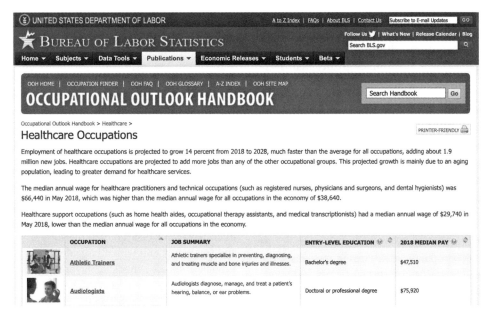

FIGURE 10.4 BLS Healthcare Occupations
U.S. Bureau of Labor Statistics.

an agent of personal economic self-interest or as a patient-focused moral agent. As a moral agent, the physician acts in the patient's best interest despite the economic consequences of the directed plan of care.

Payment

While moral agency is the position most physicians seek to maintain, economic self-interest does play a part in their diagnostic and treatment decisions. Physicians are paid through a fee-for-service model where they are paid for the amount of work they perform, or through a capitation model where they are paid a predetermined amount per month to keep patients healthy, regardless of the number or types of services provided. The incentives associated with fee-for-service are to do more and thus, earn more money, whereas the incentives associated with capitation are to do less and thus, keep more money. The impact of these incentives on physician decision-making were tested by Brosig-Koch, Hennig-Schmidt, Kairies-Schwarz,

and Wiesen (2016) who chronicled the work of other scholars and tested physician responses to ordering incentives in lab and practice settings. When given the same patient scenarios, practicing physicians, residents, and medical students all ordered (statistically) significantly more tests under fee-for-service payment than under capitation. The historical trend in physician payment evolution finds physicians maximizing their economic potential and payers progressively seeking to impose risk and accountability on them in return for payment.

Physicians are generally well paid, with their incomes on the low end putting them in the top quintile of income earners (2015 quintile mean $202,366) and many, especially specialists, in the top 5% of income earners (2015 quintile mean $350,870) (Brookings Institute, 2017). Another way to understand their income is comparing their earnings as a ratio to the average wage of workers, with primary care physicians earning 3.5 times greater than average wage earners and specialists earnings five times greater than average wage earners.

While those numbers may seem high, they are comparable to similar Western European OECD countries, with the mean for primary care physicians at 3.3 times greater than average wage earners and specialists at 5.2 times greater than average wage earners (Fujisawa & Lafortune, 2008).

Another factor that could potentially influence physician payment is physician density or number of physicians per population. Related to this is the economic relationship of low density or scarcity with higher price. The United States has 1.0 primary care physicians per 1000 population, as compared to the OECD mean of 0.8 primary care physicians per 1000 population. Regarding specialists, the United States has 1.0 specialists per 1000 population, as compared to the OECD mean of 1.4 specialists per 1000 population (Fujisawa & Lafortune, 2008). Other factors that influence physician pay include hours worked, with primary care physicians and specialists both working 50–60 hours per week. Gatekeeping functions are significant for primary care physicians. Finally, payment types with mixed methods and fee-for-service payment positively affect their pay.

Business Model

Economics of payment and practice administration have driven the evolution of physician practice models. The general evolution of physician practice models, from solo practices to private group practices to health system group practices, closely correlates with the evolution of increased requirements for receiving payment, complexity, managerial sophistication, and economies of scale necessary to meet the payment requirements. These evolutionary changes in physician practice have transformed physician office visits from a counselor, transformational type of visit, to a transactional business encounter focused on productivity.

Barriers to Entry

This increased need for sophistication in practice management is a barrier to entry for new physicians who, in a previous time, sought to set up a practice and now find themselves looking for a job. Other barriers to entry physicians encounter begin with the preparation that minimally includes earning a bachelor degree while maintaining a high grade point average and can include earning a graduate degree, entry into medical school that includes preparation for and successfully taking the Medical School Admissions Test and the added cost of interview travel, delayed earnings for 4–7 years, and frequently end with a large debt of around $250,000. Finally, medical malpractice or liability insurance is a cost barrier that generally ranges from $4000 to $40,000 per year and can run as high as $200,000 depending on specialty and location. Mello, Chandra, Gawande, and Studdert (2010) calculated the national cost of medical liability as $55.64 billion, or 2.4% of total national medical costs. These scholars came to this figure through the use of MEPS data that they segmented into four categories: (1) indemnity payments, $5.72 billion or 10.3%; (2) administrative expenses, $4.13 billion or 7.4%; (3) defensive medicine, $45.59 billion or 81.9%, (a) hospital defensive medicine, 38.8% or 69.7% and (b) physician, $6.8 billion or 12.2%; and (4) other, 0.20 billion or 0.4%.

Licensure

From an economic lens, licensure is a regulatory tool used by states to control entry into an occupation to individuals who have met a basic set of educational and professional requirements and thus ensure a basic level of quality. Physicians move through a series of licensing exams as they progress through medical or osteopathic training and residency. If a physician decides to relocate to another state, 45 states provide either licensure reciprocity or endorsement, and only 5 provide neither.

▶ Allied Health Professionals

The Bureau of Labor Statistics (BLS) 2016 data indicates there are a total of 11,918,100 healthcare professionals in the United States, with 11,209,800 (94%) being non-physicians or allied health professionals. This is a group of dedicated individuals whose education ranges from secondary to professional doctorate degrees and who in some way interact with physician-directed care. At the lower end, these individuals include various aides and assistants who have educational requirements ranging from high school diplomas to postsecondary non-degree training and whose median annual wage is $25,250. The next group consists of registered nurses and other technical occupations, such as dieticians and radiology technicians, whose educational requirements range from associate's to bachelor's degrees and who earn a median annual wage of $63,420. Finally, there is a group of limited license physicians, such as podiatrists, and an array of clinical providers-professionals, such as physician assistants and advance practice nurses, whose education ranges from master to professional doctorate and who earn a median annual income of $117,503. These individuals are vital to supporting the U.S. health system, with many of them being specialists who operate our technologically sophisticated diagnostic equipment and associated treatment regimes. Registered nurses are the largest allied health group, constituting 23.1% of total healthcare professionals. When registered nurses are coupled with advance practice nurses, LPN/LVNs, nursing assistants, and medical assistants to form a larger group of nursing care providers, they constitute 48.5% of all healthcare professionals. The remaining 45.6% of allied healthcare professionals are primarily technical professionals, such as radiology technicians and physical therapists. Most allied health professionals require either a professional certification or a license. While the BLS considers health professions a growth area with a forecasted 2014–2024 growth rate of 19%, many in these fields find earning educational degrees a barrier to entry, due to lack of capacity by certification and degree programs.

Health policy supports the allied health professionals through the financial support of research that results in the medical technologies they support and through educational financial aid. All allied health professionals are paid by the providers or organizations they support at a minimum of 10%–20% above the mean national income, giving them solid middle-class incomes, with some of these professionals at the top of their clinical specialty or providing independent care earning in the six-figure range.

▶ Provider Organizations

Provider organizations are all organizations that provide healthcare services and minimally include hospitals, ambulatory and outpatient care centers, physician offices, and long-term care centers. Healthcare policy has incented the building of these organizations and systems through the development of payment systems.[10] The first incentive was when health insurance premiums became deductible in 1951, thus encouraging employers to provide employees with health insurance. Cost-plus fee-for-service payment incented hospitals to expand service since they could pass along the cost of their expansion to the payers. Next, this model was expanded with the passage of Medicare in 1965, adding a new source of income to providers.

The first substantial attempt to control costs was the enactment of the Prospective Payment System for Medicare that forced

---

10   With the exception of the Hill-Burton Act that supported the building of hospitals throughout the country.

hospitals to examine how they were organized and added a new utilization review role. This payment model was founded on the idea of regular, predictable pricing based on historic costs, resulting in the bundling of payment for diagnoses. During the 1990s, provider organizations faced two payment changes that affected their organization. First was the call for improved quality of care and incentives, although limited, that resulted in the addition of staff to monitor and track quality initiatives. Next was the burst of managed care onto the payment world that fueled vertical and horizontal health system integration, including the development of insurance companies owned by health systems. Over the first decade of the 2000s, system integration continued, although at a slower pace. These integrations were primarily for economies of scale, access to capital, and ensuring a larger patient base for admissions and referrals. The PPACA (2010) and Medicare Access and CHIP Reauthorization Act (2015) are the most recent policy and payment changes that have fueled further provider reorganization with a sharp uptick in vertical and horizontal integration. These integration activities include joint ventures and mergers of hospitals with health systems, purchase of physician practices,[11] and systems integrating with systems. Over the past 50 years, hospitals and other providers have continually added staff as a result of the increasing complexity of their systems due to multiple, and sometimes conflicting, regulatory requirements.

▶ Technology and Pharmaceuticals

The federal government has supported technological and pharmaceutical research and development by awarding grants to research labs and through basic scientific research performed by the National Institutes of Health (NIH). The NIH's roots go back to a single lab established in 1887 and expanded significantly through the Public Service Act of 1944, and then again through almost every subsequent decade. Once the basic research is completed, commercial firms take these results and develop them into commercial medical products generally categorized as durable medical equipment, pharmaceuticals, imaging equipment, surgical equipment, and other apparatus. The federal government gets involved with these products through actions of the Food and Drug Administration that certifies durable medical equipment and pharmaceuticals are safe for use in humans. The length of development time and cost associated with developing a new product, including the six research testing stages,[12] add considerable cost to product development, reaching the billions of dollars. Commercial firms producing new technical apparatus provide access to them through providers and negotiate prices with both providers and insurance companies. Due to the structure of the current payment system, consumers often are not aware of prices that are passed along to them through their third-party payer. As a result, consumers often do not recognize how high costs are due to defrayal or absorption of the cost by their health insurance.

Smith, Newhouse, and Freeland (2009) estimate that medical technology explains 27%–48% of healthcare spending growth since 1960. When this estimate is coupled with the highest density of technological products such as advanced imaging (CT, MRI, PET scanners), laparoscopic and robotic surgical devices, and advanced pharmaceuticals, we see the major sources that drive the intensity of services delivered in the United States.

---

11 Up from 25% of physicians in integrated systems pre-ACA to greater than 50% post-ACA.

12 *Preclinical* testing on non-humans for efficacy, toxicity, and pharmacokinetics, *Phase 0* testing on humans in very small trials for drug half-life and oral bioavailability, *Phase 1* testing on humans for dosing ranges, *Phase 2* testing on humans for efficacy and side effects, *Phase 3* testing on humans for efficacy and safety, and *Phase 4* post marketing surveillance.

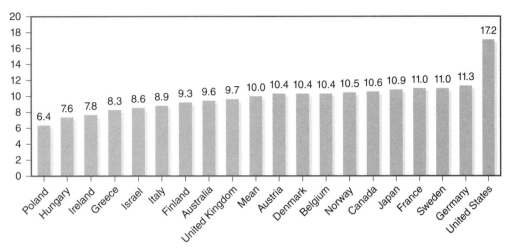

Note: None of these values have changed by more than 0.5 percentage points over the past 5 years

FIGURE 10.5 2016 Healthcare Expenditures as Percentage of GDP-Selected OECD Countries
OECD.

It is the intensity of services that drives our higher prices and is a major reason for healthcare costs per GDP being two to three times higher than any of our peer OECD countries (**FIGURE 10.5** and **TABLE 10.3**) (Peterson & Burton, 2007).

▶ Demographics and Cost

The demographics of age and gender are closely correlated with the cost of healthcare services (**FIGURES 10.6** and **10.7**). Both males and females begin life with high cost at birth that quickly and dramatically drops to minimal. A slight upward cost trend begins in the pre-teen to teen years, with males costing slightly more than females. Throughout the childbearing years, females have a significantly higher cost of healthcare services than males, with the largest gap occurring around 30 years age. From 30 to 45 years age, the cost of healthcare services for women plateaus while remaining higher than the cost of healthcare services for men, whose cost of care continues its own upward escalation. From 60 to 90 years age, the cost of healthcare services for both men and women continues to escalate at

a similar rate, with the rate for men exceeding women and increasing at a slightly faster rate. At 90 years age, the cost of healthcare services for women plateaus for 5 years, then begins to decline, whereas the cost for men continues to increase through age 95 years before plateauing.

When considering the projected present value of future healthcare costs for retirees, the cost of healthcare services is considerably higher for those who retire early (**TABLES 10.4** and **10.5**). The projected present value of healthcare costs for an individual who retires at 55 years age and lives for 20 years to 75 years of age is nine times higher than an individual who retires at 70 years of age and lives 5–75 years of age. This same comparison holds when the projected present value of healthcare costs for a 55-year-old retiree and a 70-year-old retiree are compared at 20 years post retirement, with the 55-year-old's projected cost 1.4 times higher than the 70-year-old's projected cost. It takes the 70-year-old retiree 25 years (90 years of age) to equal the projected present value costs of the 55-year-old retiree in 20 years (75 years of age). At 90 years of age, the projected present value costs of the 55-year-old retiree are three times higher

TABLE 10.3 Selected OECD Health Funding and Expenditure Characteristics

Country	Primary Insurance Type	Funding	Private Insurance	HC as % GDP 2000	HC as % GDP 2010	HC as % GDP 2015
Denmark	National Health System	Income tax	37% Complimentary	8.7	11.1	10.6
England	National Health System	General tax	11% Supplemental	6.9	9.5	9.8
Italy	National Health System	Corporate, VAT, general and regional taxes	7% Complimentary	7.9	9.4	9.1
New Zealand	National Health System	General taxes	35% Complimentary	7.5	11.2	9.4
Norway	National Health System	General taxes	7% Complimentary	8.3	9.3	9.9
Sweden	National Health System	General taxes	5% Complimentary	8.2	9.5	11.1
Australia	National Health Insurance	General revenue & income taxes	48% Complimentary	8.1	9.0	9.3
Canada	National Health Insurance	General tax (provincial & federal)	67% Complimentary	8.7	11.2	10.1
Israel	National Health Insurance	General taxes	Several plans	7.1	7.4	7.8
Japan	Statutory Health Insurance	General taxes and insurance	70% Cover cost-sharing	7.5	9.6	11.2
France	Statutory Health Insurance	Payroll and general revenue taxes	90% Complimentary (government vouchers)	9.8	11.2	11.0
Germany	Statutory Health Insurance	Payroll and general revenue taxes	11% Complimentary and cover cost-sharing	10.1	11.3	11.1

Netherland	Statutory Health Insurance	Payroll and general revenue taxes	84% Complimentary	7.4	10.5	10.8
Singapore	Statutory Health Insurance	General taxes	Several plans	2.7	4.0	4.9
Switzerland	Statutory Health Insurance	General taxes	Several plans	9.9	11.1	11.5
United States	Statutory Health Insurance, National Health Insurance, National Health System	Payroll and general revenue taxes	56% Private insurance	13.7	17.0	16.9

Commonwealth Fund (2016).

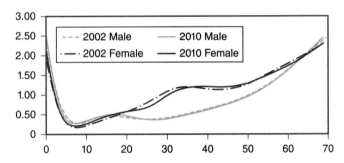

FIGURE 10.6 Aggregate Commercial Costs by Age, 2002 and 2010

Reproduced with permission from Yamamoto, D. H. (2013). *Health care costs—From birth to death*. Sponsored by Society of Actuaries, Part of the Health Care Cost Institute's Independent Report Series—Report 2013-1.

than the projected present value costs of the 70-year-old retiree. When this same comparison is made for the 55-year-old and 70-year-old using Medicare costs, both total dollar amounts are 60% higher, with the projected costs for the 55-year-old retiree continuing to be three times the projected costs for the 70-year-old retiree.

Medicare claims data from 1976 to 2006 analyzed by scholars consistently found payments for the last year of life ranging from 25% to 30% of lifetime medical expenditures, with the last 60 days of life responsible for 52% of the last year's cost (Lubitz & Riley,

1993; Hogan, Lunney, Gabel, & Lynn, 2001; Riley & Lubitz, 2010). Aldridge and Kelley (2015) posit that, while this claim to high end-of-life Medicare spending is true, the alarm drawn by it is out of context. These two authors first find that any analysis of high spending is incomplete due to the lack of a national data repository of all claims. Despite the incompleteness of the data set, they compiled a data set from the Medical Expenditure Panel Survey (MEPS) and the Health and Retirement Survey data. Next, they analyzed spending of the highest 5% of annual health spenders. Their analysis segmented

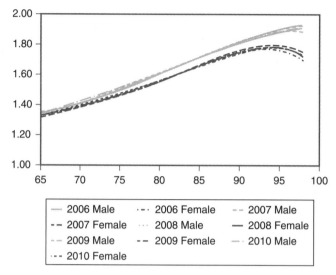

FIGURE 10.7 Medicare Allowed Charge by Age, 2006 Through 2010

Reproduced with permission from Yamamoto, D. H. (2013). *Health care costs—From birth to death*. Sponsored by Society of Actuaries, Part of the Health Care Cost Institute's Independent Report Series—Report 2013-1.

TABLE 10.4 The Present Value of Future Expected Healthcare Costs in Not Paid by Medicare

Retirement Age	75	80	Life Expectancy 85
55	$206,200	$276,300	$37,240
60	$123,400	$176,500	$24,930
65	$50,900	$91,200	$14,640

Office of Actuary, at www.CMS.gov

these spenders into three groups: (1) 49% of the total were individuals with a discrete, short-term but expensive medical event; (2) 40% of the total were individuals with persistently high cost due to chronic illness; and (3) 11% of the total was end-of-life spending. Further analysis of the end-of-life spending cohort found 80% were in the high-spending group, with the remaining 20% opting for less expensive care.

As medical care has technologically advanced, we have seen death from chronic illnesses that were rare 100 years ago. Individuals become more expensive to care for due to the prevalence and course of chronic disease(s). The high cost of end-of-life care is at least in part correlated with the hospitalization of end-of-life care. These scholars (Aldridge & Kelley, 2015) found that 63% of the end-of-life population were hospitalized in their last year of life,

TABLE 10.5 Projected Medicare Costs for Single Retiree in 2013

Retirement Age			Life Expectancy		
	75	80	85	90	95
55	$130,100	$250,700	$433,900	$705,400	$1,092,900
60	$61,000	$153,800	$292,700	$498,500	$792,200
65	–	$72,600	$178,600	$334,500	$557,100
70	–	–	$83,700	$202,600	$371,300

Office of Actuary, at www.CMS.gov

with 27% having several hospitalizations (25% increase since 1978) and 33% being admitted to an intensive care unit (22% increase since 1980). Only recently have changes in Medicare policy been enacted to encourage palliative and hospice care in the final months of life over prolonged inpatient stays. The CMS finds that hospice admissions have doubled since 1998 and the average length of stay has increased from 48 days in 1998 to 73 days in 2009, or a 52% increase.

The continual frenzy over Medicare solvency is due to people living 10–12 years longer than when Medicare was enacted, the increased size of this population, and the increased cost of care due to medical advancements since 1965. Besides the cost control policies already discussed earlier, Medicare's two most significant changes have occurred as a result of the Medicare Modernization Act (MMA) of 2004 that provided for prescription drug coverage, a private HMO option, and the Affordable Care Act's closure of the MMA prescription drug donut hole.

Finally, one-third of end-of-life cost covered by both Medicare and Medicaid is for long-term care that occurs in a variety of venues, including both institutional and home care. Depending on the provider, the annual cost of long-term institutional care ranges from $30,000 to $80,000 per year. Unless the family is of substantial financial means, most people requiring institutional care end up on Medicaid during their last months of life.

The most recent attempt to address the high cost of long-term care was the Community Living Assistance Services and Supports (CLASS) Act in the PPACA that was repealed. A required review (contained in administrative rules drafted after passage) by CMS actuaries of the structure of long-term care insurance in the Act determined they would not be able to price the services within the limits of the law. The minimum PPACA premium requirement was $5 per month for those below the poverty line. An additional actuarial requirement reported under the same review was the need for a 75-year actuarially sound program with a $50 per day room charge. The PPACA original premium estimate was $65 per month, while CMS actuaries calculated a premium of $110 per month at $50 per day and $160 per month at $75 per day that closely aligned with CBO's estimate of $123 per month. One final requirement was that individuals could be fully vested after 5 years. Concerns from the actuaries focused on the unsustainability of the program over time due to adverse selection (there was no individual mandate for this insurance) and the inability to meet a sustainable premium under PPACA requirements. These actuarial concerns caused the Obama administration to deem the Act unworkable in October of 2013 and support its repeal on January 1, 2013.

▶ Behavioral Economics

Neoclassical economics, what most people think of when hearing the term economics, is based on the model of a rational man making all decisions based on logical and rational criteria. Behavioral economists find this approach is ideal, rather intriguing, and appealing. After all, does anyone like to think they are not a rational decision maker? The unfortunate truth is that we all are prone to failings and inaccuracies in our information, most notably the unrealistic failure to recognize the nonrational and emotional aspects of decision-making.

In an effort to differentiate between these two approaches, we need to compare and contrast their assumptions (**TABLE 10.6**). As noted earlier, neoclassical economics treats every decision as if it were *rational*, or thought through thoroughly with all positive and negative consequences considered. However, even neoclassical economists recognize this approach as idealistic, as acknowledged by Milton Friedman (with Savage) in an influential paper they published in 1948 in which they argued it was sufficient for people to act "as if" they were rational and obeying the neoclassical assumptions. In contrast, behavioral economics acknowledges that people are not always rational and builds upon other *nonrational and emotional* aspects of decision-making.

Neoclassical economics contends that people understand their *preferences* and in doing so, seek to maximize that *utility* or happiness, whereas behavioral economics contends that if there are preferences, they are built upon *experiences* and not utility. *Complete or full information* prior to decision-making is another neoclassical assumption that without discussion lacks face value. The contrasting behavioral economic assumption is the *lack of complete information* in decision-making. The concept of lack of complete information falls

TABLE 10.6 Neoclassical and Behavioral Economic Assumptions	
Neoclassical Economic Assumptions	**Behavioral Economic Assumptions**
■ Everyone is *rational*	■ Everyone is NOT *rational*
■ Known *preferences*	■ No *preference* utility function rather *experience*
■ *Full information*	■ Incomplete *information*
■ Preferences and decisions *path independent*	■ Preferences and decisions *path dependent*
■ *Mistakes random* NOT systematic	■ *Mistakes systematic* NOT random

Modified from Hough, D. E. (2013). *Irrationality in health care: What behavioral economics reveals about what we do and why*. Stanford, CA: Stanford University Press.

within the realm of Herbert Simon's work on decision-making and the concept of *bounded rationality*, or the idea of there being a limit to how much information even the brightest of us can rationally consider when making a decision. Simon is also responsible for the term *satisficing*, or having or knowing when you have enough information to make a decision. *Path independence* is another neoclassical assumption that contends all preferences and decisions are isolated, independent events not influenced by context or circumstance. In contrast, behavioral economics assumes the exact opposite contending that *preferences and decisions are dependent* upon and influenced by their context and circumstances. Finally, neoclassical economics contends that *mistakes are random* and not systematic events, thus implying no patterns or causative preemptive elements to mistakes. Behavioral economics again contends the exact opposite, that *mistakes are systematic* and not random. The systematic assumption of mistakes aligns with current management and quality improvement theory that interprets individual and organizational behavior through a systems lens. System errors are frequently rooted in efforts by management to control behaviors and outcomes.

Behavioral Economics Axioms

There are at least 10 axioms that provide insight into how behavioral economics is demonstrated in decision-making and opinion development (Table 10.7). *Loss aversion yielding an endowment* effect carries with it the idea of taking for granted something you currently possess or will possess in the future until this possession is challenged with either a revision (that could be positive) or revocation. Once this possession is challenged, it suddenly becomes something that has been endowed to the owner. The phenomenon here is one of valuing a current possession over the uncertainty of a future possession. A good example of this is the public opinion of the PPACA. While the public opinion of the PPACA has been relatively steady with the favorable and unfavorable opinion around 40% for either opinion with a delta ranging from 0% to 11% points, the unfavorable opinion was higher from January 2011 to January 2017. This positive public opinion trajectory is easily seen in **FIGURE 10.8** that graphs the deltas between the two opinions. When the Republicans took control of both chambers of Congress and the presidency, the opinion began to shift, and from January 2017 to October 2017 has grown

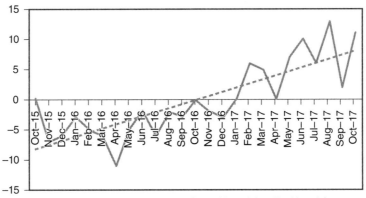

Notes: Negative delta equates to unfavorable opinion. Positive delta equates to favorable opinion.

FIGURE 10.8 PPACA Favorable/Unfavorable Delta

Kaiser Family Foundation.

steadily in favor of the PPACA. This shift in public opinion is correlated with the potential repeal of the PPACA with PPACA favorability increasing as Congress gets closer to passing repeal legislation.

Framing and anchoring is another behavioral economics axiom that revolves around decision-making based on how the information is presented. The classic example of this is provided by Johnson, Hershey, Meszaros, and Kunreuther (1993), who describe how consumers view insurance rebates more favorably than deductibles. When an insurance company prices a policy, consumers are more willing to pay a little more and receive a rebate for "positive" behaviors than pay a lower premium price plus a deductible that they view as a segregated loss of (1) the cost of accumulated insurance premiums and (2) additional out-of-pocket deductible costs. In this example, the rebate is framed as a positive gain that is anchored against the insurance premium, whereas the deductible is framed as a segregated loss anchored against a lower premium.

Projection bias and hyperbolic discounting are phenomena associated with how people view the future. Neoclassical economics posit that people's views of the future accommodate an exponential, declining performance over time similar to the phenomenon of entropy that describes a gradual, proportional, or time consistent, decline of function. Hyperbolic discounting is time inconsistent including the project bias that causes a quicker, steeper time discount that levels off quicker. From a health lens, hyperbolic discounting and projection bias can be described by an individual's rationale for engaging in any unhealthy behavior. If an individual engaging in an unhealthy behavior viewed the effects of the behavior through a lens of exponential discounting, the individual would recognize how the behavior would result in a gradual, time consistent loss of function. However, if the unhealthy behavior is viewed through the lens of hyperbolic discounting, a quicker, time inconsistent loss of function would be recognized, followed by

a very gradual decrease, almost plateauing, of function.

Hot and cold decision-making can otherwise be framed as emotional and rational decision-making. Hot decisions are characterized as decisions made in emotional haste, whereas cold decisions are made following collective deliberation. Healthcare leaders frequently encounter these phenomena with end-of-life decisions. Cold decisions occur when individuals with chronic or terminal illnesses have rational discussions with their physician(s) regarding the circumstances of their impending death and how they would like those circumstances handled. This discussion often results in the completion of advance directives that clearly delineate the end-of-life wishes of the individual. Hot decisions occur when end-of-life circumstances occur the individual or family member(s) reverse prior cold decisions in the panic of impending death.

Choice overload occurs when people are given more choices than are cognitively meaningful to them. This axiom takes on the ideas from bounded rationality, developed by Herbert Simon, and embraces the concept of there being a limit to the amount of information any individual can process in a meaningful way. Choice overload is present throughout healthcare decision-making, ranging from a physician seeking to engage a patient in plan of care and providing multiple treatment choices without a recommended path to offering individuals multiple insurance plans to choose from. When choice overload results in an individual having trouble making a final decision, we hire agents such as physicians to help make sense of multiple options and make recommendations for the options that make most sense for us.

System 1 and system 2 thinking are opposite ways of addressing decision-making, with neither approach being the only way to make decisions; rather, they are two methods of decision-making that are appropriate at different times for different circumstances. System 1 thinking occurs in an effortless manner that is normally associated with some type of rules and easy to define criteria. In decision-making theory, system 1 thinking leads to programmed decisions, often with algorithms, decision trees, and if–then statements. System 2 thinking is more deliberative and slower, taking into consideration an array of circumstances and possibilities. Each of these types of thinking have a potential for abuse and misuse. For example, physicians working under a rigid productivity model can make incorrect diagnoses as a result of system 1 thinking when a more deliberate system 2 approach, while slower and not rewarded by the productivity model, would allow the physician time to process the information and correctly diagnosis a patient's problem.

Action bias is a phenomenon when watchful waiting is overruled by a need for some type of action. A frequently cited example of action bias occurs when individuals present to their physician with a viral infection that is best treated by watchful waiting and demand an antibiotic that will do nothing to treat the problem and may lead to additional future problems associated with antibiotic resistance. Action bias can also be associated with the intensity of services when diagnostics tests are performed without a strong clinical need and frequent negative or inconclusive results.

Hedonic and decision efficiency are opposite approaches to coupling payment with purchase decisions. A few terms that need defined prior to engaging in the differences of these two approaches are vividness, salience, coupling, and decoupling. *Vividness* is associated with how well an object or thought presents itself. Often times, text describing an object or thought that is rather bland becomes vivid when the text is transformed into a graphic. *Salience* is associated with prominence, outstanding, or notable an object or thought presents itself. The differences between these two are important to distinguish, with vividness associated with what an object or thought represents and salience associated with why an object or thought exists. *Coupling* occurs when a price or payment is directly associated

with a purchase. *Decoupling* occurs when a price or payment is not directly associated with a purchase. *Decision efficiency* is a neoclassical concept and occurs when price or payment are tightly linked or coupled with a purchase and when system 1 thinking overpowers system 2 thinking. *Hedonic efficiency* is a behavioral concept and occurs when price or payment are not linked or decoupled with a purchase and when system 2 thinking overpowers system 1 thinking.

The importance of these concepts is evident in how consumers pay for and use healthcare services. In all healthcare systems, access to healthcare services is linked to payment for those services. When a third party pays the premium on an insurance policy and pays for the consumption of healthcare services, the payment for those services has been decoupled from the purchase, with the consumer often stating that their healthcare services are free. The greatest concern with this attitude is moral hazard when the consumer indiscriminately uses or overuses healthcare without regard to cost or payment. A 1974 Rand study demonstrated that even a slight coupling of payment such as a modest copay causes consumers to be more judicious in their use of healthcare services.

Heuristics and bounded rationality are decision-making concepts about the use of limited information in decision-making. Heuristics are by definition a path to follow, surface when decisions need to be made rapidly and in quick succession, and are often referred to as decision-making shortcuts. Bounded rationality is a concept developed by Herbert Simon and is associated with the cognitive limits individuals have on the amount of information we can process in the decision-making process, recognizing that no one will ever have or be able to consider all information relative to any given decision. These concepts are closely associated with system 1 and system 2 thinking. Heuristics are often a by-product of system 1 thinking and are frequently used by professionals who have to make rapid decisions with limited information. As noted earlier, caution should be deployed when using this type of decision-making process to ensure that enough information has been gathered to avoid making erroneous decisions. The question of how much information is enough is closely associated with bounded rationality. Decision makers need enough information to make sound judgments and, depending on the circumstances, may have the opportunity of deliberating over the information in a system 2 thinking style before coming to a deliberate, sound decision.

Getting to zero is an illusionary and complex concept of how consumers react to and value product and service pricing. Everyone loves a bargain; in fact, studies on how consumers react to product or service pricing demonstrate that the lower the price, the greater the perceived bargain, and ultimately the greater the number of purchases as the price nears or reaches zero. As intuitive as this concept seems, it has two underlying problems: (1) over purchase or overuse—the insurance equivalent of moral hazard—and (2) a perceived loss of value. The overuse or moral hazard problem is a result of price being decoupled from the product or service. When there is no price associated with a service, there is no incentive to hold back on its purchase or use. Concomitantly, a price of zero frequently correlates with a value of zero. Even when a purchaser knows a product or service is of high quality, the purchaser questions the value of the product or service with questions such as, "What am I not getting that I would normally get with a full priced product or service?"

A classic example of this concept is illustrated by the 1974 Rand Insurance experiment. In this experiment, Rand researchers enrolled 7700 people over six sites, randomly assigning them to 14 different fee-for-service plans or an HMO. The fee-for-service plans had coinsurance rates of 0%, 25%, 50%, and 95%, with annual out-of-pocket costs of 5%, 10%, and 15%. The Rand researchers found that those with free care or no out-of-pocket costs generated 45% greater health expenses that those with a 95% coinsurance plan. Those with zero coinsurance generated 67% more physician office visits than those with 95% coinsurance, as compared to those with 25% coinsurance that generated 22% more physician office

⌕ CASE EXAMPLE

A salient current policy example of employing behavioral economics to influence behavior is the required elements of health insurance emanating from the PPACA. The law now requires the inclusion of covered services often absent from coverage in order to reduce premium costs. One element of particular interest is "preventative and wellness services" that are to be provided at no additional cost to the consumer. From the behavioral economics lens, these services are decoupled from payment or are perceived as free. The rationale for these services being of "no cost" to consumers is to encourage their use and decrease the cost of health care by treating medical and behavioral health problems discovered during preventative screenings earlier and at a lower cost.

A caution associated with the zero cost is that the services become undervalued. In an effort to control moral hazard, policy makers and insurance providers couple cost to desired behaviors. Frequently, wellness program couple the reward of lower premium cost to participation in wellness activities. Similarly, state legislators in Michigan couple the rewards of lower or no out-of-pocket costs to the development and follow through on healthy behavior goals in their design of the Healthy Michigan Plan (expanded Medicaid waiver). Deductibles, viewed negatively by most consumers, are used to encourage loss aversion and discourage moral hazard or the overuse of services.

visits than those with 95% coinsurance. Hospital admission rates for coinsurance cohorts were 10.3% (0 coinsurance), 8.4% (25% coinsurance), and 7.9% (95% coinsurance). Finally, these researchers calculated that moving from a policy providing 95% coinsurance to zero would generate a 18%–30% welfare loss.[13] The final conclusion of this study is that health insurance needs to deter moral hazard and avoid unnecessary expenses by increasing price salience and vividness through minimal coupling payment to the purchase of a product or service. All of the earlier behavioral economic axioms can be employed by policy makers in efforts to encourage or "nudge" (Thaler & Sustein, 2009) healthcare providers and consumers to make judicious and cost conscious use of healthcare resources.

References

Aldridge, M. D., & Kelley, A. S. (2015). The myth regarding the high cost of end-of-life care. *American Journal of Public Health, 105*(12), 2411–2415. doi:10.2105/AJPH.2015.302889

Brookings Institute. (2017, September). Household Income quintiles. Retrieved from http://www.taxpolicycenter.org/statistics/household-income-quintiles

Brosig-Koch, J., Hennig-Schmidt, H., Kairies-Schwarz, N., & Wiesen, D. (2016). Using artefactual field and lab experiments to investigate how fee-for-service and capitation affect medical service provision. *Journal of Economic Behavior and Organization, 131*, 17–23. doi:10.1016/j.jebo.2015.04.011

Fujisawa, R., & Lafortune, G. (2008). OECD Health Working Papers No. 41. The Remuneration of General Practitioners and Specialists in 14 OECD Countries: What are the Factors Influencing Variations Across Countries?

Grytten, J. (2017). Payment systems and incentives in dentistry. *Community Dentistry and Oral Epidemiology, 45*(1), 1–11. doi:10.1111/cdoe.12267

Hogan, C., Lunney, J., Gabel, J., & Lynn, J. (2001). Medicare beneficiaries' costs of care in the last year of life. *Health Affairs, 20*(4), 188–195. doi:10.1377/hlthaff.20.4.188

Hough, D. E. (2013). *Irrationality in health care: What behavioral economics reveals about what we do and why.* Stanford, CA: Stanford University Press.

Lubitz, J. D., & Riley, G. F. (1993). Trends in medicare payments in the last year of life. *The New England Journal of Medicine, 328*(15), 1092–1096. doi:10.1056/NEJM199304153281506

Johnson, E. J., Hershey, J., Meszaros, J., & Kunreuther, H. (1993). Framing, probability distortions, and insurance decisions. *Journal of Risk and Uncertainty, 7*(1), 35–51. doi:10.1007/BF01065313

Mello, M. M., Chandra, A., Gawande, A. A., & Studdert, D. M. (2010). National costs of the medical liability system. *Health Affairs (Project Hope), 29*(9), 1569–1577. doi:10.1377/hlthaff.2009.0807

Peterson, C. L., & Burton, R. (2007). *U.S. health care spending: Comparison with other OECD countries (RL34175).* Washington, DC: Congressional Research Service. Retrieved from http://digitalcommons.ilr.cornell.edu/crs/310/

Rice, T. H., & Unruh, L. (2015). *The economics of health reconsidered* (4th ed.). Chicago, IL: Health Administration Press.

Riley, G. F., & Lubitz, J. D. (2010). Long-term trends in medicare payments in the last year of life. *Health Services Research, 45*(2), 565–576. doi:10.1111/j.1475-6773.2010.01082.x

Smith, S., Newhouse, J. P., & Freeland, M. S. (2009). Income, insurance, and technology: Why does health spending outpace economic growth? *Health Affairs, 28*(5), 1276. doi:10.1377/hlthaff.28.5.1276

Squires, D., & Anderson, C. (2015). U.S. health care from a global perspective: Spending, use of services, prices, and health in 13 countries. *Issue brief (Commonwealth Fund), 15*, 1–15.

Starr, P. (1982). *The social transformation of American medicine.* New York, NY: Basic Books.

Thaler, R. H., & Sustein, C. (2009). *Nudge: Improving decisions about health, wealth, and happiness.* London: Penguin Books.

Yamamoto, D. H. (2013). *Health care costs—From birth to death.* Sponsored by Society of Actuaries, Part of the Health Care Cost Institute's Independent Report Series—Report 2013-1.

---

13   Welfare loss is a situation where marginal social benefit is not equal to marginal social costs and society does not achieve maximum utility.

Appendix

APPENDIX TABLE 10.7 Major U.S. Health Policies

Year	Bill	President	Sponsored	Legislation Introduced	Passed Congress	Signed by President	Type of Justice	Access	Cost	Quality
1854	Bill for the Benefit of the Indigent Insane	Franklin Pierce	No	Yes	Yes	No	Social	X	X	
1912	Party Platform	Theodore Roosevelt	Yes	No	No	No	Social	X	X	
1933	Healthcare provisions as part of Social Security legislation	Franklin Roosevelt	Yes	No	No	No	Social	X	X	
1946	Mental Health Act	Harry Truman	Yes	Yes	Yes	Yes	Social	X	X	
1946	Hospital Survey and Construction Act (Hill-Burton Act)	Harry Truman	Yes	Yes	Yes	Yes	Social	X	X	
1948	Federal Water Pollution Control Act	Harry Truman	Yes	Yes	Yes	Yes	Social			X
1949	Fair Deal	Harry Truman	Yes	Yes	No	No	Social	X	X	
1951	Health Insurance premiums declared tax deductible by businesses	Harry Truman	Yes	Yes	No	No	Market	X	X	
1960	Kerr Mills Bill	Dwight Eisenhower	Yes	Yes	Yes	Yes	Social	X	X	

(continues)

APPENDIX TABLE 10.7 Major U.S. Health Policies   *(continues)*

Year	Bill	President	Sponsored	Legislation Introduced	Passed Congress	Signed by President	Type of Justice	Access	Cost	Quality
1962	Medicare	John Kennedy	Yes	Yes	No	No	Social	X	X	
1963	Clean Air Act	Lyndon Johnson	Yes	Yes	Yes	Yes	Social			X
1965	Medicare and Medicaid	Lyndon Johnson	Yes	Yes	Yes	Yes	Social	X	X	
1964	Food Stamps	Lyndon Johnson	Yes	Yes	Yes	Yes	Social	X	X	
1965	Cigarette Labeling and Advertising Act	Lyndon Johnson	Yes	Yes	Yes	Yes	Social			X
1966	Fair Packaging and Labeling Act	Lyndon Johnson	Yes	Yes	Yes	Yes	Social			X
1971	Private Health Insurance Employer Mandate and Federalization of Medicaid	Richard Nixon	Yes	Yes	No	No	Social	X	X	
1972	Social Security Amendments of 1972 (Disability and End Stage Renal Disease)	Richard Nixon	Yes	Yes	Yes	Yes	Social	X	X	
1972	Clean Water Act	Richard Nixon	Yes	Yes	Yes	Yes	Social			X
1973	HMO Act of 1973	Richard Nixon	Yes	Yes	Yes	Yes	Market	X	X	
1974	Employer Mandate and Replacement of Medicaid by state-run plans	Richard Nixon	Yes	Yes	No	No	Social	X	X	

1979	Employer mandate, federalization of Medicaid, and Medicare catastrophic coverage	Jimmy Carter	Yes	No	No	No	Social	X	X	
1983	Social Security Amendments of 1983 (Prospective Payment System)	Ronald Reagan	Yes	Yes	Yes	Yes	Market		X	
1985	EMTALA	Ronald Reagan	Yes	Yes	Yes	Yes	Social	X	X	
1993	Health Security Plan	Bill Clinton	Yes	No	No	No	Social	X	X	
1996	HIPAA	Bill Clinton	Yes	Yes	Yes	Yes	Social	X	X	
1997	CHIP	Bill Clinton	Yes	Yes	Yes	Yes	Social	X	X	
2004	Medicare Prescription Drug, Improvement, and Modernization Act	George W. Bush	Yes	Yes	Yes	Yes	Social	X	X	
2009	American Recovery and Reinvestment Act	Barak Obama	Yes	Yes	Yes	Yes	Market		X	X
2010	Patient Protection and Affordable Care Act	Barak Obama	Yes	Yes	Yes	Yes	Social	X	X	X
2010	Health Care and Education Reconciliation Act of 2010	Barak Obama	Yes	Yes	Yes	Yes	Social	X	X	X

Office of Actuary, at www.CMS.gov

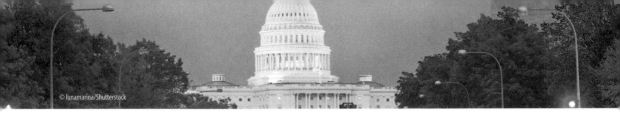

CHAPTER 11

Access, the Uninsured, and Health Policy

This chapter is designed to give healthcare leaders an understanding of how access affects health policy by covering the following topics:

- Brief history of access to healthcare services
- Access and payment
- Government efforts to expand access and the beginning of the "uninsured"
- Access and race/ethnicity
- Access and geographic location
- Access to mental health and public health services
- Nonprofit hospitals and charity care

Understanding how individuals access healthcare services will assist the healthcare leader in gaining perspective on how their organization is positioned within the paradigm and the effects of health policy on access. First and foremost, access to health services is inextricably linked to payment for services. While the nature of the payment for services and who provides this payment has changed over the years, one seldom finds either access or payment in isolation. Keeping in mind the cost-quality-access triangle, if access is low, most likely cost (payment) is high, thus limiting access. Conversely, if access is high, cost (payment) is likely low. As noted in the previous chapter, the cost recognized by most people is the transaction cost (payment) at the point of service.

▶ Brief History of Access

Up until the 20th century, the cost for health service was borne as an out-of-pocket expense by the individual or family receiving the services. Consequently, access to health services was limited to what an individual or family could afford to pay whether in cash or noncash payment. During this period, medical training was limited and often times took the form of apprenticeship without the benefit of formal medical school. Other types of providers include individuals who were naturalistic in their approach or what we would call today naturopaths and homeopaths—who often had no formal schooling. Thus, people had their access to health services limited to the types of providers who were within their geographic area, with care providers concentrated in more densely populated geographic areas.

▶ Access and Payment

Beginning in the 20th century, people began to have access to medical insurance for use in accessing services, with the first formal plan coming out of Baylor Hospital in 1929. This first plan was developed for the Texas Teachers Union and provided medical insurance for 50 cents per month. Soon, these types of plans began to develop around the country primarily in the form of Blue Cross plans to cover hospital costs and Blue Shield plans to cover physician costs. These plans began to take the financial pressure off people, shield them from the true costs of services, and resulted in more people accessing medical services. One result of the two World Wars was that a large number of people gained access to regular medical services for the first time in their lives—and found they liked the access. Thus, there was pressure to continue this access once they completed their military service post war. In addition, the first half of the 20th century produced some of the first significant scientific medical advancements that resulted in higher quality services, which increased demand for services. From the middle to the end of the 20th century, scientific, medical advancements exploded, pushing the growth in demand for access to health services. This growth in demand was due in part to an increase in access to medical insurance that both ensured payment to providers and shielded patients and providers from the true costs of services.

The beginning of serious discussion about how involved our federal government should become in the provision of health services commenced during the first years of the 20th century. Several European countries had begun to provide health services to their population (Germany) or at least the poor

(England). In the United States, increased government involvement came in the form of three pieces of legislation: the Mental Health Act, the Hill-Burton Act, and the Water Pollution Control Act. The Mental Health Act and the Hill-Burton Act began a trend of the federal government getting involved in providing access to health services for vulnerable populations.[1] As western European countries implemented national health plans that ensured access to all residents, the focus of most efforts in the United States was on how to control rising costs. This focus had the goals of controlling costs without decreasing access, reducing racial/ethnic disparities, and increasing access for the uninsured.

▶ Government Efforts to Expand Access and the Beginning of the "Uninsured"

During this period, 18 pieces of legislation were introduced on the federal level, with 12 enacted. Of these 12 statutes that were enacted, 8 were medical focused and 4 were public health focused, with 7 of the 8 medical focused statutes directed at increasing access for vulnerable populations (see **TABLE 11.1**). Cost increased as demand for services increased from a limited pool of providers and supplies. With the medically insured public shielded from the cost of services and the perception that new means "improved and better (i.e., perceived higher quality)," demand continued to grow. It was during the early part of this period that the norm of possession of medical insurance equaling access to high-quality health service began to develop. As a corollary to this norm, individuals who did not possess medical insurance became known as the uninsured. The entry of this term into common use is viewed as an

---

1   The Mental Health Act provided access to services for the mentally ill and the Hill-Burton Act provided for the building of hospitals in less densely populated areas.

TABLE 11.1 Major Changes Affecting Community Benefit and Charity Care Contained in PPACA and HCEARA

Provision	Description	Effect on Nonprofit Community Benefit
T. I, Subtitle A, 2712	Prohibition of rescission	Reduced a component of charity care (in states where rescission was legal).
T. I, Subtitle A, 2714 (amended by 2301 of Reconciliation Act)	Dependent care coinage extended to age 26	Reduced uninsured and thus overall pool of candidates for charity care (where not already in practice).
T. I, Subtitle B, 1101	Pre-existing conditions	Reduced uninsured and thus overall pool of candidates for charity care (in states where denial was legal).
T. I, Subtitle C, 2702	Guaranteed issue	Reduced uninsured and thus overall pool of candidates for charity care (in states without guaranteed issue).
T. I, Subtitle C, 2703	Guaranteed renewal	Reduced uninsured and thus overall pool of candidates for charity care (in states without guaranteed renewal).
T. I, Subtitle F, 5000A (amended by 1002 Reconciliation Act)	Individual, mandate	Reduced uninsured and thus overall pool of candidates for charity care.
T. II, Subtitle A, 2001	Medicaid expansion	Reduced uninsured and thus overall pool of candidates for charity care while adding to "Medicaid loss" (for those systems that DO NOT claim this shortfall as a component of total charity care).
T. III, Part I, 3001	Hospital value-based purchasing	Increase in community benefit operations and services.
T. III, Part III, 3022 and 3025	ACOs share in Medicare cost savings under readmission reduction program	Increase in community benefit operations and services.
T. IX, Subtitle A, 9007a (IRS 501(r)(3)	Conduct community health needs assessment and implement triennial improvement plan	Increase in community benefit operations and services.

(continues)

TABLE 11.1 Major Changes Affecting Community Benefit and Charity Care Contained in PPACA and HCEARA   *(continued)*

Provision	Description	Effect on Nonprofit Community Benefit
T. IX, Subtitle A, 9007a (IRS 501(r)(5)	Charge parity for financial assistance patients (those identified as charity care)	Reduced a component of charity care for those systems that "converted" some portion of bad debt for inclusion as a part of total charity care.
T. IX, Subtitle A, 9007a (IRS 4959)	$50,000.00 excise tax for failure to comply with 5601(r)(5)	Increase in community benefit operations and services.

Notes: IRS—Internal Revenue Service, ACO—Accountable Care Organization, Medicaid loss—revenue lost as determined by subtracting Medicaid reimbursement from actual cost (generally found on the organization "charge data master," "converted" bad debt—moving uncollectable patient debts from a revenue loss (a negative) to charity care (a positive) on the organizational balance sheet).

Congress.gov.

unfavorable status with at best limited access to health services.

The uninsured can be broken up into three categories: (1) those of substantial financial means who viewed medical insurance as a poor economic decision, consisting of about 5%; (2) the acutely uninsured who were generally married individuals with children aged 30–50 years who were between jobs and normally had new jobs and medical insurance within 6 months, consisting of about 45%; and (3) the chronically uninsured who were generally single minority males without children with low-paying jobs, consisting of about 50%. What needs to be pointed out is that virtually all of these people were employed or had the likelihood of re-employment within 6 months.

One of many federal attempts to improve access for the uninsured was through the development of Federally Qualified Health Centers (FQHCs).[2] Throughout the 1970s, several types of health centers were developed, targeting vulnerable populations that ultimately resulted in the Health Centers Consolidation Act of 1996.

The FQHCs target low-income populations of people who are either uninsured or on Medicaid and are funded through federal grants under section 330 of the Public Health Service Act.

Throughout this period, a great divide began to develop between the Democrats and Republicans as each party attempted to maintain their philosophical view of what was best for America. Democrats held the social justice view and sought to increase federal governmental involvement in the provision of health services, and Republicans held the market justice view that individuals, not the federal government, should be responsible for their health services. Both parties realized that neither would attain their goals with large, grand programs. Instead, each pursued incremental approaches focusing on federal government provision of services for vulnerable populations. The Democrats were successful in seeing Medicare and Medicaid enacted and incrementally increasing access through the broadening of eligibility criteria for both of these programs. While the Republicans believe those who can provide for themselves,

---

2 These began life as Neighborhood Health Centers during the "War on Poverty" in 1965.

should, they have also come to see a place for government providing for those with no alternative means. Their objection to the expansion of the federal government in the provision of health services is both philosophical and fiscal. Philosophically, they question if the federal government should be involved in providing any social service, and fiscally, they question the federal government's ability to pay for services without limiting funds for other programs.

At the beginning of the 21st century, the concerns of the 20th century only increased with the percentage of GDP consumed by health care growing from 15% to 17% and projected to go to 25% by mid-century. Crippling costs continue to constrain access due to cost of service provision. The first major health statute of the 21st century was the Medicare Modernization Act of 2004 that provided for prescription drug coverage and reformulated the Medicare Advantage program, allowing Medicare recipients the option of purchasing a health maintenance organization (HMO) product on the private market instead of enrolling in traditional Medicare. The passage of this act continued the trend of the federal government providing health services for vulnerable populations. The next two major acts make up the Patient Protection and Affordable Care Act (PPACA) and, for the first time, sought to include the federal government in the provision for non-vulnerable or less-vulnerable populations.

▶ **Expansion of Current Federal and State Programs**

Reimer (2003) and Garfield, Orgera, and Damico (2019) found, through analysis of current federal and state program enrollments, that current programs could be expanded if all eligible adults and children were automatically enrolled. The result

of this automatic enrollment would be decreased stigma and increased access to physician and healthcare services. A descriptive and multivariate analysis of survey data by Dubay and Kenney (2004) indicates there is unused funding in current State Children's Health Insurance Program (SCHIP) that could be used to enroll parents of children in the same program.[3] Analysis of telephone survey data found strong support for this expansion of federal and workplace health insurance programs using these leftover funds (Blendon, Benson, & DesRoches, 2003).

▶ **Premium Subsidies, Tax Credits, and Decreased Regulations**

Federal- and state-sponsored programs have taken a variety of approaches to expanding access, including expanding private sector coverage, expanding public sector coverage, targeting specific populations (e.g., college students), targeting health delivery programs, and developing new programs. Research has shown the most effective programs were federal and state government sponsored premium subsidies (e.g., subsidizing employer-sponsored coverage and tax credits). Other programs deemed effective include building on existing programs and structures, streamlining eligibility and enrollment requirements, and allowing family members to enroll in the same program (Garfield et al., 2019). Kapur and Marquis (2003) analyzed panel survey data and found that subsidies of COBRA premiums would benefit only a small portion of the uninsured and would not be cost-effective; however, tax credits or other subsidies to low-income workers who become involuntarily jobless were effective (Health Insurance: Premiums and Increases, 2018). A cost-benefit analysis of the cost of healthcare regulations

---

3 SCHIP was reauthorized in 2009 and renamed Children's Health Insurance Program (CHIP).

versus the cost of providing health insurance coverage for the uninsured by Brostoff (2004) found the cost of regulations to be three to six times greater than the cost of providing health insurance coverage for the uninsured. The regulations quantified include costs related to the tort system, Food and Drug Administration, and health facilities regulations. These regulations yielded a net cost of $128 billion, while the cost of health insurance coverage for the uninsured is estimated to be between $34 and $69 billion. Another recent deregulatory movement is allowing advanced practice nurses to perform traditional physician tasks, with the quality of outcomes at least equal to that of physicians at a markedly lower cost (Zweifel, 2018).

▶ Why Not Universal, Single-Payer Coverage?

Whether or not the United States should enact a universal, single-payer healthcare system was first introduced in 1912 as a national policy question by Theodore Roosevelt in the presidential election of that year. It was not acted upon legislatively due to vigorous lobbying by manufacturing groups. Subsequently, Presidents Franklin Roosevelt, Harry Truman, and William Clinton have all unsuccessfully considered or proposed that the United States enact a universal, single-payer healthcare system (Starr, 1982). Scholars' and practitioners' views on enacting a universal, single-payer healthcare system in the United States range from embracing to deploring the idea. The most common arguments for such a system are financial (i.e., lack of financial resources by the poor) and resource allocation, while the most common arguments against such a system are lack of timely access to healthcare services and poor quality of care (Hinkel, 2005; Relman, 2005). The Affordable Care Act (ACA) requires that all Americans are mandated to

possess a health insurance policy purchased either by their employer or on the private market (Title I(F)(1)(1501-1502)). Others contend that switching the U.S. healthcare system to a single-payer system would be cost neutral to the U.S. economy due to decreased insurance overhead and decreased bureaucracy (Hadley & Holahan, 2003; Himmelstein, 2003). Reinhardt (2003) contends that while a universal, single-payer system may seem reasonable and desirable, it is not a viable solution for the ills of the U.S. healthcare system due to lack of political will by the actors involved. Recent research found mixed results regarding the cost of a single-payer health system (Fox & Poirier, 2018; Petrou, Samoutis, & Lionis, 2018). While polling data demonstrated 56% of Americans are in favor of a single-payer health system, that percentage dropped to 37% when confronted with the possibility of having to pay increased taxes for such a system (Kaiser, 2019).

▶ The Importance of Access

Those who have health insurance coverage are more likely to seek preventive care and follow through on prescribed treatments (e.g., diagnostic procedures, pharmaceuticals, specialist physician care, and hospital care). The importance of preventive and follow-up treatments is directly related to decreased morbidity and mortality, increased worker productivity, increased family stability, and decreased societal cost of medical care (Fairbrother, Gusmano, Park, & Scheinmann, 2003; Hadley & Holahan, 2003; Proser, 2004; Sudano, 2003). Individuals who do not engage in preventative treatment behaviors or chronic treatment regimens live shorter lives and are more expensive to care for due to their chronic medical problems exacerbating into acute medical problems that are difficult and expensive to treat (Fairbrother et al., 2003; Hadley & Holahan, 2003; Proser, 2004; Sudano, 2003).

Researchers have studied why the uninsured fail to seek preventative and follow-up treatments from several viewpoints, using several research methods. In 2003, Fairbrother et al. mailed a survey to internal medicine physicians and analyzed using a chi-square technique "to determine statistical significance of differences in proportions." These physicians reported that patients' inability to pay for office visits was the main reason patients gave for failing to return for follow-up care. This survey also found that patients who were unable to pay for office visits were also unable to secure laboratory or other diagnostic tests (90%) and unable to secure pharmaceuticals (75%). Additional findings in this study indicated that 35% of the internists provided free care to these patients, with the remaining 65% providing care with some type of deferred payment.

Community health centers (CHCs) are government supported outpatient clinics primarily serving uninsured adults—discussed in more detail later in this chapter. Forty-three percent of the patients seen in CHCs are uninsured and, while no payment for services is required, a sliding payment scale is available for those with some means to pay. CHC administrative staff and physicians are successful securing secondary physician and medical care through their professional networks only 30% of the time. CHC staff's inability to secure pharmaceuticals for patients is also a major barrier to adherence to prescribed medical regimens. Proser found a 68.5% increase in the volume of patients seen by CHCs nationally from 1998 to 2004 and indicates that CHCs are successful in providing primary, preventative, and chronic disease management; however, he did not indicate if or how CHCs provide for pharmaceutical, laboratory and diagnostic tests, and the need for specialist care (2004).

Studies using the National Health and Retirement Study have demonstrated that 40% of the respondents were without health insurance at some period during the study periods (Sudano, 2003). He tested the use of five preventative services (mammography, cholesterol test, influenza vaccine, prostate examination, and breast examination) during the study period and found the uninsured population had a usage rate that was approximately 20% lower than a similar insured group. These studies indicate that all uninsured individuals have access to some level of primary physician care, but virtually all lack access to pharmaceuticals and diagnostic or secondary healthcare services. The primary reason indicated for patients' lack of access to care is their inability to pay for the services out-of-pocket.

Uninsured African Americans and Latinos, as a group, avoid accessing the healthcare system due to cost (Becker, 2004). Others have found that due to this avoidance of the healthcare system, the uninsured are often sicker than if they had sought care earlier, thus requiring more expensive care. This leads to a quickly deteriorating financial situation that often leads to medical bankruptcy (Daly, Oblak, Seifert, & Shellenberger, 2002). Researchers have also shown that medical expenses are the leading cause of bankruptcy in the United States (Himmelstein, Warren, Thorne, & Woolhandler, 2005).[4]

▸ Access and Race/Ethnicity

Since 2003, the Agency for Healthcare Research and Quality has produced a healthcare disparities report that has tracked both the quality and disparities of access to healthcare services. Since the inception of the report, there has been some improvement in quality, with little shift in disparities of access and quality for populations of low socioeconomic

---

4 The researchers' most compelling finding was that 75.7% of the respondents had health insurance at the onset of their illness and that 42% had a lapse of health insurance coverage sometime during their bankruptcy saga.

status, racial and ethnic minority groups, and selected geographic areas. There is some hope that these disparity groups will have increased access through expanded Medicaid and the Health Exchanges as part of the ACA. The numbers reported by the U.S. Department of Health and Human Services (HHS) indicate that the uninsured rate has dropped from 16.8% to 13.4%, or that approximately 10 million people now have access to health care through either expanded Medicaid or policies through the Health Exchange.

African Americans are less likely to pursue health care than whites. African Americans deselect themselves from the system due to real and perceived racial discrimination within the system. Immigrants are 10% less likely to have health insurance than their U.S.-born counterparts. Meanwhile, Hispanics are overtaking African Americans as the minority with the largest percentage of uninsured. Finally, in addition to cost barriers, they also avoid the healthcare system due to real and perceived racial and financial discrimination.

▶ Access and Geographic Location: The Role of the HRSA

A fair proportion of the access barriers faced by racial/ethnic minorities also conforms to access barriers defined by geography. While we most often think of limits to healthcare access in terms of rural areas, access is also constrained in urban areas. Federal policy addresses geographically constrained access through three separate, but linked, policy measures. First, an application is made for a geographic area to be designated a shortage area for healthcare professionals OR a

population that is underserved. These applications are submitted by private sector healthcare organizations in concert with approval and support of the state Medicaid agency. After the area designation is awarded, the area then qualifies for federally qualified health centers (FQHCs) and for healthcare provider student loan repayment programs to encourage providers to practice in areas with low access.

The story of how government policy has responded to these twin problems is a textbook example of incremental theories of policy change. Two approaches were taken with near simultaneity. One approach was to develop infrastructure—clinics for the uninsured/underserved. The other approach was to entice providers to practice in these underserved areas (either at the clinics or as independent practitioners). Alongside these two policy approaches to the problem of access defined by geography was a separate, but closely linked, process to develop a common definition of geographic underservice.

The first few decades, the policy activity was confined almost wholly within the Health Resources and Services Administration (HRSA) located within the HHS. Government efforts to address these two frames for defining the access problem (barriers defined by geography and minority groups) began in 1965 with the first federal funding for CHCs. The policy decision authorizing the funding of CHCs was taken in the executive branch through the interpretation of administrative rules governing the Office of Economic Opportunity (OEO).[5] This decision led to the first attempts to define Health Manpower Shortage Areas (HMSAs) and then define the operationalization of CHCs. The success of these federally funded health centers in increasing access to underserved, uninsured adults led to steady increases in funding, the founding of more

---

5   The OEO had been created the year prior as a part of the Great Society programs signed into law by President Johnson. It resided in the Department of Health Education and Welfare (DHEW), which was superseded by the Department of Health and Human Services (HHS) after President Carter established a separate Department of Education in 1979.

centers, and attempts to better define areas with constrained access.

The first legislative involvement to increase the supply of providers in underserved areas was in 1970, with the establishment of the National Health Service Corps (NHSC). In 1972, the NHSC created the student loan repayment methodology for the attraction of healthcare providers to underserved areas. The NHSC is administratively under another unit of the HRSA, the Bureau of Clinician Recruitment and Service.

In 1973, disagreements over methodologies for defining HMSAs led to Congress requiring the development of an Index for Medical Underservice (IMU). The work to create the index led to the creation of two new definitions of access barriers—Medically Underserved Areas (MUAs) and Medically Underserved Populations (MUPs)—thus linking the twin issues of geography and race/ethnicity in law. Two years later, Congress required CHC funding changed with the enactment of the 1975 Special Health Revenue Sharing Act. This mandated that funding for CHCs follow the IMU, which also qualified underserved areas for HMOs, federal investments in healthcare professionals, and other federal health funds. This act also caused an increase in funds to flow to rural MUAs.

The shift in funding focus to rural communities grew over time as a part of a broader government concern over steady population loss and lowering of income levels in rural areas driven by job losses and farm consolidations, which led to losses of healthcare providers and infrastructure. The establishment in 1987 of the Office of Rural Health Policy (ORHP) inside of the HRSA followed with programming aimed at strengthening existing healthcare organizations within rural areas and

stemming the loss of access to services.[6] At this time, links across these different units inside of the HRSA were not established; the ORHP organized rural supports while the Bureau of Primary Care implemented the designation of shortage areas and funding for FQHCs. It would not be until the late 1990s and then, more fully, after the passage of both the American Recovery and Reinvestment Act of 2009 (ARRA) and the PPACA that the connections between these two became regularized.

The last piece of federal policy enacted to address the under supply of healthcare providers (as defined by shortage areas) is the Conrad 30 J-1 Visa Program.[7] In 1994, Senator Kent Conrad of North Dakota led the drafting of the law that bears his name. Administered by U.S. Citizenship and Immigration Services within the Department of Homeland Security, qualified foreign physicians may travel to the United States for graduate medical education (normally for residency training). Upon completion of the program of study, these healthcare providers may apply to waive a waiting period for permanent residency. Each state healthcare agency may annually support up to 30 waivers (hence the policy name), provided each applicant is (and will continue to) work in a defined shortage area.

The remainder of the policy innovation in this area is a story of *payment*. Medicare payment became available to FQHCs in 1991—an important new revenue stream for these financially straightened health centers. Wrangling over refining the definition of shortage areas began in 1995 and was not complete until 2008, although the use of the prior definitions remained in force. In 1996, after the failure of his signature healthcare reform plan, President Clinton signed into law the Health Center Consolidation Act, a necessary reorganization and rationalization of

---

6 The primary infrastructure focus was on sustaining rural critical access hospitals (CAHs) by supporting the development of rural healthcare provider networks, at the center of each was a CAH. These networks are now in the process of converting to Accountable Care Organizations (ACOs).

7 Originally titled "Conrad 20," when reauthorized in 2003 it was expanded to 30.

oversight and funding across all federally funded health centers for the uninsured. In 2001, George W. Bush followed this with a dramatic expansion in funding and authorizations for more health centers. To bring us to the present, in 2009, the ARRA further expanded the number of health centers, while the PPACA expanded upon this again just 1 year later. Lastly, under the PPACA, Medicare's prospective payment system was opened to FQHCs in 2014.

The story of healthcare policy addressing access by geography, involving three separate subunits of the HRSA, the Centers for Medicare and Medicaid Services, and the Department of Homeland Security (and as you will see, the Indian Health Service [IHS]) may appear disjointed and awkward when viewed from the federal level. At the state level, though, the appearance is largely opposite. These programs are normally housed within one state agency responsible for health, often within one branch of the agency, so one state agency coordinates the programmatic work at the state level, thus making the policy implementation more coordinated and "seamless" across communities receiving supports (**FIGURES 11.1** and **11.2**).

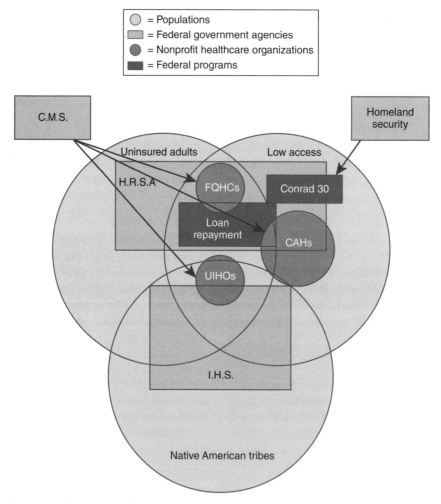

FIGURE 11.1 Federal Programming for Increasing Access: Population, Agencies, and Organizations

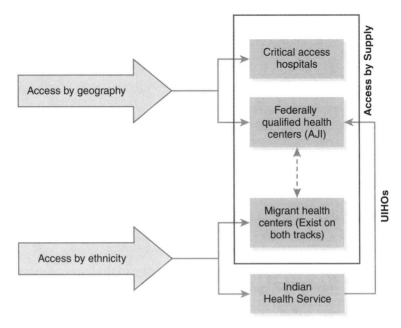

FIGURE 11.2 Federal Programming for Increasing Access: Geography, Ethnicity, and Supply

▶ Access and American Indian/Alaskan Natives

American Indians and Alaskan Natives (AI/AN) also suffer access problems similar to African Americans and Latino Americans. Unlike other ethnicities, these two groups have access to health care on tribal lands from the IHS. Founded in 1955 (taking over services provided by the Bureau of Indian Affairs and the Public Health Service), the IHS is a separate healthcare system located on the tribal lands of federally recognized tribes.

Beginning in the 1970s, the IHS began to extend healthcare services to AI/AN populations that had relocated from tribal lands to urban areas in search of employment. In 1992, Congress recognized the change in needs of AI/AN populations by amending the Indian Health Care Improvement Act. By the new millennium, Urban Indian Health Organizations (UIHOs) were operating in 33 locations

across the United States, serving both persons from federally recognized tribes as well as non-members that meet the eligibility for care standards of FQHCs. Thus, UIHOs fall under the IHS while coordinating closely with the Bureau of Primary Care and being eligible for payments from Medicare.

▶ Access to Mental Health and Public Health Services

Access to mental health and public health services remains almost entirely a state and local government function. Two agencies are in place at the federal level for these services, the Substance Abuse and Mental Health Services Administration (SAMHSA) and the Centers for Disease Control and Prevention (CDC). Both agencies perform clearinghouse functions and disperse grant funding to encourage innovation in care delivery and organization.

The CDC also coordinates active disease surveillance with state and local public health agencies. However, the day-to-day organization and funding of these services is a state-level activity often in conjunction with local government agencies.

Government coordination of mental health and substance abuse services tends to be focused around the effective and efficient provision of these services to the Medicaid population. Public health services are similarly focused at the state and local levels, although sometimes with the inclusion of offering additional safety net services (e.g., dental care) where resources are available.

▶ Nonprofit Hospitals, Charity Care, and Community Benefit

Lastly, we should also note that nonprofit hospitals are obliged to provide community benefit (until this century conceptualized almost solely as charity care) in order to maintain tax-free status for the 501(c)3 designation. Although the creation of nonprofit status dates back to the first federal tax code in 1913, separate rules governing the fulfillment of this requirement specifically for nonprofit hospitals date to 1969. The concept of "community benefit" was then first used in federal law regarding nonprofit hospitals for the purpose of expanding beyond charity care what "counts" toward the maintenance of a hospital's tax-free status. Implementation and oversight are responsibilities of the Internal Revenue Service (IRS). These rules—even today—contain no clearly articulated formula or methodology for defining the minimum cumulative annual value of community benefit a hospital must provide in order to maintain this status.

State laws mostly follow federal law with few, if any, enhancements. Barely half (26) of states require annual reporting of community benefit activities—with just eight making those reports publicly available. Few states set a more stringent standard than the federal standard (Nelson, Tan, & Mueller, 2015). Those states that require reporting and/or have more stringent standards have been found to result in higher proportions of community benefit dollars spent (James, 2016).

After decades of reporting to the IRS under vague definitions and the absence of a formula or methodology, no observer should be surprised that nonprofit hospitals devoted little attention to careful documentation of community benefit activity. It should come as no less a surprise that those outside of the IRS and nonprofit health care paid even less attention. However, after a decade of slowly growing attention and pressure from government agencies (federal and state) and advocacy groups regarding lax oversight and thin rules governing community benefit, in 2004, Senator Charles Grassley (R-Iowa), then Chair of the Senate Finance Committee, spearheaded hearings regarding the matter. A few years prior to the Finance Committee attention, the Catholic Health Association (CHA) and the Voluntary Hospital Association (VHA) formed a joint committee to develop standards for their members, regardless of a specific outcome from Congressional hearings.[8] The completion of both processes—Congressional hearings and the publication of the first edition of the CHA-VHA *A Guide to Planning and Reporting Community Benefit*—was nearly simultaneous. Upon review, Senator Grassley accepted the CHA-VHA publication as the starting point for the IRS to develop new administrative rules for reporting community benefit. A key component of the new rules was the creation of IRS Schedule H, a separate community benefit tax form for nonprofit hospitals.

Language codifying the recently drafted administrative rules and expanding upon these rules was included in the PPACA, passed in

---

8 VHA is no longer an acronym. In 1994, the Voluntary Hospital Association formally changed its name to VHA, Inc.

March 2010. Additional changes were passed later the same year in the Health Care and Education Affordability Reconciliation Act of 2010 (HCEARA) (see Table 11.1). The IRS was also required to use the initial rules as a starting point—not an end point. Over the ensuing years, the IRS has reviewed in aggregate annual Schedule H reporting and both further defined existing reporting rules and added new rules to better measure community benefit—and to discourage "lip service" reporting.

Although the implementation of an increasingly more complex and defined Schedule H has drawn, mostly, praise from all interested parties, calls for a federally mandated formula and methodology that produces a minimum percentage of revenue for maintenance of 501(c)(3) status continue. Opponents to such calls argue that the definition of qualifying community benefit expenditures are too narrow and should be broadened prior to developing such a methodology. While we cannot predict the outcome of this current struggle over defining and reporting community benefit, we encourage the reader to compare this process to the same described regarding settling on a common agreed upon methodology for defining geographic access barriers. Over a period of several decades, a difficult to define problem was led slowly—with the involvement of many different (and not always aligned) stakeholders—to consensus on common measurements applied by all.

🔍 CASE STUDY

The Superior Department of Health and Human Services[1] (SDHHS) had placed coordination of these separate federal programs and funding streams in the Bureau of Health Policy and Legislation. In addition to federal funds, two decades prior, the Superior state legislature decided to provide supplemental funding for federal loan repayment entitled the State Loan Repayment Program (SLRP). Around the same time as the creation of the SLRP, the state legislature decided to fund 10 additional safety net clinics, eight qualified as CHCs and the two others served underserved populations. Lastly, the Superior state legislature also funds the State Office of Rural Health (SORH) to augment federal supports to better coordinate rural health resources statewide, including support for rural Critical Access Hospitals and Certified Rural Health Clinics.

Elizabeth Paisley is the administrator tasked with coordinating the use and pass through of these funds. Not surprisingly, Ms. Paisley found that ensuring communities produce smooth, seamless delivery of healthcare services from the apparent chaos of federal programming required her to not just master program management, but also to coordinate efforts with multiple agency partners, to frequently assess the potential effects of future changes, and to maintain a close working relationship with the healthcare committees in both chambers of the state legislature.

Ms. Paisley found that federal agencies regularly implement small changes to ongoing programs and occasionally legislation is passed by Congress that introduces both large and small programmatic changes. She determined that staying on top of both sources of policy change while always remaining flexible in how to best respond is an ongoing process. Only through such ongoing attention and flexibility could she maximize the effectiveness of coordinated federal programming delivered to her state's communities. This attention begins with the partners in coordination, the Superior Primary Care Association (SPCA), the statewide association for all HRSA-funded clinics, and the Superior Center for Rural Health (SCRH), the statewide representative for all rural hospitals. Formal coordination with partners occurs quarterly, at a minimum, in regularly scheduled workforce meetings. Informal coordination occurs much more frequently, using email and phone.

Ms. Paisley has, over the past several years, coordinated and overseen multiple state-level policy changes to maximize the positive impact of all resources in a changing policy environment. These

(continues)

CASE STUDY *(continued)*

policy changes included altering the mix of funding sources for SLRP, removing state fees for Conrad 30 applicants, and moving qualifying Conrad 30 primary care provider applicants to a separate visa waiver program enacted under the HHS. She also led the push to promote efficiency through the removal of bureaucratic barriers. These included the elimination of her department as the pass through of ORHP funds to the SCRH, moving to a three-share funding model for SLRP (now each provider contract is funded by a mix of federal, state, and the facility employing the provider). Lastly, with the efficiencies gained within her office, she brought the Health Professional Shortage Area designation process back to her staff, saving the expense of the external contractor that had performed this function.

1. Within what political context might we anticipate federal policy change altering the level of match funding states are required to provide for uninsured and underinsured programs?
2. Why do you think Elizabeth Paisley lobbied to remove the state fees for Conrad 30 applicants to address uninsured and underinsured concerns?
3. Which of the uninsured and underinsured policy changes by the Superior legislature or Elizabeth Paisley's office required a pre-existing context of close collaboration, both with multiple agencies and across political parties?

[1] This case study, although fictionalized, is based on real events. The fictional state of Superior was once formally proposed for inclusion as a separate state of the United States.

References

Becker, G. (2004). Deadly inequality in the health care "safety net": Uninsured ethnic minorities' struggle to live with life-threatening illness. *Medical Anthropology Quarterly, 18*(2), 258–275.

Blendon, R. J., Benson, J. M., & DesRoches, C. M. (2003). Americans' view of the uninsured: An era for hybrid proposals. Retrieved from http://content.healthaffairs.org/cgi/content/full/hlthaff.w3.405v1/

Brostoff, S. (2004). One way to cover the uninsured? Trim health services regulation costs. *National Underwriter, 108*(4), 323.

Daly, H. F., III., Oblak, L. M., Seifert, R. W., & Shellenberger, K. (2002). Into the red to stay in the pink: The hidden cost of being uninsured. *Health Matrix, 12*(1), 39–61.

Dubay, L., & Kenney, G. (2004). Addressing coverage gaps for low-income parents. *Health Affairs, 23*(2), 225–234.

Fairbrother, G., Gusmano, M. K., Park, H. P., & Scheinmann, R. (2003). Care for the uninsured in general internists' private offices. *Health Affairs, 22*(6), 217–224.

Fox, A., & Poirier, R. (2018). How single-payer stacks up: Evaluating different models of universal health coverage on cost, access, and quality. *International Journal of Health Services, 48*(3), 568–585. doi:10.1177/0020731418779377

Garfield, R., Orgera, K., & Damico, A. (2019). The uninsured and the ACA: A primer. Henry J. Kaiser Family Foundation.

Hadley, J., & Holahan, J. (2003). Covering the uninsured: How much would it cost? *Health Affairs*, Chevy Chase, MD. Web Exclusive June 4, 2003, pp. 250–265. Retrieved from https://www.healthaffairs.org/doi/10.1377/hlthaff.W3.250

Himmelstein, D. (2003). National health insurance or incremental reform: Aim high or at our feet? *American Journal of Public Health, 93*(1), 102–105.

Himmelstein, D., Warren, E., Thorne, D., & Woolhandler, S. (2005). Illness and injury as contributors to bankruptcy. Retrieved from http://content.healthaffairs.org/cgi/content/full/hlthaff.w5.63/

Hinkel, J. (2005). A proposal for universal coverage. *New England Journal of Medicine, 353*(1), 96.

James, J. (2016, February 25). Nonprofit Hospitals' Community Benefit Requirements. Under the Affordable Care Act, many nonprofit hospitals must meet new requirements to retain their tax-exempt status. *Health Affairs*, Health Policy Brief.

Kaiser Family Foundation polling data. (2019). The public on next steps for the ACA and proposals to expand coverage. Retrieved from https://www.kff.org/health-reform/poll-finding/kff-health-tracking-poll-january-2019/

Kapur, K., & Marquis, M. S. (2003). Health insurance for workers who lose jobs: Implications for various subsidy schemes. *Health Affairs, 22*(3), 203–213.

National Council of State Legislatures. (2019). Health insurance: Premiums and increases. Retrieved from http://www.ncsl.org/research/health/health-insurance-premiums.aspx

Nelson, G. D., Tan, B., & Mueller, C. H. (2015, January). *Community benefit state law profiles.* Baltimore, MD: The Hilltop Institute, UMBC.

Petrou, P., Samoutis, G., & Lionis, C. (2018). Single-payer or a multipayer health system: A systematic literature review. *Public Health, 163,* 141–152. doi:10.1016/j.puhe.2018.07.006

Proser, M. (2004). *A nation's health at risk II: A front row seat in a changing health care system.* Bethesda, MD: National Association of Community Health Centers.

Reimer, D. (2003). What other programs can teach us: Increasing participation in health insurance programs. *American Journal of Public Health, 93*(1), 67–74.

Reinhardt, U. E. (2003). Is there hope for the uninsured? Retrieved from http://content.healthaffairs.org/cgi/content/full/hlthaff.w3.376v1/

Relman, A. (2005). A proposal for universal coverage. *New England Journal of Medicine, 353*(1), 96.

Starr, P. (1982). *The social transformation of American medicine.* New York, NY: Basic Books.

Sudano, J. (2003). Intermittent lack of health insurance coverage and use of preventative services. *American Journal of Public Health, 93*(1), 130–137.

Zweifel, P. (2018). Energy, insurance, and health: Viewpoints of a microeconomist. *International Journal of the Economics of Business, 25*(1), 191–204. doi:10.1080/13571516.2017.1374562

Appendix

APPENDIX TABLE 11.2 Uninsured Rate Among the Nonelderly, 2013–2017					
	2013 Uninsured Rate (%)	2016 Uninsured Rate (%)	2017 Uninsured Rate (%)	Change Uninsured Rate 2013–2017 (%)*	Change in Uninsured Rate 2016–2017 (%)
Total— Nonelderly[a]	16.8	10.0	10.2	−6.6	0.2*
Age					
Children—Total	7.5	4.7	5.0	−2.6	0.3*
Adults—Total	20.6	12.1	12.3	−8.2	0.2*
Adults 19–25	26.8	14.6	14.8	−11.9	0.2
Adults 26–34	26.3	15.6	15.6	−10.7	0.0
Adults 35–44	21.2	13.6	13.6	−7.6	0.0
Adults 45–54	17.4	10.4	10.7	−6.7	0.3*
Adults 55–64	13.4	7.5	7.9	−5.5	0.4*
Annual Family Income					
<$20,000	28.0	17.1	17.2	−10.8	0.0
$20,000–$39,999	27.4	16.8	17.3	−10.1	0.5*
$40,000+	11.4	7.1	7.5	−3.9	0.4*

(continues)

APPENDIX TABLE 11.2 Uninsured Rate Among the Nonelderly, 2013–2017				*(continued)*
	2013 Uninsured Rate (%)	**2016 Uninsured Rate (%)**	**2017 Uninsured Rate (%)**	**Change Uninsured Rate 2013–2017 (%)***	**Change in Uninsured Rate 2016–2017 (%)**
Family Poverty Level[b] (%)					
<100	26.2	16.5	16.6	−9.6	0.1
100–199	28.4	17.0	17.2	−11.2	0.3
200–399	17.7	11.3	11.7	−5.9	0.4*
400+	6.8	4.1	4.5	−2.3	0.3*
Household Type					
1 Parent with children[c]	11.5	6.8	7.1	−4.4	0.3
2 Parent with children[c]	10.8	6.9	7.2	−3.6	0.3*
Multigenerational[d]	20.5	11.8	11.6	−8.9	−0.2
Adults living alone or with other adults	20.1	11.6	11.8	−8.3	0.3*
Other	22.5	13.5	13.6	−8.8	0.1
Family Work Status					
2+ Full-time	13.4	8.2	8.5	−5.0	0.3*
1 Full-time	16.5	10.2	10.4	−6.1	0.2*
Only part-time[e]	26.2	14.4	14.6	−11.6	0.2
Non-workers	21.2	12.7	13.0	−8.2	0.3*

Race/Ethnicity					
White only (non-Hispanic)	12.3	7.1	7.3	−5.0	0.3*
Black only (non-Hispanic)	18.8	10.7	11.1	−7.7	0.5*
Hispanic	30.0	19.1	18.9	−11.1	−0.2
Asian/Native Hawaiian and Pacific Islander	15.8	7.2	7.2	−8.6	0.0
Am. Indian/Alaska Native	30.4	22.0	22.0	−8.4	0.1
Two or more races[f]	13.5	7.7	7.9	−5.6	0.2
Citizenship					
U.S. citizen—native	13.8	7.9	8.2	−5.6	0.3*
U.S. citizen—naturalized	20.3	9.8	10.0	−10.3	0.2
Non-U.S. citizen, resident for <5 years	38.5	26.4	27.2	−11.3	0.8
Non-U.S. citizen, resident for 5+ years	51.4	37.0	36.0	−15.4	−1.0*

*Statistically significant difference from 2017 at the $P < 0.05$ level.
[a]Nonelderly includes all individuals under age 65.
[b]The U.S. Census Bureau's poverty threshold for a family with two adults and one child was $19,730 in 2017.
[c]Parent includes any person with a dependent child.
[d]Multigenerational families with children include families with at least three generations in a household. Other families include those with adults caring for children other than their own (e.g., a niece living with her aunt).
[e]Part-time workers are defined as working <35 hours per week.
[f]Respondents can identify as more than one racial or ethnic group. The hierarchy we use for determining racial/ethnic categories places all respondents who self-identify as mixed race who do not also identify as Hispanic into the "Two or More Races" category. All individuals who identify with Hispanic ethnicity fall into the Hispanic category regardless of selected race.
Modified from Kaiser Family Foundation analysis of the 2013–2017 American Community Survey (ACS).

APPENDIX TABLE 11.3 Major U.S. Health Policies

Year	Bill	President	Sponsored	Legislation Introduced	Passed Congress	Signed by President	Type of Justice	Access	Cost	Quality
1854	Bill for the Benefit of the Indigent Insane	Franklin Pierce	No	Yes	Yes	No	Social	X	X	
1912	Party platform	Theodore Roosevelt	Yes	No	No	No	Social	X	X	
1933	Healthcare provisions as part of Social Security legislation	Franklin Roosevelt	Yes	No	No	No	Social	X	X	
1946	Mental Health Act	Harry Truman	Yes	Yes	Yes	Yes	Social	X	X	
1946	Hospital Survey and Construction Act (Hill-Burton Act)	Harry Truman	Yes	Yes	Yes	Yes	Social	X	X	
1948	Federal Water Pollution Control Act	Harry Truman	Yes	Yes	Yes	Yes	Social			X
1949	Fair Deal	Harry Truman	Yes	Yes	No	No	Social	X	X	
1951	Health Insurance premiums declared tax deductible by businesses	Harry Truman	Yes	Yes	No	No	Market	X	X	
1960	Kerr Mills Bill	Dwight Eisenhower	Yes	Yes	Yes	Yes	Social	X	X	
1962	Medicare	John Kennedy	Yes	Yes	No	No	Social	X	X	
1963	Clean Air Act	Lyndon Johnson	Yes	Yes	Yes	Yes	Social			X

1965	Medicare and Medicaid	Lyndon Johnson	Yes	Yes	Yes	Yes	Social	X	X	
1964	Food Stamps	Lyndon Johnson	Yes	Yes	Yes	Yes	Social	X	X	
1965	Cigarette Labeling and Advertising Act	Lyndon Johnson	Yes	Yes	Yes	Yes	Social			X
1966	Fair Packaging and Labeling Act	Lyndon Johnson	Yes	Yes	Yes	Yes	Social			X
1971	Private health insurance employer mandate and federalization of Medicaid	Richard Nixon	Yes	Yes	No	No	Social	X	X	
1972	Social Security amendments of 1972 (disability and end stage renal disease)	Richard Nixon	Yes	Yes	Yes	Yes	Social	X	X	
1972	Clean Water Act	Richard Nixon	Yes	Yes	Yes	Yes	Social			X
1973	HMO Act of 1973	Richard Nixon	Yes	Yes	Yes	Yes	Market	X	X	
1974	Employer mandate and replacement of Medicaid by state-run plans	Richard Nixon	Yes	Yes	No	No	Social	X	X	
1979	Employer mandate, federalization of Medicaid, and Medicare, catastrophic coverage	Jimmy Carter	Yes	No	No	No	Social	X	X	
1983	Social Security amendments of 1983 (prospective payment system)	Ronald Reagan	Yes	Yes	Yes	Yes	Market		X	

(continues)

APPENDIX TABLE 11.3 Major U.S. Health Policies   (continued)

Year	Bill	President	Sponsored	Legislation Introduced	Passed Congress	Signed by President	Type of Justice	Access	Cost	Quality
1985	EMTALA	Ronald Reagan	Yes	Yes	Yes	Yes	Social	X	X	
1993	Health Security Act	Bill Clinton	Yes	No	No	No	Social	X	X	
1996	HIPAA	Bill Clinton	Yes	Yes	Yes	Yes	Social	X	X	
1997	CHIP	Bill Clinton	Yes	Yes	Yes	Yes	Social	X	X	
2004	Medicare Prescription Drug, Improvement and Modernization Act	George W. Bush	Yes	Yes	Yes	Yes	Social	X	X	
2009	American Recovery and Reinvestment Act	Barak Obama	Yes	Yes	Yes	Yes	Market		X	X
2010	Patient Protection and Affordable Care Act	Barak Obama	Yes	Yes	Yes	Yes	Social	X	X	X
2010	Heath Care and Education Reconciliation Act of 2010	Barak Obama	Yes	Yes	Yes	Yes	Social	X	X	X

Country	Primary Insurance Type	Funding	Private Insurance	2014 Overall Rating	HC as % GDP 2011	HC as % GDP 2012
Denmark	National Health System	Income tax	40% complimentary		10.87	10.98
England	National Health System	General tax	11% supplemental	1	9.23	9.22
Italy	National Health System	Corporate, VAT, general and regional taxes	15% complimentary		9.25	9.19

Japan	National Health System	General taxes	70% cover cost-sharing		10.05	10.28
New Zealand	National Health System	General taxes	35% complimentary	7	10.00	
Norway	National Health System	General taxes	7% complimentary	7	9.28	9.28
Sweden	National Health System	General taxes	5% complimentary	3	9.47	9.58
Australia	National Health Insurance	General revenue and income taxes	50% complimentary	4	9.08	
Canada	National Health Insurance	General tax (provincial and federal)	67% complimentary	10	10.94	10.93
France	Statutory Health Insurance	Payroll and general revenue taxes	90% complimentary (government vouchers)	9	11.52	11.61
Germany	Statutory Health Insurance	Payroll and general revenue taxes	70% complimentary and cover cost-sharing	5	11.25	11.27
Netherlands	Statutory Health Insurance	Payroll and general revenue taxes	85% complimentary		12.10	
Singapore	Statutory Health Insurance	General taxes	Several plans			
Switzerland	Statutory Health Insurance	General taxes	Several plans	2	11.05	11.43
United States	Statutory Health Insurance, National Health Insurance, National Health System	Payroll and general revenue taxes	56% private insurance	11	17.02	16.09

Commonwealth Fund.

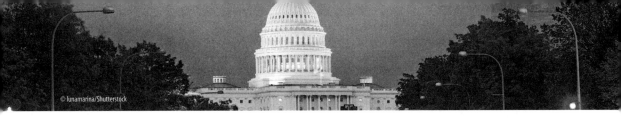

CHAPTER 12

Payment and Quality

This chapter is designed to give healthcare leaders an understanding of how payment and quality affect health policy by covering the following topics:

- Brief history of payment in healthcare services
- Brief history of quality in healthcare services
- How payment and quality became linked in federal healthcare policy
- Value-based purchasing
- Government policy focused on quality
- Private sector efforts focused on quality

As initially discussed, in part, in the previous chapter, payment and access are inextricably linked and, until recently, have been linked with the **absence** of quality. Referring back to Chapter 3, the cost/quality/access triangle remains the basic theoretical (and practical) construct for assessing the inextricable link between these three healthcare concerns. It is only this century that the Centers for Medicare and Medicaid Services (CMS) has begun to pay for quality through pay-for-performance programs that rewarded providers for the provision of what was deemed to be quality care; although, even these programs were not directly linked to payment models. The Affordable Care Act (ACA) has strengthened the payment-quality link by directly linking payment to quality of performance through Accountable Care Organization (ACO) delivery models and value-based purchasing. When payment becomes linked

to delivery or outcomes of services provided, a discussion of risk and risk sharing also has to be introduced. While financial risk has traditionally been born by payers, all payment reform has resulted in shifting more risk from the payer to the provider (**TABLE 12.1**).

▶ Brief History of Payment for Health Services as Related to Quality

Until very recently, most health services have been provided and paid for by some variation of a fee-for-service model. Prior to the development of health insurance, those who received health services paid the provider out of pocket

TABLE 12.1 Timeline of Major Healthcare Quality Actions

Year	Actor	Action
1847	Semmelweis	Hand disinfection or hand washing that reduced mortality in obstetrical wards to less than 1%
1847 and 1911	Medicine's transformation to a sovereign profession	(1847) Organization of physicians through the American Medical Association and (1911) the Flexner report resulting in reorganization and resetting professional medical education
1951	Joint Commission on Accreditation of Healthcare Organizations (JCAHO)	Established to ensure standardization of practice; today accredits health organizations as adhering to Medicare Conditions of Participation
1965	Credentialing in Medicare/Medicaid initial legislation—utilization review begins under National Center for Health Research	Seeks to improve the quality of medical and public health through vetting research-based programs and policies
1966	Donabedian	Developed a framework for evaluating health delivery quality through the categories of structure, process, and quality
1970	National Academy of Medicine (Institute of Medicine)	Provides unbiased, evidence-based, and authoritative health policy advice
1972	Congress established pilot organizations entitled "Experimental Medical Care Review Organizations."	A criteria-based review of physician diagnostic and medical management through use of insurance claims data
1972	Professional Standards Review Organizations (PSROs)	Established by PL 92-603; through peer review evaluates the medical necessity and appropriateness of hospital care, evaluates medical care for quality and improvement of utilization, and analyzes practitioner, institutional, and patient care
1983	Peer Review Organizations (PROs)	Established by the PL 97-248; an organized group of local physicians who evaluates quality, necessity, cost, and adherence to medical standards for Medicare patients
1989	Agency for Healthcare Research and Quality (Agency for Health Care Policy and Research)	Established under PL 101-239 and reauthorized under PL 106-129 as a department under Health and Human Services; charged with ensuring the quality, effectiveness, and appropriateness of healthcare services and access to care through research, demonstration projects, and evaluations; guideline development; and disseminating information on healthcare services and delivery systems; under reorganization, guideline development moved to the National Guideline Clearinghouse

1990	National Committee for Quality Assurance (NCQA)	A non-profit established to improvement of healthcare quality through evidence-based standards, measures, programs, and accreditation
1991	Health Effectiveness Data and Information Set (HEDIS)	Established in 1991 as the HMO Employer and Data Information Set that, after 3 revisions, was renamed in 2007 the Health Effectiveness Data and Information Set; a tool used by health plans to measure quality of care performance through 5 domains and 81 measures
1992	HCFA's Quality Improvement Initiative	Moved the focus of PROs from individual physicians to monitoring patterns based on national and regional trends
1994	National Surgery Quality Improvement Project (NSQIP)	Established by Congress to address poor surgical outcomes in VA hospital but found unreliable due to lack of risk-adjusted data. Once data was risk adjusted, mortality risk decreased by 27%–45% and program was adopted by the American College of Surgeons (2004)
1995	Consumer Assessment of Healthcare Providers and Systems (CAHPS)	Established to assess the health consumer's experience of care through a standardized set of surveys and to generate tools and methods for use of this information for public use and improvement of healthcare services
2003	Medicare Prescription Drug, Improvement, and Modernization Act and the Hospital Inpatient Quality Reporting Program	Collects quality data from hospitals through the Inpatient Prospective Payment System that is provided to consumers through the Hospital Compare website allowing consumers to compare the quality of health service delivery by hospitals; hospitals that choose to not participate are penalized by an established reduction in annual payments

Congress.gov.

with cash or some form of cash equivalent. This personal transaction cost often caused people to forego accessing health services until they became severely ill.

In 1912, the National Convention of Insurance Commissioners developed a model for how states could regulate health insurance. The Commissioners' development of this model was a proactive step for an insurance product that was not prevalent in our society but that they understood was on the horizon as evidenced by its presence on Teddy Roosevelt's Bull Moose party platform and what they observed happening in Europe with the development of social insurance programs. While there were some isolated attempts to make pre-payment arrangement with providers, the first organized and sustained program to provide health insurance was in 1929 when Baylor Hospital provided the Texas Teachers Union with pre-paid hospital insurance for 50 cents per month. Eventually, this program was organized as the first Blue Cross plan, became highly popular, and was replicated in several other states,[1] with physicians organizing themselves a decade later in 1939 under Blue Shield plans.

Up through 1940, several bills were introduced in Congress and papers were issued declaring the need of comprehensive national health insurance, yet the mood of the nation was not in step with this call for national coverage. One of many reasons for this national resolve against a national health insurance plan was the public's association of such plans with German socialism. As the United States had just ended the second of two wars with Germany, the nation was in no mood for policies perceived as connected to Germany. A second outcome of this period was the economic strain the country was under after financing these two World Wars while still becoming accustomed to the multiple social support programs enacted early in the Great Depression. As a result of wartime economic strains in 1943, the War Labor Board implemented wage and price controls that did not include controls on health insurance benefits. With employers unable to increase cash wages, they increased employee compensation through non-cash wages in the form of health insurance benefits. These plans paid physicians and hospitals on a fee-for-service basis with little, if any, questioning of the quality or necessity of the services provided. Six years later, in 1949, the Supreme Court agreed that employer-provided health insurance could be included in collective bargaining. Finally, in 1954 employer-provided health insurance was solidified by the Revenue Act of 1954 that provided a tax exemption for employer-provided health insurance premiums.

The next major payment development is associated with the increased access Medicare and Medicaid provided for approximately 5 million people (at time of enactment). While the American Medical Association (AMA) was resistant to Medicare, physicians very quickly found its payment arrangement agreeable and have become ardent supporters of Medicare, although they are not as sanguine toward Medicaid due to its low payment rates and variability from state to state. Medicare was modeled on 1960s era Blue Cross and Blue Shield plans—paying on a cost-plus mechanism. This mechanism allowed providers to charge the usual and customary cost for their services, plus the cost of capital associated with the provision of care.

As costs continued to increase at approximately twice the rate of the consumer price index, several feeble attempts were made to control the rise in costs; such as wage and price controls including limited price increases to hospital and physicians, the Health Maintenance Organization (HMO) Act of 1973, and ultimately, the Prospective Payment System in 1983. The Prospective Payment System is a fee-for-service model that bundles payment based on diagnosis(es) and resulted in significant models of care changes, an increased focus on documentation and coding, and the development of utilization review. Eventually, providers learned how to work within this system and the cost savings quickly evaporated.

The other significant payment action that occurred during the middle of the 20th century was the development of HMOs beginning with the development of Kaiser-Permanente in 1945, when industrialist Henry J. Kaiser partnered with the Permanente medical group to provide comprehensive, integrated medical care for his employees. While this model was copied in a few other progressive areas in the country, it was not widespread. The unique aspect of early HMOs was that they sought to hold down medical costs through the provision of health maintenance or preventive treatments, they paid their physicians a salary (the original staff-model HMO), and they paid the medical group a capitated fee. The AMA reacted bitterly to the development of HMOs, seeing them as the practice of corporate medicine, and expelled the physicians who participated

---

1   Blue Cross plans were all originally non-profit plans chartered by the states.

in them from the county medical societies. The AMA's opposition to HMOs became very choleric and violent, with the Supreme Court ultimately stepping in and telling them to cease and desist with their disruptive activities.

Capitation is the opposite of fee-for-service. In capitation, the medical group is given a set amount of money per member per month (PMPM) and agrees to take care of the group of assigned patients (panel) regardless of the cost. This model laid rather dormant until 1973 when President Nixon was convinced that it could help hold down costs, and is the rationale for the HMO Act of 1973 that required all employers to provide an HMO option to their employees. Despite less than inspiring results with few employees acting on the HMO offer, they did prove to be effective in holding down costs. As a result of this success, the U.S. Department of Health and Human Services allowed several states to sponsor demonstration projects in which they enrolled their Medicaid population into Managed Care programs. As a result of these programs, states saved a considerable amount of money, allowing them to loosen eligibility requirements and to enroll more people in coverage. This success was followed by a second roll out of managed care to the general population in the late 1990s and early 2000s in an effort to control increasing healthcare costs. The cost control mechanisms imposed by the managed care plans were draconian, resulting in a dramatic decrease in healthcare expenditures across the nation and over 1000 state and federal laws that directed them to loosen or to discontinue their cost control tactics. The managed care companies responded as directed and redeveloped their plans to more consumer-friendly plans with Preferred Provider Organizations (the current managed care product) replacing the Indemnity plans of the pre-1990 era.

Up through the end of the 20th century, we had two competing payment models, with fee-for-service incenting volumes and all of the associated disincentives, such as overtreatment and fraud, and capitation incenting too little treatment. Both of these models ended up being payer-centric as opposed to patient-centric, neither incenting concern over quality of care delivery or patient outcomes, and neither incenting the coordination of care. Thus, we have a fragmented and expensive system that rewards activity (either too much or too little) at the cost of quality outcomes.

▶ Government Policy and Quality

Although the manner in which payment and quality have become closely linked has been discussed in prior chapters, it is important to also understand how government policy became more focused on healthcare quality (as expressed through Medicare—and later Medicaid—payment models as well as through the government funded organizations discussed in Chapter 11). This quality focus was originally independent of payment models. In 2003, two quality-related events happened in an effort to measure and encourage quality practice. First was the initiation of the national health disparities and health quality report published annually by the Agency for Healthcare Research and Quality (AHRQ).[2] The second was the Medicare Modernization Act of 2003, signed into law by George W. Bush. Under this Act, the CMS formally launched the formation of (largely nonprofit) quality improvement organizations. These entities' purpose is to educate, train, and assess outcomes of efforts to introduce quality innovations.

From the patient lens, they generally associate good quality and outcomes with the efficacy of the treatment[3] and being treated with

---

2 These reports have not been published since 2017.
3 If they feel better and have recovered from their illness.

respect and dignity. This perception of quality has resulted in providers surveying their patients through customer satisfaction surveys. From the clinical lens, quality and outcomes have been judged from adherence to evidence-based practice. Evidence-based practice is based on research of treatment methods developed through clinical research published in medical journals and debated in clinical meetings. The primary problem most clinicians have with evidence-based standards is the dynamism of their development and implementation. Two often-quoted statistics are that (1) it takes 17 years for medicine to adopt evidence-based standards and (2) practice standards become obsolete in 10 years.

▶ The Joining of Payment and Quality: NCQA, HEDIS, and Leapfrog

The story of when the joining of payment and quality became an inevitability in the United States begins in the private sector with the formation of the National Committee for Quality Assurance (NCQA). Initially formed by a consortium of HMOs and private foundations in 1979, it went dormant in the early 1980s after operational funding dried up. The healthcare foundation sector remained interested in the concept of an independent review organization able to assess and publicly report on the quality of healthcare services covered by managed care organizations. Interest turned to action in 1990, led by the Robert Wood Johnson Foundation. The NCQA was resurrected with a new governing board broadened to include employers and consumer advocacy organizations. This reorganization of board membership endowed

the second incarnation of the NCQA as independently able to perform quality assurance over managed care services. NCQA rapidly became, in effect, the accrediting body for HMOs in the United States.

The following year, the NCQA released its initial quality measures entitled the Healthcare Effectiveness Data and Information Set (HEDIS). From those initial nine measures, the HEDIS data set has grown to 81 and has become the gold standard for measuring the quality of services paid for under managed care arrangements. As of 2017, the NCQA reports that accredited health plans cover 109 million Americans, accounting for over 70% of all enrolled in health plans. Perhaps as important, if less heralded, is the substantial proportion of public health measures included—primarily those measuring disease prevention, health promotion, and population-based screening.[4]

Since the 1950s, employers have been agreeable to providing health insurance as an employee benefit; however, when employers began providing health insurance as an employee benefit, the cost was rather meager and insignificant for what they were providing. Following the passage and implementation of Medicare in 1965, the cost of medical care (medical inflation) began to increase about twice as much as consumer price inflation. As a result of the rapid increase in medical inflation, health insurance premiums subsequently increased at a rapid rate that was no longer meager nor insignificant. This concern about premiums was what prompted the managed care surge of the 1990s.

Around this time (1998), a group of industry CEOs were having dinner together discussing their healthcare cost and quality concerns and by the end of dinner had sketched out the structure of what in 2000 was organized as the *Leapfrog Health Group*. The Leapfrog Health Group began with 60 corporate members and funding from the Business Roundtable, the

---

4 Although an unintended outcome, the wide adoption of HEDIS measures led to increased collaboration with state and local public health agencies (Harris, Caldwell, & Cahill, 1998).

Robert Wood Johnson Foundation, and the Commonwealth Fund. Since their inception, they have added numerous members and corporate sponsors (no member count is available), have provided influence through their Hospital Survey and Hospital Safety Guide, and recently developed a Value-Based Purchasing platform providing pay-for-performance incentives. Leapfrog has been very effective at influencing hospital quality and safety reporting over the past 20-plus years, with hospitals marketing their Leapfrog rating as evidence of delivering high-quality and safe healthcare services.

A more recent organization to enter this field is the *Health Transformation Alliance* founded in 2016 by a group of 40 employers seeking to positively influence the healthcare system. They cite their purpose as "… a large group of employers working together to find innovative ways to provide high-value and high-quality health benefits to their employees, retirees, and their families."[5] As opposed to Leapfrog's approach of quality and safety reporting, the Health Transformation Alliance provides its members group buying solutions. They do this through (1) analyzing data to identify the most effective and efficient medical solutions, (2) working with pharmacy benefit managers to influence formularies and incent savings, (3) influencing medical solutions focusing on improved health outcomes and optimal quality of care, and (4) consumer engagement solutions seeking to assist employees in finding solutions from difficult medical solutions.

▶ State and Federal Governments Follow

The beginning of the 21st century began with more soul-searching regarding care delivery and payment and improving outcomes. Every year when Organisation for Economic Co-operation and Development (OECD) countries are rated on delivery and cost of health services, the United States is always highest in cost (double) and lowest in overall quality. The conundrum has always perplexed the healthcare and governmental communities. How can we have the largest global economy; be the research, innovation and production hub for innovative medical techniques, products, and pharmaceuticals; spend the most money; and yet have the lowest overall quality and poorest overall outcomes? While we have always been concerned about quality of services, we have never tied outcomes or quality to payment. With this debate, two contentious questions arise. How do we define good outcomes? How do we define good quality? There are two sides to the answers to these questions. First, what does the patient perceive as good quality and a good outcome? Second, what do clinicians perceive as good quality and good outcomes? (**TABLE 12.2**).

Next was the pay-for-performance program that rewarded providers for adhering to evidence-based standards. Pay-for-performance programs have resulted in less-than-stellar outcomes while providing significant increases in payment to providers. The national health quality report demonstrates increases in overall quality without any significant changes noted in disparities of care.[6] Throughout the last half of the 20th century, a couple of practice experiments caught the attention of providers and policy makers. In 1967, pediatrics implemented a patient-centered medical home model whose purpose was to provide children and their parents one place to go for care and one place who would coordinate their care with other providers and services. This has proved to be an effective model for pediatrics and is currently being adopted around the country in primary care practices. The difficulty with this model is that it is patient-centric and our payment models

---

5 Retrieved from http://www.htahealth.com/faqs/
6 Retrieved from https://www.ahrq.gov/research/findings/nhqrdr/index.html

TABLE 12.2	State and Federal Policy Milestones for Payment and Quality
Year	**Federal or State Action**
1999	State of Maryland establishes permanent Healthcare Commission for the annual comparison and reporting of hospital quality and performance
2006	Tax Relief and Health Care Act of 2006 (TRHCA)/Physician Quality Reporting Initiative (PQRI)
2008	American Recovery and Reinvestment Act (ARRA) with Health Information Technology for Economic and Clinical Health Act (HITECH)
2010	ACA and Health Care and Education Reconciliation Act (HCEARA)—Patient-Centered Outcomes Research Institute (PCORI) and Comparative Effectiveness Research (CER)
2011	Physician Quality Reporting System (PQRS) as of 2011
2011	Final ACO rules released
2012	Medicare Access and CHIP Reauthorization Act (MACRA)

Congress.gov

are physician-centric. Additionally, implementing these models requires a redesign of the office practice and the addition of staff that have not traditionally been a part of physician practices. The ACA has provisions to encourage the development of these practice models and has provided additional practice development funds to bring up these practices and pay based on the type of care provided.

The other model under development is the ACO, which was initially based on a Medicare waiver project that coordinated care for cardiac care and resulted in several million dollars in savings. Currently, there are several hundred ACOs around the country, with successful models being those that reimburse based on either no risk sharing or positive risk sharing. The original ACO model organizations found that positive and negative risk sharing was more than most systems could organizationally tolerate, and while committed to the ACO model, requires a different

and more gradual progression in risk-sharing models. As a result of this feedback, the CMS plans on rolling out risk-sharing models at a slower pace and will ultimately result in positive and negative risk-sharing options. In 2015, the CMS established targets for moving all payments to quality links with 2016 goals of 85% of fee-for-service payments linked to quality and within that amount, 30% linked to alternative payment models including ACOs. For 2018, the goals are 90% of fee-for-service payments with a quality link and within that amount, 50% linked to alternative payment models, including ACOs.

Value-based purchasing—another method of linking payment to quality of care delivery—has also been implemented through the ACA. Much of the details contained in the ACA regarding the moves by the CMS toward value-based purchasing were derived from extensive waiver demonstration opportunities completed by the CMS during the administration of George

W. Bush. (See Figure 12.1 for the progression of CMS programs.) In value-based purchasing, providers are rewarded based on how they score on quality measures. These quality measures have been dynamic since implementation and have continually moved to increased levels of complexity. The elements of the quality equation have always had one-third based on patient satisfaction, with the remaining two-thirds based on variations of quality and process improvement measurements. One characteristic that distinguishes this payment program from other pay-for-performance programs is its revenue neutral methodology. In older programs, providers were rewarded with additional money at the rate of 1%–5% based on their performance, whereas the value-based purchasing program withholds 1%–5% and returns the money to providers based on their performance.

Episode of care-based payments is the other method that is currently being tested. While there are a couple of variations of this model, the basic model is the payer sends one payment for the episode of care that is to cover all care provided within an episode. One variation of this model withholds payment if the patient is readmitted for any reason within 30 days. This payment method has resulted in massive consolidation of healthcare providers in an effort to limit administrative costs and enhance coordination of care. This model has demonstrated limited success, with the primary marker of success being the geographic location of the providers within the community.

The current payment models coming out of the ACA have resulted in massive changes in how healthcare providers organize themselves and how they deliver care. Two major problems that have surfaced during this transition are uncertainty in delivery model and payment. Traditionally, payment changes have driven model changes, whereas now, model delivery changes have preceded payment, thus putting providers in a difficult financial position as they seek to fund two models of care while building the infrastructure for the newer models. Payment based on outcomes is an innovative approach to payment and is impelling a major paradigm shift in how medical care providers organize themselves. Even the often-touted OECD countries, with national costs per GDP half of ours, pay providers either by salary or fee-for-service. If this payment change is successful, it may revolutionize how healthcare services are paid for around the world.

Medicare Access and CHIP Reauthorization Act (MACRA) of 2015 is the most recent federal attempt at linking payment to quality. MACRA was passed to fix the problems associated with the Sustainable Growth Rate statute for physician payment. The statute provides physicians two options for receipt of payments from the CMS: (1) Merit-based Incentive Payments (MIPS) and (2) Advanced Alternative Payment Models (APMs). The MIPS option is a consolidation of three previous quality reporting programs: the Physician Quality Reporting System, the Physician Value-based Payment Modifier, the Medical Health Record Incentive Programs for Eligible Professionals and Improvement Activities. Alternative Payment Models are risk-bearing models such as ACOs that require (1) providers to use a certified electronic health record, (2) payment based on quality measures similar to those under MIPS, and (3) providers to bear risks for monetary losses or use a medical home model. In the final rule published on November 2, 2017, the CMS was generous to the concerns voiced by physicians and other provider organizations[7] providing adjustments to reporting times and a delay in use of the cost provision until 2020. Throughout the entire process of developing MACRA, Congress and the CMS

---

7   The CMS reviewed 1300 comments and had over 100,000 physicians and other concerned parties in attendance at their outreach meetings across the country.

have sought to balance the provision of quality care to patients with concern for not providing undue administrative burdens for physicians. The CMS displays this attitude in the opening paragraphs of the Final Rule Executive Summary:

> Our goal is to support patients and clinicians in making their own decisions about health care using data driven insights, increasingly aligned and meaningful quality measures, and innovative technology. To implement this vision, the Quality Payment Program emphasizes high-value care and patient outcomes while minimizing burden on eligible clinicians. The Quality Payment Program is also

designed to be flexible, transparent, and structured to improve over time with input from clinicians, patients, and other stakeholders.

In today's healthcare system, we often pay doctors and other clinicians based on the number of services they perform rather than patient health outcomes. The good work that clinicians do is not limited to conducting tests or writing prescriptions, but also taking the time to have a conversation with a patient about test results, being available to a patient through telehealth or expanded hours, coordinating medicine and treatments to avoid confusion or errors, and developing care plans.

🔍 CASE STUDY

DISCIPLES[8] health system was formed in 2000 from two separate faith-based health systems to achieve three overarching goals. The primary goal of the merger was to create a new entity with the capital to become a recognized lead innovator in both service delivery and management innovations. The secondary goal was to design, test, and implement across all 50 subordinate health systems a "first in the nation" (FIN) integrated information system across all clinical, financial, and enterprise resource planning (ERP) systems. The third goal was to become a leader in "smart" community benefit operations.

Just 5 years later, DISCIPLES had made substantial progress on all three goals. It led one of the (then) 15 partnerships in AHRQ's Accelerating Change and Transformation in Organizations and Networks (ACTION) initiative—"a model of field-based research designed to promote innovation in healthcare delivery by accelerating the diffusion of research into practice."[9] It had successfully tested its FIN, starting implementation across all subordinate health systems. A senior community benefit analyst from DISCIPLES chaired the Religious Health Association community benefit committee.

Near the same time that DISCIPLES began implementation of FIN, the George W. Bush administration had the CMS begin a series of waiver demonstrations seeking to increase quality while reducing costs—with some savings being returned to any partner health systems meeting the goals of each demonstration. While DISCIPLES did not bid on these CMS waiver demonstrations, senior leadership tracked the goals and methods of each as a way to anticipate future CMS policy change on cost and quality as measured by outcomes. By 2009, DISCIPLES

---

8 This case study, although fictionalized, is based on real events.
9 Retrieved from https://www.ahrq.gov/research/findings/factsheets/translating/action/index.html

leadership determined that the outcomes from the CMS waiver demonstrations would eventually result in new legislation tying Medicare reimbursement to quality—and that, while these changes would begin with carrots, eventually these would become sticks. The leadership team decided that developing solutions for avoiding future penalties should begin well in advance of the penalties coming into force.

DISCIPLES leadership (including Board members) determined that community benefit activities could play a role in developing solutions. This was termed "smart" community benefit and would consist of innovations to further all three goals. With a long history of community benefit operations, the system leadership had learned the value of collaborating with community-based social welfare organizations, local public health departments, etc. as a part of improving healthcare service outcomes. An internal competitive funding initiative was created to foster competition amongst subordinate health systems for community benefit innovations—especially those emphasizing collaboration beyond healthcare service providers. The program was entitled Programs to Policy. The long-term goal of Programs was to build an inventory of successful community benefit projects that could be replicated across interested subordinate systems. To receive Programs to Policy funding, proposed projects needed to address access, quality improvement, return on investment, and relevance for future health policy advocacy.

By 2016, the Programs to Policy funded innovations began producing second-generation innovations—capitalizing on learning from prior innovations by combining components from earlier successful projects. One important second-generation innovation focused on reducing readmissions among vulnerable Medicare patients—where in 2012, "carrots" had already changed to "sticks" (see **FIGURE 12.1**).

One of the most recent Programs to Policy innovations demonstrating the success of iterative innovations that build on prior successes is one that targeted vulnerable Medicare patients. After an 18-month trial, the partnering community-based organization and its extensive use of community health workers conducting home visits yielded demonstrated savings of $7000–$20,000 for each Medicare patient through avoided readmissions. Most surprising, almost all of the "unnecessary variation" in services and negative health outcomes had disappeared among the treatment group.[10] The government affairs team of DISCIPLES health began using the findings from this study to advocate for receiving some share of the savings to the CMS—arguing that CMS savings were also lost revenue for health systems that deliver high-quality, low-cost services.

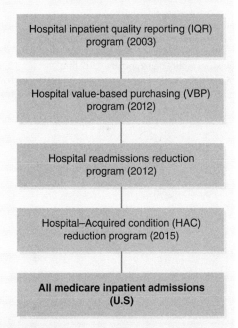

FIGURE 12.1 Progression of CMS Quality and Value-Based Purchasing Initiatives

---

10 "Unnecessary variation" comes from the manufacturing world, referring to excess activity and variation in outcomes eliminated by the application of rigorous quality control analysis. The use of the term in health care stretches back as far as 1989. JAMA. 1989; 262(20), 2869–2873.

Discussion Questions

1. Is the CMS at risk of not providing an equitable return to innovators like DISCIPLES that produce savings well above those from avoided readmissions?
2. Should the CMS replicate this system of increasing accountability for quality outcomes to state Medicaid programs?
3. What might cause the CMS to ask Congress for additional legislation supporting the broadening of this successful quality—cost initiative that has produced unexpected improvements in other health outcomes?
4. What policy changes might be suggested by the findings encouraging the linking of community-based social support agencies?

References and Useful Links

Harris, J. R., Caldwell, B., & Cahill, K. (1998). Measuring the public's health in an Era of accountability: Lessons from HEDIS. *American Journal of Preventive Medicine, 14*(3S), 9–13.

http://kaiserpermanentehistory.org/latest/birth-of-the -national-committee-for-quality-assurance/

http://www.ncqa.org/about-ncqa

https://www.cms.gov/medicare/quality-initiatives-patient -assessment-instruments/hospitalqualityinits/hospital -compare.html

http://www.phc4.org/reports/fyi/fyi17.htm

https://www.cms.gov/medicare/quality-initiatives-patient -assessment-instruments/hospitalqualityinits/hospital compare.html

https://archive.ahrq.gov/cahps/surveys-guidance/hospital /about/The-Hospital-Quality-Alliance.html

https://www.cms.gov/Medicare/Quality-Initiatives-Patient -Assessment-Instruments/HospitalQualityInits/index .html?redirect=/HospitalQualityInits/33_Hospital -QualityAlliance.asp

http://www.qualitynet.org/dcs/ContentServer?cid =112178350618&pagename=QnetPublic%2FPage% 2FQnetTier2&c=Page

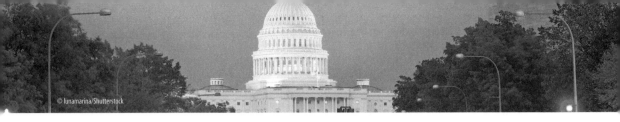

CHAPTER 13

How to Influence the Policy Process

This chapter is designed to give healthcare leaders an understanding of how to influence the policy process by covering the following topics:

- Developing an understanding of the influence of political philosophies on policy development
- Developing an understanding of policy theories and the opportunities to influence policy throughout the policy development process
- Keeping abreast of policy activities through interest groups, professional associations, and legislative briefs
- Developing relationships with legislators, key administrators, and their staff
- Developing effective lobbying skills and tools
- Making a policy case
- Rules on presentation

This chapter briefly summarizes the material from the preceding chapters and provides healthcare leaders with additional understanding, resources, and tools to facilitate their influencing the policy process. Despite the long list of tools and resources that follow, the most important single action healthcare leaders can take is to develop trusting relationships with legislators.

▶ Developing an Understanding of the Influence of Political Philosophies on Policy Development

In order to understand how to influence a legislator, healthcare leaders need to understand the political philosophy that guides and influences the legislator's views and priorities. Most Republicans work under a market justice philosophy that emphasizes personal responsibility and limited government intervention, whereas most Democrats work under a social justice philosophy that emphasizes government largess and social support interventions. It is obvious that these two philosophies are opposites and can be the source of conflict when legislators seek solutions to an agreed upon social problem. As an example, when the Patient Protection and Affordable Care Act (PPACA) was being debated in 2009, both Republican and Democratic caucuses agreed that America's healthcare weaknesses could be diagnosed as cost, quality, and access problems; however, that was where their agreement ended, with both caucuses having different approaches on how to address these problems that were in alignment with their differing philosophies. Many in the Democratic caucus would have preferred to have taken a Paine-like approach by abolishing the current system and replacing it with a single payer system, whereas the Republican caucus preferred an approach that would increase personal responsibility and make incremental adjustments to the current system.

Another way to frame this is by examining the table of *presidents*, healthcare bills, and actions. Of the 95 bills and actions listed, 64% of them have taken place under Democratic presidents, with social justice attributed to 97% of these actions. In contrast, 36% of these actions have taken place under Republican presidents, with social justice attributed to 68% of these actions. When comparing the type of justice attributed to these actions, 82% are social justice and 18% market justice, with 76% of the market justice actions attributed to Republican presidents. It is noteworthy that only three of the market justice actions have been restrictive, with most of these actions seeking to redirect or correct inequities in the market.

▶ Developing an Understanding of Policy Theories and the Opportunities to Influence Policy Throughout the Policy Development Process

Understanding how policy theories and frameworks describe and predict policy actions is another area the healthcare leader needs to understand before delving too far into advocacy. In this book, we have categorized theories into process-oriented and interest group–oriented theories. Understanding where a policy is in the policy process will help the healthcare executive better focus the type of influence offered to policy makers. For example, if the policy is in the agenda-setting stage, broad ideas and plans are appropriate for proposals, with these proposals becoming more refined and specific as the agenda-setting transitions into the phase where specific legislation is developed. In contrast, during the operations phase, finely focused rules need to be developed and understood in finite detail with influential comments very tailored to specific actions and potential consequences. Another process-oriented concept specific to agenda-setting is depicted in Multiple

Streams and Punctuated Equilibrium theories that describe the policy process as primarily incremental with a few larger policies enacted when the "equilibrium is punctuated" and "the policy streams come together moving through the policy window." Examination of the policy data demonstrates that 36% of the 12,000 proposed bills enacted since 2000 have been healthcare bills, with only three of these bills rising to the level of major legislation. The final policy concept that can be drawn from the process-oriented policies is that it normally takes 10–20 years for a policy idea to move from initial germination of an idea to enacted legislation. Thus, the healthcare leader must be patient and persistent when advocating for policy ideas.

From interest group-oriented theories, the healthcare leader learns the value of collective action when proposing policy ideas and concepts. Interest groups are organized in a variety of ways, ranging from topical to professional. The many great values of interest groups include their strength in numbers and unity in action, specialists with deep issue knowledge, and relationships with legislative, administrative, and professional peers (Network Approach & Advocacy Coalition). It is through the strength and diversity of these groups that effective policies are developed and proposed to legislators. Through Institutional Rational Choice, the executive learns the importance of understanding the action area or where the influential policy action is taking place. The official and unofficial rules governing the policy process should assist healthcare executives in where and how to focus their influence.

Along with an understanding of the action arena, the healthcare leader needs to understand the participants in the policy process. First, all participants have goals or objective they would like to achieve in the public arena based on who they are, what they believe, and the philosophy behind their beliefs. Second, as initially posited by Simon, we all have a limited ability to process large quantities of information or bounded rationality. Third, we develop ways to process, understand, and interpret this data. Finally, despite the rationality we seek to impose on our decisions, we are all emotional beings who are affected by our emotions when making decisions (Weible, Heikkila, deLeon, & Sabatier, 2012). All of the above provide healthcare executives an opportunity to build trusted relationships with legislators by building on the legislator's interests, providing legislators with resources and topical data they are unaware of as well as an interpretation of impact and consequences of this data, and finally, providing the legislator with trusted counsel and friendship.

▶ Keep Abreast of Policy Activities Through Interest Groups, Professional Organizations, and Legislative Briefs

Healthcare leaders are busy people who do not have time to intimately follow legislative developments and thus need to rely on others to assist them in understanding the current issues and proposed policy solutions. Despite time constraints, healthcare leaders have a personal, professional, and organizational responsibility to keep up with current events, especially those that affect the healthcare profession and organizations. One way to keep up is through reading national newspapers, such as the *Wall Street Journal*, that provide regular coverage of prominent events. Topic-specific information can be obtained through interest groups such as the American Hospital Association, the American College of Healthcare Executives, the American Public Health Association, and the American Heart Association on the national level, as well as state and regional professional and disease-specific associations that provide regular news and legislative updates. Finally, regular interaction with business, professional, and governmental leaders is another important avenue to current legislative and professional news and developments.

▶ Develop Relationships with Legislators, Key Administrators, and Their Staff

While there is no single influential act that a healthcare leader can engage in to affect policy change, developing meaningful relationships with legislators, key administrative officials, and their staff should be considered the closest. An often-overlooked characteristic of the policy process is that the people involved in it are human beings who respond to acts of kindness, consideration, and genuine interest in policy-related topics.

It is not uncommon to hear the government and government officials vilified publicly because whatever the current matter at hand is has not gone "our way." However, before we go too far down the vilification route, we need to (1) separate government from people, (2) introspectively ask what we have done to influence the outcome, and (3) evoke the Covey maxim by "seeking to understand before seeking to be understood." Legislative and governmental leaders understand that they are public servants serving at the will of the public and have a responsibility to them and their concerns, and seek what they believe to be the best solutions for America.

In order to develop good interpersonal relationships that build trust over time, it is important that relationships be built on the characteristics of honesty, integrity, sincerity, friendliness, listening skills, the ability to see things from another view, and being able to disagree without being disagreeable. While all of these characteristics are important, the most important two are honesty and integrity. The legislator needs to be able to trust the data and program ramifications provided, since these have the potential of being used in legislative

debates and even affecting how a law is written, thus having long and lasting ramifications. As several legislators and administrators have said, "You will only lie to me once." The ramifications of false information are too severe and long lasting to tolerate, and the trust lost is too hard and time consuming to rebuild.

Next, there are some common assumptions that apply to all legislators regardless of party affiliation or political-philosophical view. First, all legislators want to develop and enact good public policies, all legislators care about their community, and all legislators are interested in producing and enacting policies that they believe are the best answers for America's problems. Few, if any, legislators are narcissistic, rather they see themselves as public servants providing a public voice for concerns of their constituency and as seekers of public solutions for their concerns. Most legislators are also interested in the activities and organizations in their community and are always interested in learning about the needs of their community and the creative solutions community leaders are developing. Getting the attention of a legislator can be as simple as attending the legislator's community meetings or inviting them to meet with your organization. When presenting a legislator with a potential problem or solution, always make certain to use verifiable facts, since every solution will have someone lobbying for an opposing view. Do not assume that legislators are not interested in your organization or that they are aware of your organization's concerns, rather use the communication method that works best for the legislator to keep informed of your organizational and constituency needs and potential solutions for these problems.

Finally, among the potpourri of actions that strengthen relationships with legislators is the importance of building relationships with staffers. These are often as important as building relationships with legislators. The importance of staffers to legislators cannot be overstated; it is through developing these relationships that the healthcare leader can develop longer and deeper influence, as staffers have the ear of the legislator. Second, learn about the legislator's interests as identified by the legislator's committee assignments. Provide meaningful comments on those interests as a gateway to topics that are of more concern to you and your organization. Third, learn to effectively listen to the legislator and your constituency. One maxim states that if you are talking more than listening, you are not engaging in effective advocacy. Fourth, remember that legislators are busy, so make certain to be concise with your request, provide clear rationale for your concern, provide a clear "ask" for what you are seeking from them, and provide them with a one-page handout that summarizes your concern and ask. Finally, provide the legislator with a friendly audience of constituents when hosting meetings and, if possible, public recognition of the legislator's service to your community.

▶ Developing Your Political IQ and Effective Lobbying Skills

The development of both your political IQ and effective lobbying skills is two parts of one whole: successfully advocating for policy change. You must learn the political context AND build skills at the same time. Sometimes you will use your new skills when you identify the correct moment in the political context for policy change. In other times you will use your new skills to slowly alter the existing political context to make it possible to later press for policy change.

You should note that these skills are not all that different than the development of good relationship skills. First, speak with unity on issues within your sector and/or geographic region. There are few actions that will drive legislators to move on from your issues than a diversity of opposing views. Legislators are

frequently called to defend their views on many topics, thus they do not seek to multiply this problem! To avoid this, be aware that healthcare executives have the potential to speak for at least four different groups, including themselves, their organization, their community, and their professional or topical interest group. Each of these groups could have different opinions and the healthcare executive needs to be very clear at all times regarding whose opinion is being represented. Do not bring an issue up to a legislator until your organization or interest group is unified in defining the problem and proposed solutions. Make certain your data are truthful and accurate and that your arguments are sound. Next, develop good working relationships with legislators, legislative staffers, committee staffers, and local members working on the issues of concern.

As a part of developing good working relationships, keep lines of communication open to both legislators and your partners in your community with calls, emails, and newsletters that tell personal stories about constituents illustrating the issues and potential solutions. Note that the least effective form of advocacy is from letters or emails—legislators want to know that you have a personal interest in the issue and have taken time to think through the details of the problem and potential solutions. Always, always, always tell the truth. Always know what you are seeking to gain from proposed legislation—enunciate the potential outcomes.

Understand the difference between the legislative chambers. The House of Representatives is designed to be closer to the people and have more raucous, dynamic, and quick debates and action, whereas the Senate is designed to take a more deliberative pace with longer debates and slower legislative turnaround times. For the healthcare leader, this means they need to act quickly when a topic is coming up in the House of Representatives, before the debate is over and the legislation is voted on. In contrast, if legislation is being debated in the Senate, there is normally more time to respond with opinions about the problem and potential solution.

Also keep in mind that the differences between the chambers causes friction—including between members of the same party. If in your first approach you have no familiarity with the presence or absence of tensions between same party Representatives and Senators, be sure NOT to initiate any discussions you have had with opposite chamber legislators until asked. Generally, if you are asked by the legislator (or, more likely, office staff) about discussions with opposite chamber legislators, this means that tensions do not exist and you should feel free to share those discussion. If you are not asked, then, generally, that means you should not offer the information. Once you have engaged with your legislators across both chambers a few times, you will be able to pick up on the presence or absence of same-party tensions between Representatives and Senators.

Make certain to stand behind a legislator who makes a stand for your cause by showing support through op-eds in local news programs and organizational newsletters, funding, and assistance with outreach campaigns. Know that if you fail to stand behind a legislator who has taken a stand for you, it will be the last time the legislator will take a stand for you.

Next, understand and remain abreast of changes in the political landscape that constrain what is politically achievable. Understand that achieving policy change in health care is incredibly difficult except along narrow margins. The only exceptions would be in moments of extraordinarily punctuated equilibria—Medicare, Medicaid, Medicare Part D, and the PPACA being clear examples. Changes in party control of the executive or legislative branches are the most obvious, followed by any changes in the makeup of upper-level courts.

Changes in the political landscape include any alterations in the private sector that affect political clout. The best way to explain this is with an example. Prior to the passage of the PPACA, the American Medical Association (AMA) had strenuously (and with success) resisted all

efforts at expanding healthcare coverage beginning under FDR and up to the Clinton Health Security Act, especially any policy seeking universal or near universal coverage. Just 16 years later, the AMA made no effort to obstruct the PPACA, while several subgroups of physicians actively supported passage. What happened? As described in Chapter 2 (and detailed further in Chapter 9), physicians experienced a precipitous decline in market power—and thus also in political power. By 2009, physicians were faced with payment models that restricted cost-shifting. These same models compelled participation in group practices (at a minimum) and both changes in the market and in public policy led to steep increases in capital costs. By the time the PPACA arrived, physicians needed to stabilize revenue more than they needed to ensure their independence—something that would be achieved with fewer uninsured. Referring back to Chapter 11, a large proportion of nonprofit health systems (represented by Catholic Health Association [CHA] and VHA) had already identified and worked to produce a guide on community benefit definitions and standards for adherence. Senator Grassley (R) used the first edition of the guide wholly unchanged as the basis for the Internal Revenue Service to implement as new administrative rules. These rules were eventually updated and codified in the PPACA—a clear and successful example of the power of established partnerships with legislators.

Even though achieving policy change in health care is difficult in the short term, it is useful to step back and recall where the United States was in 1963, the year before the passage of Medicare. Most elderly persons had no healthcare coverage, nor did children in lower income families. Most employees that had employer-based coverage had coverage that did not include family members. As of this writing, the elderly have comprehensive coverage with high standards of quality in Medicare, and between Medicaid and the Children's Health Insurance Program, most children under 200% of poverty have comprehensive coverage. With the healthcare exchanges of the PPACA, over 20 million additional persons have obtained relatively comprehensive coverage. So, despite the extreme difficulty all sides experience when attempting to change healthcare policy, it is possible, as evidenced by the 50+ year time span described here in which large policy change has, in fact, occurred.

Become a topical expert and resource for your legislator.[1] There is nothing more effective for building a relationship for later lobbying than to have your legislator see you as a trusted and expert source on a topic or variety of topics upon which they can summon for advice at any time. Make certain when you bring up social problems and potential solutions that they get to the bottom of the problem and do not function as temporary, inadequate, or incomplete solutions. Provide your legislator with regular updates and keep up with what is going on through reliable sources. "The best individuals can do is to place themselves in a position to have a chance to make a difference, which includes developing the following strategies: (1) develop deep knowledge, (2) investing in networks, and (3) participating for long periods of time" (Weible et al., 2012).

Finally, there are a series of effective lobbying cautions that all healthcare leaders should be aware of and include in their lobbying efforts. First, more money does not equate to better policy or outcomes. More money poured into ineffective solutions is only going to yield more ineffective solutions. Legislators are looking for political solutions that yield positive outcomes. As noted earlier, incrementalism is the way of American politics, thus it is easier for legislators to back small changes to existing law or small pilot projects than large disruptive changes to public programs and policies. The

drivers of change in increments is that public preferences and budgets change over time. Again, it is much easier for a legislator to back a program update than a dramatic change; therefore, it is wise to enfold new program ideas into existing programs when possible.

Be aware that there are two political views to every story. Healthcare leaders need to recognize where legislative members are politically and philosophically and propose solutions that legislators are able to support. When a proposal is directly in opposition to a legislator's views, the proposal should be put forward only if it can be framed in such a way that it highlights the benefits of the solution that are most agreeable to the legislator—while not hiding or diminishing the aspects of the policy that are less agreeable. Note that all facts will be debated as to their reliability, variability, and pertinence to the public question at hand. Therefore, be prepared to defend the data and its pertinence in the most agreeable terms. Also, note that most of the time, legislators work within a bipartisan spirit.

Be cautious to not be publicly or privately seen as closely tied to a political party. Rather, make certain to position yourself as a bipartisan problem solver. Next, be cautious about the potential shallowness of talking points and that they do not turn into stereotypes. Finally, do not go asking for legislative support for an issue when you have not previously supported the legislator. The reason for developing relationships with your state and federal legislators prior to asking for policy change (or resisting a policy change) is that your chance of success with an "ask" is virtually zero when you first make the "cold" contact in the form of a request. To learn how to make an effective case, we recommend the Toulmin Model.[2]

---

1 Topics frequently of interest to CEOs include organizational context and position in healthcare market, delivery of care, and payment; COOs and other internal leaders include internal organization of care delivery and its link to payment and quality of care; and physicians, nurses, and other allied healthcare practitioners include care delivery models and payment.

2 This model is widely used and replicated in many open source online publications. We suggest https://owl.excelsior .edu/argument-and-critical-thinking/organizing-your-argument/organizing-your-argument-toulmin/for a user-friendly interface.

🔍 *MAKING A POLICY CASE*

Structuring Your Case

The structuring of any case for policy change (or resisting policy change) is best based on Toulmin's formula. Citing Aristotle, Toulmin makes the "case" for his methodology of structuring a case:

> As a start, we must say what this inquiry is about and to what subject it belongs; namely, that it is concerned with the way in which conclusions are to be established and belongs to the science of their establishment.[3]

Before proceeding to presenting Toulmin's structure, it must be stated that when making a claim, you have the option of making an ethical claim or a solely fact-based claim. Ethical claims include beliefs drawn from religion, culture, and/or societal norms. While there is nothing "wrong" with incorporating ethics into a claim as you construct your case, you need to remain aware that by doing so, you will exclude some proportion of the individuals you seek to convince from ever accepting your case. This also is best demonstrated with examples.

- Is health care a right?
- Is contraception a right?
- Is abortion murder?

For each of these three possible ethical components of a claim, you can easily see that the inclusion of any of these in your case will immediately delineate who may be convinced by your case and who will never be convinced of your case.

Claim

A claim is a statement that you are asking the other person to accept. This includes information you are asking them to accept as true or actions you want them to accept and enact.
For example:

You should use a hearing aid.

Many people start with a claim, but then find that it is challenged. If you just ask me to do something, I will not simply agree with what you want. I will ask why I should agree with you. I will ask you to prove your claim. This is where grounds become important.

Grounds

The grounds (or *data*) are the basis of real persuasion and are made up of data and hard facts, plus the reasoning behind the claim. It is the "truth" on which the claim is based. Grounds may also include proof of expertise and the basic premises on which the rest of the argument is built. The actual truth of the data may be less than 100%, as much data are ultimately based on perception. We assume what we measure is true, but there may be problems in this measurement, ranging from a faulty measurement instrument to biased sampling.

It is critical to the argument that the grounds are not challenged because, if they are, they may become a claim, which you will need to prove with even deeper information and further argument.
For example:

Over 70% of all people over 65 years have a hearing difficulty.

---

3 Ibid.

Information is usually a very powerful element of persuasion, although it does affect people differently. Those who are dogmatic, logical, or rational are more likely to be persuaded by factual data. Those who argue emotionally and who are highly invested in their own position will challenge it or otherwise try to ignore it. It is often a useful test to give something factual to the other person who disproves their argument, and watch how they handle it. Some will accept it without question. Some will dismiss it out of hand. Others will dig deeper, requiring more explanation. This is where the warrant comes into its own.

Warrant

A warrant links data and other grounds to a claim, legitimizing the claim by showing the grounds to be relevant. The warrant may be explicit or unspoken and implicit. It answers the question, "*Why* does that data mean your claim is true?"

For example:

A hearing aid helps most people to hear better.

The warrant may be simple and it may also be a longer argument, with additional sub-elements including backing and qualifiers. Warrants may be based on values that are assumed to be shared with the listener. In many arguments, warrants are often implicit and, hence, unstated. This gives space for the other person to question and expose the warrant, perhaps to show it is weak or unfounded.

Backing

The backing (or *support*) for an argument gives additional support to the warrant by answering different questions.

For example:

Hearing aids are available locally.

Qualifier

The qualifier (or *modal qualifier*) indicates the strength of the leap from the data to the warrant and may limit how universally the claim applies. They include words such as "most," "usually," "always," or "sometimes." Arguments may range from strong assertions to generally vague and uncertain kinds of statement.

For example:

Hearing aids help most people.

Another variant is the *reservation*, which may give the possibility of the claim being incorrect.

Unless there is evidence to the contrary, hearing aids do no harm to ears.

Qualifiers and reservations are often used by advertisers who are constrained not to lie. Thus, they slip "usually," "virtually," "unless," and so on into their claims.

Rebuttal

Despite the careful construction of the argument, there may still be counterarguments that can be used. These may be rebutted either through a continued dialogue, or by pre-empting the counterargument by giving the rebuttal during the initial presentation of the argument.

For example:

There is a support desk that deals with technical problems.

Any rebuttal is an argument in itself, and thus may include a claim, warrant, backing, and so on. It also, of course, can have a rebuttal. Thus, if you are presenting an argument, you can seek to understand both possible rebuttals and rebuttals to the rebuttals.

(continues)

⌕ *MAKING A POLICY CASE* *(continued)*

Rules on Presentation

It is our unhappy task to pass on an unpleasant fact—only about half of making a strong case (at least in written or presentational form) is how well you construct your argument. The other half is solely tied to how attractive it is to the eye. While this fact, if new to you, is difficult and disappointing, you save yourself a great deal of heartbreak by approaching your cases with this in mind. Here are a few rules for both written and presentation work:

- Avoid adjectives and adverbs (if you can't make your case without these, perhaps your case is weak).
- Do not fear graphs, charts, etc., especially for drawing comparisons (see Chapter Appendix).
- Photographs or videos at opening and closing are excellent for getting attention at the start and summarizing and cementing what was presented at the end.
- With the exception of slides with footnotes at the end, all words must be legible from the back of any room within which you expect to present.

Remember, being visually appealing is also only half of the story—it can be overdone as easily as too much drab narrative.

Reference

Weible, C. M., Heikkila, T., deLeon, P., & Sabatier, P. (2012). Understanding and influencing the policy process. *Policy Science, 45,* 1–21. doi:10.1007 /s11077-011-9143-5

Appendix

Example of dialogue of reasoning[4]

The claimant makes a **claim**.

The interrogator questions whether this claim is true.

Claim

The claimant produces **grounds** for the claim (perhaps a single ground or several grounds).

Grounds → Claim

The interrogator questions whether these grounds support the claim.
After all,

1. the grounds might not be *relevant* to the truth of the claim, or
2. the grounds might not be *sufficient* to show the truth of the claim.

Grounds → Claim
Warrant ↑

The claimant produces a **warrant** that the claim follows from the grounds.

The interrogator questions whether this warrant is valid. After all,

1. the warrant might not be *relevant* to these grounds and claim, or
2. the warrant might not be *sufficient* in the context of this argument.

Grounds → Claim
Warrant ↑
Backing ↑

The claimant produces **backing** for the warrant (a single backing or several backings, all supporting its validity).

The interrogator questions whether the backing supports this warrant.
After all,

1. the backing might not be *relevant* to the truth of this warrant, or
2. the backing might not be *sufficient* to support the claimed strength of the warrant (see Qualifying the strength of an argument).

---

4 https://owl.excelsior.edu/argument-and-critical-thinking/organizing-your-argument
   /organizing-your-argument-toulmin/

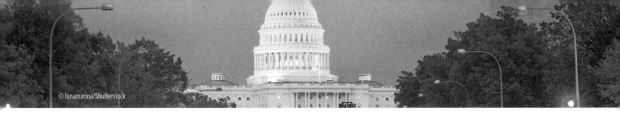

CHAPTER 14

Applied Theory for Professional Advocates

This chapter is designed to give healthcare leaders intending to take a more active role in government advocacy a nuanced understanding of policy making to better understand when, where, and how private sector influence may best be applied. This will be accomplished by covering the following topics:

- Diffusion of innovation theory
- Government agencies and foundations as social change agents
- The environment for change and the connection to market and policy entrepreneurs
- Decision theory modeling and a model for innovation and entrepreneurship within this framework

The concepts of *the diffusion of innovation*, *policy entrepreneurs*, and *change agents* are shared across most social science disciplines. Policy entrepreneurs are individuals who advocate for innovation in policy, and may be found in both the private sector and government. Change agents are organizations that encourage (and often fund) innovations with the intent that these innovations will be willingly adopted elsewhere. Depending on the innovation proposed, change agents may also seek to influence change in government policy with an innovation's success. Change agents exist in the private sector and at all three levels of government.

There are similarities in the characteristics and activities of both change agents and

policy entrepreneurs, which likely explains the application of the term "agent of change" to policy entrepreneurs by some researchers (Schneider, Teske, & Mintrom, 2000). In retrospect, it is perhaps a little surprising that the linking of potential interactions between philanthropic foundations and/or government agencies acting as change agents and policy entrepreneurs has not been extensively studied, given this congruence. Regardless, these two types of actors appear to have a congruence of characteristics and activities, including the perception of possibilities or innovations not previously given "air time," separation from elected constituencies, and willingness to attempt to bring innovative possibilities into the real world. Grant-making change agents (both government agencies and private sector entities) support national-, state-, and community-level change through citizen participation and planning, and policy entrepreneurs go about change through the building of coalitions broad enough to support transformative innovation.

▶ Diffusion of Innovation Theory

Diffusion of innovation theory explains why innovations (good or bad) either succeed or fail to be adopted. Examples of innovations in the field of healthcare administration would include new government policy (e.g., introduction of accountable care organizations [ACOs] for bundled Medicare reimbursement), new organizational policy (e.g., staffing models), and new technology (e.g., integrated electronic health records). Although it may seem this text is concerned with only one of these three types (government policy), the other two types are often components of policy (e.g., licensed nursing home minimum staffing rules and the adoption of electronic health records in the Health Information Technology for Economic and Clinical Health Act).

The theory has four elements—innovation, communication, time, and society (within which the diffusion does/does not occur) (Rogers, 1995). Innovation is described in the previous paragraph. Communication refers to the two-way communication between the change agent (person, persons, organization, or groups of organizations) attempting to diffuse the innovation and the adopters (persons and/or organizations to whom the innovation is to be diffused). Time refers to the amount of time necessary to diffuse the innovation—to successfully communicate to potential adopters what it takes for the innovation to be adopted.

Innovations have five characteristics—relative advantage, compatibility, complexity, trialability, and observability (Rogers, 1995).

Relative advantage refers to the improvement of the innovation over what it would displace. Compatibility is the fit of the innovation to the social setting. Complexity is the perception of the difficulty in incorporating the innovation. Trialability is the extent to which an innovation can be tested before it is fully adopted. Observability is the extent to which the innovation is observed beyond its user and is adopted.

A reinvention of past practice/policy/technology is also an "innovation" that fits the theory of diffusion. Innovations that do not "catch on" do not necessarily die. Often, these innovations resurface after re-examination. The following two examples demonstrate the five characteristics of an innovation across time. The health insurance exchanges in the Affordable Care Act (ACA) are descended from a similar innovation tested in Massachusetts's "An Act Providing Access to Affordable, Quality, Accountable Health Care" passed in 2006, better known as RomneyCare. These exchanges were drawn directly from policy research by the Heritage Foundation, which refined these from the proposal for exchanges in President Clinton's Health Security Act of 1993 (which did not pass). An earlier example of this is the little-known Kerr-Mills Act of 1960 that was the direct precursor to Medicare (passed just 5 years later).

▶ Foundations as Social Change Agents

At the end of the 19th century, large foundations in the United States discovered their ability to influence public policy at all levels of government by funding specific research projects and educational programs (Rabinowitz, 1990). However, these contributions were relatively insignificant until the period after World War II, when American foundations began to take on a more activist role, and the proliferation of foundations as well as the growing endowments of existing large foundations permitted this sector to reach a critical mass that could be seen to have an effect as compared to the comparatively much larger amounts of funding produced by federal and state governments (Faber & McCarthy, 2005).

A foundation change agent's goals include (1) discovering new knowledge; (2) encouraging excellence; (3) enabling individual and group potential; (4) relieving misery; (5) preserving and enhancing democracy; (6) building better communities; (7) nourishing the human spirit; (8) creating tolerance, understanding, and peace; and (9) remembering the dead (O'Connell, 1987). O'Connell and other researchers of foundations agree that foundations often combine a number of these roles when engaging in grant-making decisions (Rabinowitz, 1990).

All change agents, including foundations, must identify leadership for proposed innovations (Ospina & Foldy, 2010). According to Perlstadt, Jackson-Elmoore, Freddolino, and Reed, a "… traditional procedure for finding community leadership [for a project] is for a small group of influentials to approach an individual with prior volunteer activities or service who would be able to call upon his or her business or organization for staff support, and encourage him or her to become the project champion" (1999). However, "… coalitions or partnerships … created by granting agencies face the dual challenge of identifying leaders and creating a local organization since the individuals who might spontaneously organize in response to specific community problems have not voluntarily done so" (1999). We believe that the search for leadership is in reality a search for a policy entrepreneur who may be supported by the change agent in the collaborative development and launch of some innovative solution(s) to the social problem(s) identified by the change agent (Cline, 2001).

Examples of private foundations acting as change agents abound in the field of health care and healthcare policy (Roelofs, 2007). The Robert Wood Johnson Foundation is the leader in terms of funding, number of projects, and breadth of healthcare issue areas addressed. The Kaiser Family Foundation acts as a diffuser of knowledge of innovations primarily funded by government agencies acting as change agents. An early study of foundation efforts to influence healthcare policy decision-making through conscious funding strategies identified a typology of four types of foundation strategies for influencing public policy (Knott & Weissert, 1995). These strategies were identified across two dimensions: (1) when a foundation enters an issue area with funding (early or late), and (2) how long a foundation continues funding within an issue area (continuous or sporadic). Knott and Weissert contended that these two dimensions provided a useful typology of foundation behavior, and defined the types of behaviors consistent with the four types of strategies exhibited across these two strategies. Pioneers were identified as foundations that entered issue areas early and maintained consistent funding patterns. Explorers were those foundations that entered issue areas early but were less consistent in their funding, perhaps because of lower resource levels. Foundations that entered issue areas late but were consistent funders were termed ranchers. Lastly, foundations that were late entrants into an issue area and had less consistent funding were termed itinerants; they routinely entered issue areas late, funded for just a few years, and then moved onto another issue area.

▶ Government Agencies as Social Change Agents

Private foundations are not the only organizations that act in the role of change agent. Government agencies at all levels also sometimes assume this role, and some government agencies have as a key part of their mission the pursuit of goals that are typical of change agents (Bach, Niklasson, & Painter, 2012).

As discussed earlier, it is not just resources that are important to change agents; the flow of relevant information and the encouragement of the growth of information networks are perhaps just as important (Bloomquist, n.d.). Mossberger and Hale (1999) tie theories of information diffusion with the role that federal agencies play in intergovernmental networks that promote federally funded innovation. Mossberger and Hale argued, "[F]ederal agencies promote the diffusion of information to subnational governments to encourage the adoption of certain policies and administrative processes. … [in this activity] the federal government acts as a policy entrepreneur or change agent" (1999, p. 2). Mossberger and Hale not only demonstrated that federal agencies were important primary agents of change with a central role in the formation of intergovernmental information networks, but also noted in their mixed use of terms the overlap between the behaviors of policy entrepreneurs and change agents.

Federal agencies have been directed to act as change agents in a manner similar to that taken by foundations with federal agencies' focus on citizen participation in regional health planning from the 1960s to the 1980s (Langton, 1981; Wandersman, 1984). In these efforts, their activities moved beyond the scope of the development of the intergovernmental information networks described by Mossberger and Hale (Bloomquist, n.d.).

If we examine the literature on government agencies' role as change agents, we immediately note that much of the literature is dominated by the study of federal agencies acting as change agents abroad. This is not surprising because the U.S. government funds agencies whose explicit purpose is the pursuit of social, economic, and/or administrative change and development in countries perceived to lack the domestic resources necessary to pursue change through an inside-outward approach (Kamel, 1999). Although

the scale of these change agents' efforts differs from domestic agencies acting as change agents, there exist close similarities.

Regrettably, the primary contribution of this literature is the study of failures of government agencies acting as change agents. One key reason cited by Rondinelli (1993) for failure is that the problems being addressed are intractable and plans for addressing them are not sufficiently long-term. This correlates well with historical findings of the history of American foundations, that foundations are better positioned than government agencies to begin, support, and achieve change because of their freedom and independence from external constituencies, and their ability to plan, implement, and stick to long-term change efforts. Change strategies of government agency change agents have also been accused of focusing on interests that are transient and serve short-term political interests (Kamel, 1999). Finally, a key reason for failure often cited in this literature is the change agent's inability to aggressively access and develop native expertise and intellectual capacity, instead relying heavily on international experts with little knowledge of local contexts and their associated problems (Dow, 1985; World Bank, 1992). This last distinction in overseas change agent behavior seems to counter the traditional inclusive and citizen-directed social planning approach ingrained in the American foundation community and also exhibited by federal change agents acting within the United States. It is beyond the scope of this text to assess why the difference exists.

There have been few efforts to study federal agencies acting as change agents within the United States, although it is certainly the case that some agencies do act in this manner with some of their grantmaking efforts. In the healthcare agencies, we see the movement of this role from solely grantmaking to a mix of grantmaking and direct government contracts.

We believe (based on our own anecdotal experiences observing and sometimes interacting with these agencies) that federal agencies are more successful in this role when operating in the United States. Perhaps the best example of government agency success in the role belongs to the Centers for Medicare and Medicaid Services (CMS).[1] The CMS has under many successive administrations performed an explicit change agent role. So successful had the results of these efforts been through the end of the George W. Bush administration that under the ACA, a new entity, the Center for Medicare and Medicaid Innovation, was formed in 2010. Although these change agent activities are not secret, the nature of the activities is not commonly known outside of the specific sectors of health care targeted. Many of the innovations to Medicare and Medicaid incorporated into the ACA (bundling and ACOs) were the direct results of a series of deliberate, sequential innovations begun during the George W. Bush administrations and continued under the Obama administrations.

▶ Readiness for Social Change: Context

Many researchers have highlighted the importance of context to the potential entry of a policy entrepreneur into a policy arena (Mintrom, 2000; Oliver & Paul-Shaheen, 1997). Mintrom argues that context matters and developed typologies to illustrate the possible milieus (i.e., contexts) within which we would expect to see policy entrepreneurs engaging in the development of policy innovations. Mintrom claims that no policy entrepreneur is a free agent, because there are limits placed on what he or she is able to do (specifically the matrix on the possibilities of introducing policy innovations) and these limits are based on institutional structures for policymaking, policy settings, and the behaviors of the groups and individuals around them. This milieu shapes the possibilities of action by a policy entrepreneur and allows us to develop expectations about the possibility of generating support for policy innovation.

The political context depends on the openness of political venues and the pace of change within the issue area, whereas for Wilson (1973) it is dependent on the distribution of costs and benefits of the policy. Oliver and Paul-Shaheen argued that policy entrepreneurs operating within Wilson's typology attempt to dilute concentrated benefits and create new or concentrate existing diffuse benefits to build winning coalitions (1997). Baumgartner and Jones similarly argued that the outcomes of political debates vary with the arena or venue (1991). Wilson focused primarily on federal policy change, while Mintrom examines policy change at the federal, state, and local levels.

▶ The Environment for Change and the Connection to Entrepreneurs

In the context of healthcare innovation, it is arguable that social, market, and policy entrepreneurship skills are all required for the successful implementation of an innovation, because these innovations do not exist solely in a social, market, or political context. This is not inconsistent with the literature on policy entrepreneurs, as Schneider and Teske have called for a synthesis of political and economic theory in order to develop better theories around the emergence of policy entrepreneurs

---

1 The Agency for Healthcare Research and Quality (AHRQ) also has long embraced the change agent role. Perhaps the best example of this prior to the formation of the Center for Medicare and Medicaid Innovation is AHRQ ACTION (Accelerating Change and Transformation in Organizations and Networks). Retrieved from https://www.ahrq.gov /research/findings/factsheets/translating/action11/index.html

and the nature of their activities (1992, p. 93). Similarly, Mintrom draws heavily on economic theories of market entrepreneurs to develop a milieu of the market entrepreneur (2000, 2009). It has been argued that social and policy entrepreneurship are required for successful entrepreneurs in the issue area of rural health. Baumgartner and Jones argued that both stability and punctuated change are manifestations of a process that is "the interaction of beliefs and values concerning a particular policy … [the policy image] … with the existing set of political institutions …. [venues of policy action]" (1993).

▶ The Market Entrepreneur

Mintrom developed two typologies of the entrepreneur, one derived from his observations of the behavior of market entrepreneurs, and the other derived from his observations of the behavior of policy entrepreneurs (2000, also Mintrom & Norman, 2009). As with Wilson's earlier typology (1973), explicit in both of Mintrom's typologies is that context affects the ability of both market and policy entrepreneurs to introduce innovations. Mintrom's emphasis on milieus (contexts) is echoed by Schneider and Teske, who emphasize the importance of a community's organizational milieu within which the activities of potential policy entrepreneur occur (1992). Like Mintrom, Schneider and Teske emphasize collective action restraints as the key feature of the organizational milieu.

In the milieu of the market entrepreneur, Mintrom observes that two contextual factors affect the opportunities available for profitable market entry, the pace of change (innovation) within the market, and the concentration of firms within the market. In Schneider and Teske's article on anti-growth entrepreneurs, they note that the "local growth machine" holds a privileged position vis-à-vis local politicians, in part because the market for

businesses in the growth machine is not primarily local (1993).

Within healthcare markets, the reverse is less true. The market for healthcare services for healthcare providers (hospitals and physicians) tends to either be entirely local or primarily local, depending on the size of the healthcare system(s) and the availability of similar services in surrounding communities, as well as on the geographic proximity of the majority of persons using services to providers of the services. This privileged position should be expected to vary considerably across local markets, such that in highly urbanized areas where tertiary care hospitals exist, as well as where the very specialized high-end procedures are more prevalent, the privileged position of healthcare firms will approach (but not reach) that described in this literature. In local healthcare markets where these functions are absent, the privileged role will be considerably weakened. Thus, this aspect of the external privileged position is variably reduced within healthcare markets.

However, one wrinkle to this understanding of the market players with a privileged position is raised with respect to the need to have large firms represented at the table when a local-level entrepreneur is attempting to build a winning coalition. If a substantial minority of the community's privately insured population is employed by firms that are controlled outside of the community, then any effort to engage these market actors represents an extreme version of the privileged position described by Schneider and Teske, because the growth machine is not entirely local; rather, parts of the local growth machine are controlled from outside the community.

▶ The Policy Entrepreneur

Mintrom (2000, also Mintrom & Norman, 2009) developed a milieu for the policy entrepreneur based on his observations of the milieu of the market entrepreneur and on Wilson's typology of the politics of policy issues (1973). This is consistent with Schneider and Teske's "organizational milieu," which is based on the idea that there exist varying possibilities for successful collective action (1992) and is based on two contextual factors that affect the ability of policy entrepreneurs to enter the policy arena and introduce policy innovations. The first contextual factor is the pace of change within the policy milieu and could be measured "… in terms of citizens' and interest groups' preferences, and the introduction of public sector management reforms in and around a given jurisdiction" (2000, p. 118). The second is the number of venues for political participation. Mintrom considers the venues where participation may occur to consist at all levels, from town halls to state and federal legislatures. Mintrom described the openness of these venues as a continuum stretching from direct democracy with full and equal participation by all voters to a milieu where only a few powerful interest groups interact across the venues.

▶ Combining the Roles, and the Use of Information

By drawing on the policy entrepreneur literature and the literature on policy change presented so far, it becomes possible to consider how a policy entrepreneur may combine these roles (Cline, 2001). Mintrom (2000) has argued that the roles are similar, although as Schneider and Teske tentatively point out, the role of information is dissimilar. However, Schattschneider (1975) have argued that along with traditional political venues for achieving policy change, the private market must also be considered a venue for action. Thus, postulating the combination of these roles for this research is a natural extension of previous research. See **TABLE 14.1**.

For both market and policy entrepreneurs, the issue of the openness of venue (represented by policy networks or industry concentration) constitutes one of two constraints on their activities. The other constraint relates to the pace of change within the issue area (whether market or political). Thus, it becomes relatively simple to postulate a set of expectations for entrepreneurs who must act in both realms, since the postulated constraints for both milieus are the same. We would expect that if venues and pace of change in the policy milieu present opportunities for a policy entrepreneur, but the market venues and pace of change present no opportunities, then the entrepreneurs under study here would be expected to fail. However, the discussion of the interaction of different policy venues by Baumgartner and Jones (1993) suggests that such a disjunct between a policy issue area milieu and its corresponding market issue area milieu is unlikely. In fact, we would expect that these two milieus would manifest

TABLE 14.1 Information Use by Milieu			
	Mintrom's Milieus		**Cline's Milieu**
	Market Milieu	**Political Milieu**	**Mixed Milieu**
Use of information	Guard	Disseminate	Guarded dissemination

Dissertation for PhD at Michigan State University, May 2001. Courtesy of Greg Cline.

similar constraints and/or opportunities for entrepreneurs at coincident moments in time, based on the argument that the venues are synergistic and mutually reinforcing. Adding Baumgartner and Jones' terminology to Mintrom's milieus, it can be argued that since these two sets of venues are interactive and affect each other, the openness of each venue in the milieus, as well as the milieus' pace of change, should be expected to covary. Thus, the only concern is the difference in the use of information, tightly controlled by market entrepreneurs, but disseminated widely by policy entrepreneurs.

The matrix presented in Table 14.1 illustrates the information use problem. We would expect that healthcare policy entrepreneurs operate in the mixed milieu, so we postulate that they will guardedly disseminate information as they go about building a winning coalition that may then develop and launch an innovative program or product. Guarded dissemination would represent the careful dissemination of information in the coalition building stage, perhaps by using causal arguments that do not stipulate the all of specific design aspects of some program or product to address the problem, but rather discuss the aspects of the problem, and suggest a number of possible approaches to solving or ameliorating the problem. Once the healthcare policy entrepreneur has built what is believed to be a winning coalition, he or she would then engage in more closed discussions with the minimum number of partners determined to be necessary to the successful development and launch of the program or product.

This careful information-use tightrope suggests that the healthcare policy entrepreneur must possess very high levels of the communication skills described earlier. Guarded dissemination could also be expected to draw heavily on the entrepreneur's existing social connections, such that he or she may discuss ideas, problems, and solutions with a wide number of influential people, believing these discussions will be held in confidence. It also suggests that the entrepreneur may have to engage in more "politicking" than is described in the literature, as more of the discussions that are a part of the coalition building process may have to occur in private, one-on-one settings. Thus, the task of combining the roles should be expected to be difficult—more difficult than would be expected when separately performing either role.

▶ Characteristics of Entrepreneurs

To explain the characteristics of policy entrepreneurs, we will use Mintrom's detailed description to frame this discussion. Keep in mind as you read this section that healthcare administrators quickly discover that a part of success in the field is becoming highly skilled in networking. Successful healthcare administrators arguably are already positioned to become successful healthcare policy entrepreneurs.

According to Mintrom, a policy entrepreneur must have social perceptiveness and social connectedness, and be able to creatively frame social problems and to develop widely acceptable policy innovations. Mintrom describes the characteristic of social perceptiveness as the ability to listen to others and to understand their needs. This characteristic is the starting point for entrepreneurial creativity. Entrepreneurs gain insight on a policy problem by listening to others and using this information to interpret and understand the problem in the broadest possible terms. After listening to the concerns of a variety of actors, the policy entrepreneur thinks creatively about policy in the issue area, and also thinks about what motivates these actors in their pursuit of policy goals.

Social connectedness corresponds to Oliver and Paul-Shaheen's criterion of institutional access, although it is somewhat broader (1997). Social connectedness (institutional access) is the extent to which a policy entrepreneur is already connected, or can become connected through social or political ties, to the key players in the issue area. Mintrom argues two benefits arise from high levels of social connectedness: one is the ability to detach oneself from a particular view on an issue and view it in an objective fashion, and the other is that entrepreneurs have opportunities to present arguments for policy change to all or most of the relevant actors within a policy issue area.

The ability to detach from a particular viewpoint on an issue is critical to the development of new thinking concerning the social problem. Mintrom specifically argues, "... [T]he likelihood that an entrepreneur will perceive opportunities for gain where others do not will be enhanced by his or her movement across various social and professional communities" (2000, p. 126). Oliver and Paul-Shaheen (1997) support this idea by arguing that entrepreneurs, unlike others, are not afraid of change, but rather see change as natural and positive.

The ability to creatively frame social problems in a compelling manner and then offer a solution is Mintrom's third characteristic of the policy entrepreneur. Mintrom characterizes this ability as problem-solving and the search for solutions. Policy entrepreneurs are unwilling to accept business as usual solutions, but are rather adventurous, holding their skepticism in abeyance while they incorporate information from the variety of social realms within which they operate (2000). After arriving at a policy innovation designed to address some social problem, the policy entrepreneur creatively frames the arguments supporting the development and introduction of the innovation to the variety of interests within the scope of conflict.

Mintrom observes that the perception of problems and solutions is indicative of a wider phenomenon that both problems and solutions are socially constructed (also Cobb & Elder, 1983). He notes that this line of reasoning holds implications for the way in which a policy entrepreneur must go about framing problems and solutions. Socially constructed problems and solutions may be reframed through new (or repackaged) argumentation and presentation of problems (2000). Thus, reframing an argument requires the entrepreneur to be able to understand the frames of his or her different audiences, to explain a problem, and to offer a solution that is consistent with the audiences' frameworks. Therefore, an entrepreneur must have the ability to develop a solution to a problem that is transportable across these different frameworks, yet remains consistent as it is presented across frames.

▸ Costs and Benefits: Motivating the Appearance of Entrepreneurs

In addition to the manner in which context affects the ability of a policy entrepreneur to engage in policy innovation, the notion of the personal costs and benefits to entrepreneurial activity is also addressed in the literature. The benefits and costs affect the rate at which entrepreneurs are attracted to such activities, as they have skills and talents that could be employed elsewhere (Mintrom & Norman, 2009; Schneider & Teske, 1992). The rate at which entrepreneurs are attracted to the local political environment is a function of the costs they face in entering the political arena and the benefits they garner if they succeed as political entrepreneurs. Schneider and Teske address this issue by stating that "... costs are a function of the collective action problems [context] and the ease with which problems can be solved" (1992). "... [B]enefits (or "profits") entrepreneurs reap are a function, among other things, of the budgetary slack of their local community, which affects the entrepreneur's ability to reallocate resources to achieve the policy goals held by the entrepreneur" (1992, p. 737).

A successful policy entrepreneur will reap benefits from success and these benefits would be based on the chosen career path of the individual. For politicians, the benefit of successful entrepreneurship is an increased probability of reelection, and increased influence with other local governing bodies and among the local political/power elite (Kingdon, 1995). For a civil servant, such as a city manager, the benefits of success will be increased prestige and beliefs of his or her abilities that could result in opportunities to obtain a similar position in a larger jurisdiction or continuance in office. For an entrepreneur in the healthcare sector, the benefits could be higher profits, as well as increased influence among peers within the same sector or their community. For other entrepreneurs, such as directors of nonprofit organizations, including health care, we could expect that the benefits would include increased influence in the local policy community, increased ability to attract grant funding from foundations and government agencies (both state and federal), as well as the potential for better job opportunities within and without of their community.

▶ Where Do Entrepreneurs Come From?

The preceding discussion of the costs and benefits of acting as a policy entrepreneur begs the question, "Where do entrepreneurs come from?" Most discussions in the literature begin with Kingdon, who argues that policy entrepreneurs can come from anywhere, although many of the examples he provides are from either the legislative or executive branches of government (1995).[2] Kingdon argues that

policy entrepreneurs exist essentially everywhere and are constantly attempting to tie policy innovations to existing policy problems, often without success. Policy entrepreneurs are most successful in tying solutions to problems in moments of crisis, which are what Kingdon calls "windows of opportunity" for policy innovation and change. Citing one respondent, Kingdon wrote, "You [the policy entrepreneur] keep your gun loaded and you look for an opportunity to come along. *Have idea, will shoot* (183)" (emphasis in original).

Kingdon's research was targeted at policy change at the national level. To understand where local-level policy entrepreneurs come from, we turn to Schneider and Teske. They argue that at the local level, "… there is a population of potential political entrepreneurs distributed across local governments. The size of the local population with entrepreneurial skills and ambitions is a function of the characteristics of the community, such as its income and education level" (1992, p. 737). This reasoning is appealing, although it appears that Schneider and Teske thereby restrict local-level policy entrepreneurs to elected officials and government officials. This is too restrictive and inconsistent with broader notions of who may play the role of entrepreneur at the local level (Mintrom, 2000; Mintrom & Norman, 2009; Roberts & King, 1996).

▶ Problem Complexity and Collective Entrepreneurship

The potential that a single entrepreneur would possess all of the necessary skills and assets in a complex issue area and the involved actors would seem unlikely (Shearer, 2015). Roberts

---

2 Paul Cairney (2018) provides an accessible and clarifying update to Kingdon and his theory in his article, "Three habits of successful policy entrepreneurs." *Politics & Policy, 46*(2), 199–215.

and King argue, "As issues grow more complex, constituencies more diverse, and change more discontinuous and radical, we expect groups to supplant individuals as the primary unit of analysis [of entrepreneurial activity]" (1996, p. 162). This would certainly be the case for an entrepreneur seeking to develop an innovative program or product that may (or may not) exist across all three realms: social, political, and market. Developing and launching complex innovations in diverse contexts is a difficult and multifaceted undertaking. Finding one individual with all of this knowledge who also has the characteristics of an entrepreneur would be an arduous, if not impossible, task. Thus, we would expect that in place of an individual, we may instead find a team of individuals, perhaps led by one who is primus inter pares, attacking the problem and pooling their knowledge, expertise, argumentation skills, and social connections to achieve some common end.

Katzenbach and Smith (1994) defined the look of such team as follows, "… a small number of individuals with complementary skills who are committed to a common purpose, performance goals, and approach for which they hold themselves mutually accountable" (p. 45). A collective entrepreneurship team that is complementary and diverse avoids "groupthink," promotes creativity, and is better able to build a winning coalition from diverse constituencies (Roberts & King, 1996). Roberts and King further argued that such a team "… needs support from the community to survive battles with entrenched interests" (p. 45). It is useful when thinking of linking external change agents to local-level policy entrepreneurs to also take into account that Roberts and King warn, "It is not clear who answers the phone when entrepreneurs call in … less resource-rich communities" (p. 45).

This is because innovation requires resources as coalitions need to be built to support the drive for change. Communities with low capacity will likely have few people around with the necessary skills and characteristics of policy entrepreneurs (Roberts & King, 1996). These innovators require support in order to devote significant portions of their time to entrepreneurial tasks. Interestingly, Roberts and King believe that when pursuing radical changes, the policy entrepreneurs are likely not politicians, because elected officials cannot be single-minded enough to pursue change. Thus, someone outside of government is better placed to focus on developing and launching radical change efforts than elected officials. Again, the literature on policy entrepreneurs unsuspectingly dovetails with the literature on philanthropic foundations' activities.

Why focus on market/policy/social entrepreneurs for innovative change in healthcare? By definition, these innovations require disruptive or transformative change to succeed within communities where high levels of connectedness and pre-existing strong networks are necessary to succeed (Mack, Green, & Vedlitz, 2008).

References

Bach, T., Niklasson, B., & Painter, M. (2012). The role of agencies in policy-making. *Journal of Policy and Society, 31*(3), 183–193.

Baumgartner, F., & Jones, B. D. (1993). *Agendas and instability in American politics*. Chicago, IL: The University of Chicago Press.

Bloomquist, K. (n.d.). The government's role in promoting social responsibility. Retrieved from http://csic.georgetown.edu/magazine/governments-role-promoting-social-responsibility/

Cline, G. A. (2001). *Change agents and policy entrepreneurs at the local level* (Dissertation, Michigan State University).

Cobb, R. W., & Elder, C. D. (1983). *Participation in American politics: The dynamics of agenda-building* (2nd ed.). Boston, MA: Allyn and Bacon.

Dearing, J., Larson, R., & Cline, G. (2001). *Strategic grantmaking: Lessons from CCHMs*. East Lansing: Michigan State University.

Dow, M. (1985). Science, technology and African famine. *BOSTID Developments, 5*, 16–19.

Faber, D., & McCarthy, D. (2005). *Foundations for social change: Critical perspectives on philanthropy and popular movements.* Lanham, MD: Rowman & Littlefield.

Kamel, S. M. (1999). *The minimum role of external agents in administrative reform: The case of USAID in Egypt* (Dissertation for the Degree of PhD, Michigan State University).

Katzenbach, J. R., & Smith, D. K. (1994, Winter). Teams at the top. *The McKinsey Quarterly, 1,* 71+.

Kingdon, J. (1995). *Agendas, alternatives, and public policies.* New York, NY: HarperCollins.

Knott, J., & Weissert, C. (1995, Spring/Summer). Foundations and health policy: Identifying strategies in health programming. *Policy Studies Review, 14,* 149–160.

Langton, S. (1981). What's right and what's wrong with citizen participation. In S. Langton (Ed.), *Citizen participation* (pp. 8–20). Lexington, MA: Lexington Books.

Mack, W. R., Green, D., & Vedlitz, A. (2008). Innovation and implementation in the public sector: An examination of public entrepreneurship. *The Review of Policy Research, 25*(3), 233–252.

Mintrom, M. (2000). *Policy etrepreneurs and school choice.* Georgetown: Georgetown University Press.

Mintrom, M. (2009). Promoting local democracy in education: Challenges and prospects. *Educational Policy, 23*(2), 329–354.

Mintrom, M., & Norman, P. (2009). Policy entrepreneurship and policy change. *The Policy Studies Journal, 37*(4), 649–667.

Mossberger, K., & Hale, K. (1999). *Information diffusion in an intergovernmental network: The implementation of school-to-work programs.* Conference Paper delivered at the 1999 Annual Conference of the American Political Science Association, Atlanta.

O'Connell, B. (1987). *Social change philanthropy in action.* Washington, DC: The Foundation Center.

Oliver, T. R., & Paul-Shaheen, P. (1997). Translating ideas into action: Entrepreneurial leadership in state health care reform. *Journal of Health Politics, Policy and Law, 22*(3), 721–788.

Ospina, S., & Foldy, E. (2010). Building bridges from the margins: The work of leadership in social change organizations. *The Leadership Quarterly, 21*(2), 292–307.

Perlstadt, P., Jackson-Elmoore, C., Freddolino, P., & Reed, C. S. (1999). Citizen participation in health planning: A case study of changing delivery systems. *Research in Sociology of Health Care, 16,* 75–98.

Rabinowitz, A. (1990). *Social change philanthropy in America.* Westport, CT: Quorum Books.

Roberts, N., & King, P. (1996). *Transforming public policy: Dynamics of policy entrepreneurship and innovation.* San Francisco, CA: Jossey-Bass.

Roelofs, J. (2007). Foundations and collaboration, *Critical Sociology (Sage Press), 33*(3), 479–504.

Rogers, E. M. (1995). *Diffusion of innovations* (4th ed.). New York, NY: Free Press.

Rondinelli, D. (1993). *Development projects as policy experiments: An adaptive approach to development administration.* New York, NY: Routledge.

Schattschneider, E. E. (1975). *The semisovereign people.* Hinsdale, IL: The Dryden Press.

Schneider, M., & Teske, P. (1992). Toward a theory of the political entrepreneur: Evidence from local government. *American Political Science Review, 86*(3), 737–747.

Schneider, M., & Teske, P. (1993). The antigrowth entrepreneur: Challenging the "equilibrium" of the growth machine. *Journal of Politics, 55*(3), 720–736.

Schneider, M., Teske, P., and Mintrom, M. (2000). *Public entrepreneurs: Agents for change in American government.* Princeton, NJ: Princeton University Press.

Shearer, J. (2015). Policy entrepreneurs and structural influence in integrated community case management policymaking in Burkina Faso. *Health Policy and Planning, 30*(Suppl 2), 40–53.

Wandersman, A. (1984). Citizen participation. In K. Heller, R. H. Price, S. Reinharz, S. Riger, & A. Wandersman (Eds.), *Psychology and community change: Challenges for the future* (pp. 247–272, Chapter 10). Homewood, IL: Dorsey Press.

Wilson, J. Q. (1973). *Political organizations.* New York, NY: Basic Books.

World Bank. (1992). *Governance and development.* Washington, DC: World Bank.

Appendix

Decision Theory Modeling

There are similarities in the characteristics and activities of both change agents and policy entrepreneurs, which likely explain the application of the term "agent of change" to policy entrepreneurs by some researchers (e.g., Schneider, Teske, & Mintrom, 2000). In retrospect, it is perhaps a little surprising that the linking of the potential interactions between philanthropic foundations acting as change agents and policy entrepreneurs has not been extensively studied, given this congruence. Regardless, these two types of actors appear to have a congruence of characteristics and activities, including the perception of possibilities or innovations not previously given air time, separation from elected constituencies, and willingness to attempt to bring these innovative possibilities into the real world. Grant-making change agents support community-level change through citizen participation and planning, and policy entrepreneurs go about change through the building of coalitions broad enough to support transformative innovation.

Based on the preceding discussion, we would expect that a change agent's social change funding opportunity will provide the incentive for (1) a policy entrepreneur to devote a significant proportion of his or her time to the development of a program or product and (2) the provision of the staff and information structure to support what will become a full-time information gathering, innovation search and development, and intensive political, social, and market lobbying effort culminating in the launch of the innovation. These resources are a necessary component because only a well-supported policy entrepreneur who may dedicate significant amounts of his or her time can succeed in cracking the closed political venues that may dominate policy subsystems. The change agent will attempt to ensure the flow of pertinent information to the policy entrepreneur in terms of information sharing on possible policy innovations, networking opportunities with like-minded policy entrepreneurs and health policy experts, and the potential facilitation of entry into state-level policy networks. The change agent will also provide the policy entrepreneur with sufficient discretionary spending to permit the hiring of expert consultants in the relevant areas of policy, financing, and social marketing (Dearing, Larson, & Cline, 2001).

Model Description

The model provided here illustrates the choices available to a social change agent with a predetermined community-level social change innovation opportunity determining whether or not to fund from among a variety of applications to develop and launch the innovation (see **FIGURE 14.1**). This is a model of single stage grant-making—in other words, the external change agent decides to operate a grant-making process, whereby the decision to fund or not fund the entire project is made once with whatever information can be gathered from the applicants.

The model is in the form of a lottery in which the change agent has one choice to

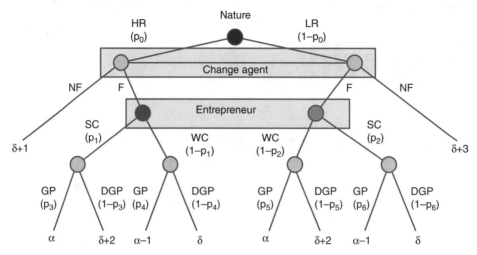

FIGURE 14.1 Single Stage Grant-Making Model

Dissertation for PhD at Michigan State University, May 2001. Courtesy of Greg Cline.

make, to fund or not to fund, after nature assigns the readiness level of the community to engage in the social change project. The outcomes are assumed to NOT be in the control of the change agent, other than the initial decision to fund/not fund. As well, there are only payoffs for the change agent. Thus, this model represents grant-making that does not include a screening process, such as a planning grant.

The model also presents an opportunity for a local policy entrepreneur to appear. As mentioned earlier, current theory holds that policy entrepreneurs are evenly distributed across populations, so the question of emergence is, first and foremost, a decision by the policy entrepreneur as to the readiness of a community for a given innovation or change. However, the appearance/absence of a policy entrepreneur in the leadership of the project is neither determined by, nor known by, the external change agent.

Lastly, the building of a community coalition for the purposes of planning and implementing the social change project must occur. The success or failure of the funded social change project is highly dependent on this effort. As pointed out in the narrative, policy entrepreneurs have been shown to be very adept at building, maintaining, and directing such coalitions.

The payoffs are related to the probabilities of (1) nature's determination of community readiness for change, (2) the appearance of a policy entrepreneur, (3) the decision to fund/not fund, and (4) the building and directing of a coalition to plan and implement the change project.

As stated previously, information is both imperfect and incomplete for the external change agent.

Model Probabilities

The first node of this model is an assignment by nature of the readiness of the community for the desired social change. The probability of assignment of high readiness is p_0, while the probability of assignment of low readiness is $1 - p_0$.

The second node is the sole decision node, where the change agent makes the decision to fund or not fund a change project. Here, the change agent is both incompletely and imperfectly aware of the readiness of the targeted community for the change project. While the change agent may make an external assessment of the project's success, it must ultimately rely on the grantee, specifically the project's lead (referred to as the "project director"), for success in building a coalition and directing the coalition to success in the change project.

If the external change agent decides not to fund, the model reaches an endpoint.

The probability of a foundation choosing to fund a high readiness community (with a policy entrepreneur as the lead) can produce either a strong (p_1) or weak ($1 - p_1$) coalition.

The probability of a foundation choosing to fund a low readiness community (with a policy entrepreneur as the lead) can produce either a strong (p_2) or weak ($1 - p_2$) coalition.

The probability that a foundation has funded a high readiness community, led by a policy entrepreneur, who forms a strong coalition that succeeds with the change project, is p_3, whereas the counterfactual is $1 - p_3$.

The probability that a foundation has funded a high readiness community, led by a policy entrepreneur, who forms a weak coalition that succeeds with the change project, is p_4, whereas the counterfactual is $1 - p_4$.

The probability that a foundation has funded a low readiness community, NOT led by a policy entrepreneur, who forms a strong coalition that succeeds with the change project, is p_5, whereas the counterfactual is $1 - p_5$.

The probability that a foundation has funded a low readiness community, led by a policy entrepreneur, who forms a weak coalition that succeeds with the change project, is p_6, whereas the counterfactual is $1 - p_6$.

The ordering of probabilities is as follows:

$$p_1 > p_2$$

$$p_3 > p_5 > p_4 > p_6$$

Payoffs

There are four payoffs associated with the eight potential outcomes of this model. These payoffs are based on the strength of the coalition formed and whether or not the change project was successfully implemented. It is proposed here that a strong coalition will support the development and launch of a successful change project that achieves the original goals of the external change agent, while a weak coalition will launch a project that is not a true change project, launch no project at all, or otherwise fail to meet the original goals of the external change agent. The other payoffs are either strong or weak coalitions that produce less innovative change projects that do not meet all of the goals of the external change agent. The payoffs vary here because the foundation could likely point to the formation of a strong coalition as a partial success, or the implementation of a partial change project as a partial success. However, the formation of a weak coalition and/or no real change project is of no benefit to the external change agent.

The payoffs are:

α: strong coalition and successful change project (best payoff)

δ: weak coalition and unsuccessful change project (worst payoff)

$\alpha - 1$: weak coalition but a successful change project (second best payoff)

$\delta + 3$: decision not to fund a low readiness community (third best payoff)

$\delta + 2$: strong coalition but suboptimal change project (fourth best payoff)

$\delta + 1$: choosing not to fund a high readiness community (fifth best payoff)

Payoff ordering is as follows:

$$\alpha > \alpha - 1 > \delta + 3 > \delta + 2 > \delta + 2 > \delta + 1 > \delta$$

Operationalization

The expected values of the decisions for the external change agent for funding (EV[F]) and not funding (EV[NF]) are as follows:

$$EV(F) = p_0 \begin{pmatrix} p_1 \left(p_3\alpha + \left(1 - p_3\right)\left(\delta + 2\right)\right) + \\ \left(1 - p_1\right)\left(p_4(\alpha - 1) + \left(1 - p_4\right)\delta \right) \end{pmatrix}$$
$$+ \left(1 - p_0\right) \begin{pmatrix} p_2 \left(p_5\alpha + \left(1 - p_5\right)\left(\delta + 2\right)\right) + \\ \left(1 - p_2\right)\left(p_6(\alpha - 1) + \left(1 - p_6\right)\delta \right) \end{pmatrix}.$$

$$EV(NF) = p_0(\delta + 1) + (1 - p_0)(\delta + 3).$$

The external change agent should choose to fund when EV(F) ≥ EV(NF).

The key questions are:

1. How do changes in the probabilities affect this decision? In other words, how does an external change agent identify a window of opportunity to fund change?

2. How do the values of α and δ affect the evaluation of this decision? In other words, what are the best and worst outcomes, should a change agent decide to fund?

▶ Results

The illustration of results will be done through several examples.

Example 1

$\alpha = 5$, $\delta = 0$, $p_0 = 0.47$, $p_1 = 0.53$, $p_2 = 0.46$, $p_3 = 0.70$, $p_4 = 0.24$, $p_5 = 0.47$, and $p_6 = 0.21$.

EV(F) = 3.3 and EV(NF) = 2.1. The decision should be to fund.

If we relax the assumption of incomplete information and permit it to be complete, the change agent will determine the probability that the community is of high readiness to be a little less than even. Keeping in mind that the latter sets of probabilities are determined by the presence of a policy entrepreneur, we can see the value of the presence/absence of such a leader for the change project.

Example 2

$\alpha = 5$, $\delta = 0$, $p_0 = 0.31$, $p_1 = 0.47$, $p_2 = 0.28$, $p_3 = 0.31$, $p_4 = 0.15$, $p_5 = 0.30$, and $p_6 = 0.02$.

EV(F) = 2.2 and EV(NF) = 2.4. The decision should be to not fund.

With only a change in probabilities, but not payoffs, the decision should be to not fund the change effort. However, this would only be in the presence of better information on readiness than is commonly held by external change agents engaged in on stage grant funding processes.

Example 3

$\alpha = 10$, $\delta = 0$, $p_0 = 0.31$, $p_1 = 0.47$, $p_2 = 0.28$, $p_3 = 0.31$, $p_4 = 0.15$, $p_5 = 0.30$, and $p_6 = 0.02$.

EV(F) = 6.6 and EV(NF) = 2.4. The decision should be to fund.

With only a change in payoffs, but not probabilities, the decision should be to fund the change effort. Here we can see that a piece of the puzzle on external change agents' decisions to fund or not fund change projects is based less on the probabilities than it is on how much value they place on α over δ. This should come as little surprise, as it would be natural that a change project that was strongly valued could be undertaken despite a belief that the associated probabilities for success were somewhat low.[3] Again, this would only be in the presence of better information on readiness than is commonly held by external change agents engaged in on stage grant-funding processes.

It will be noted that the value for δ has not been set below zero. This is purposely done, as there is no evidence that foundations engaged in social change efforts suffer negative penalties for failed initiatives, and thus do not punish directing officers.

Implications

The first and most obvious conclusion of this model (**FIGURE 14.2**) is that community readiness trumps the presence of entrepreneurial

---

3   What may come as a surprise is that there is evidence that grant-makers in foundations in fact do not always act in this manner. See Duncan (2004) for a longer discussion of the problem with the space between best and worse payoffs in grant-making.

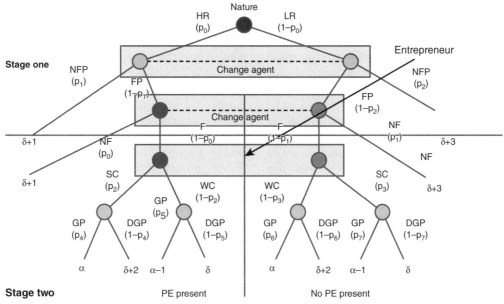

FIGURE 14.2 Two Stage Grant-Making Model

Cline, G. (2011, March 31st). *A two stage model of social change philanthropy*. Conference paper presented at the Annual Midwest Political Science Association Conference. Courtesy of Greg Cline.

leadership. This should not be taken as a signal that entrepreneurial leadership is unimportant, rather that locally based entrepreneurs "read" community readiness more effectively than external change agents. Entrepreneurial leadership should be expected to be less likely to appear in response to a social change–oriented funding opportunity in communities where readiness is indeed low. This is the premise of the model: it is easier for locally based entrepreneurs to assess the readiness of a community for social change innovations than it is for an external social change agent.

Also, it should be clear from this model that *complex change projects should not initially be undertaken through one-stage grant-making*

processes. The improvement in information gathering of external change agents from screening grant processes (e.g., planning processes and coalition forming processes) greatly improves the abilities of an external change agent to determine both community readiness and evidence of entrepreneurial leadership. It seems reasonable to assume that change projects are expensive undertakings, so maximizing the effect of funds expended would demand as close to perfect information as the external change agent can achieve. *Thus, the real decision in planning a change-focused grant process should be on determining how much of the available resources will be necessary to develop and implement a screening process that will provide enough information to adequately identify high-readiness, entrepreneurial-led applicants.*

Evidence from the grant-making world suggests that federal agencies, especially the Agency for Healthcare Research and Quality (AHRQ), have apparently learned some of these lessons and taken steps to dedicate substantial resources to developing thorough two-stage grant-making processes. Fewer foundations appear to have followed this model, with the exception of the Robert Wood Johnson Foundation, which has employed two-stage grant-making processes for large, change-focused projects for over a decade. There seems real potential for a two-stage grant-making decision theoretic model to substantially improve the outcomes of social change grant-making initiatives.

A two-stage model fielded by the AHRQ is significantly different from the common two-stage model employed by foundations and government grant-making agencies. In this model, piloted in "Accelerating Change and Transformation in Organizations and Networks (ACTION)" in 2005, the AHRQ called for innovative teams to be formed, these teams then being able to exclusively bid on future "task orders" circulated amongst the innovative teams for competitive bid.[4] Each innovative team became, in effect, a contractor to the federal government. From this initial group of applicants, winning proposals were awarded pre-qualified vendor status for the AHRQ ACTION program.

The initial process was detailed, and proposals from the groups seeking to become pre-qualified vendors frequently ran well over a thousand pages. In addition to requiring extensive detail on capacity for fielding innovations, detail on research capacity, access to a wide range of electronic data, clear and detailed memoranda of understanding across all partners, and a separate administrative structure for coordinating all AHRQ ACTION processes were also required.

Upon completion of the vendor pre-qualification process, the task order process operated at much higher speeds than normal grant-making processes as the AHRQ could then operate under the simplified rules for federal contracting. Contracting rules allowed for shorter turnaround times between the release of a task order and the order's suspense date, and as each bid came from a pre-qualified vendor, resources flowed much sooner after award than is common for federal grant-making processes.

The altered two-stage process appears to attempt to accomplish the following goals:

1. Search for innovative teams of particular capacities and a demonstrated history of innovation in health care.
2. Reduce the number of full proposals (for stage one) to be reviewed that will not be considered, thus reducing administrative costs of reviewing proposals.
3. Establish a frequent (iterative) process of fielding task orders, each of which provides information on the extent to which each responding innovation team is, in fact, innovative.[5]

The model provided in **FIGURE 14.3** illustrates the choices available to an external change agent determining whether or not to fund some community-level change effort. The model is in the form of a lottery where the change agent has two choices to make, approve a full proposal or do not, and then to fund or not to fund, after nature assigns the readiness level of the community to engage in the social change project. The outcomes are assumed to

---

4 Unlike other granting models, each task order is a contractual bid submitted to the federal government.
5 Additionally, a savvy AHRQ could, conceivably, have sent out "easier" task orders in the earliest stages to use the iterative task order process to "smoke out" the least innovative pre-qualified innovation teams, while simultaneously identifying the most innovative teams.

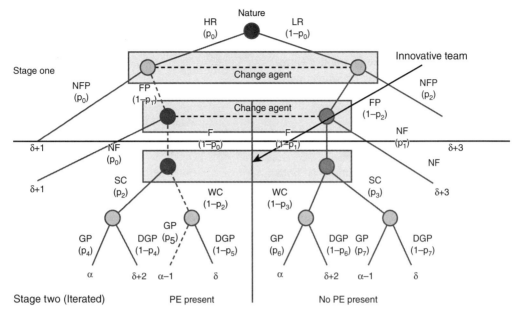

FIGURE 14.3 Two Stage Grant-Making Model with Iteration

Cline, G. (2010, April 23rd). *Should social change philanthropy search for policy entrepreneurs?* Conference paper presented at the Annual Midwest Political Science Association Conference. Courtesy of Greg Cline.

NOT be in the control of the change agent, other than the initial decisions to approve/not approve a full proposal and the second decision to fund/not fund. As well, there are only payoffs for the change agent.

The model also presents an opportunity for a local policy entrepreneur to appear. As mentioned earlier, current theory holds that policy entrepreneurs are evenly distributed across populations, so the question of emergence is, first and foremost, a decision by the policy entrepreneur as to the readiness of a community for a given innovation or change. However, the appearance/absence of a policy entrepreneur in the leadership of the project is

neither determined, nor known, by the external change agent at the first stage, although additional information in the second stage is assumed to improve the chances of eliciting that information. Additionally, as time passes, the iterative nature of stage two provides more information on each bidder.

Lastly, the building of a community coalition for the purposes of planning and implementing the social change project must occur. The success of failure of the funded social change project is highly dependent on this effort. As discussed in a previous paper, policy entrepreneurs have been shown to be very adept at building, maintaining, and directing such coalitions.

The payoffs are related to the probabilities of (1) nature's determination of community readiness for change, (2) the decision to fund/not fund, (3) the appearance of a policy entrepreneur, and (4) the building and directing of a coalition to plan and implement the change project.

Information Constraints

As stated previously, information is both imperfect and incomplete for the external change agent at stage one, with some improvement in information at stage two that continues to improve as the iterative task orders are let.

Model Probabilities

Remain the same as the common two-stage model.

Payoffs

The model payoffs remain the same as in the one stage model.

Payoff ordering is as follows:

$$\alpha > \alpha - 1 > \delta + 3 > \delta + 2 > \delta + 1 > \delta$$

Operationalization

Stage One

The expected value calculations of the decisions for the external change agent for granting pre-qualified vendor status (EV [FP]) and not (EV [NFP]) are as follows:

$$\text{EV(FP)} = p_0 \begin{pmatrix} p_1\big(p_3\alpha + (1-p_3)(\delta+2)\big) + \\ (1-p_1)\big(p_4(\alpha-1+(1-p_4)\delta)\big) \end{pmatrix}$$
$$+ (1-p_0) \begin{pmatrix} p_2\big(p_5\alpha + (1-p_5)(\delta+2)\big) + \\ (1-p_2)\big(p_6(\alpha-1)+(1-p_6)\delta\big) \end{pmatrix}.$$

$$\text{EV(NFP)} = p_0(\delta+1) + (1-p_0)(\delta+3).$$

Stage Two

The expected value calculations of the decisions for the external change agent to fund a task order bid (EV [F]) and not (EV [NF]) are as follows:

$$\text{EV(F)} = p_0 \begin{pmatrix} p_1\big(p_3\alpha + (1-p_3)(\delta+2)\big) + \\ (1-p_1)\big(p_4(\alpha-1+(1-p_4)\delta)\big) \end{pmatrix}$$
$$+ (1-p_0) \begin{pmatrix} p_2\big(p_5\alpha + (1-p_5)(\delta+2)\big) + \\ (1-p_2)\big(p_6(\alpha-1)+(1-p_6)\delta\big) \end{pmatrix}.$$

$$\text{EV(NF)} = p_0(\delta+1) + (1-p_0)(\delta+3).$$

Discussion

The differences in these three models are outlined, later. The one-stage model is a one-shot affair, one roll of the dice. The two-stage model offers real benefits over the single stage, and appears amenable to any typical grant-funded social change effort where one-shot models are employed. While more *time* is required for two-stage processes, the total *resource dedication* of the funder is likely nearly the same as in the one-stage process, or may even be less. There is no concrete evidence yet to make this assessment, although there is little reason to believe that the resource commitment would be larger. The grant-maker best known for this model is the Robert Wood Johnson Foundation, which has converted virtually all of its grant-making processes to this two-stage model.

The second two-stage process appears the same as the other two-stage process, with two improvements: the first stage is considerably more rigorous and the second stage is iterated many times each year. This iteration yields significant clues to the grantor, and also has effects on the innovative teams responding to task orders. While it would appear that the two-stage process with iteration has the most benefits for a funder, it would also appear to be restricted in its applicability. At this time, the only known use of this model is in health-care innovations, where it is known that employment of many emerging technologies for organizing care, as well as increasing quality, requires substantial social and/or cultural change in order to succeed. What isn't so clear is that most areas where grant-makers seek to encourage social change are similarly situated.

The real efficiencies in the iterated two-stage model may not be realized until iteration has proceeded. It is easy to imagine situations where competent reviewers let slip a "less than ready" innovation team into the group. However, since future resources are also competitively let, these future competitions could serve as additional information helping the administrators of the process detect lower quality innovation teams that survived the first two processes.

The iterative two-stage process does require additional resources *prior* to granting resources for social change. However, without further research, it is not possible to assume these are cost prohibitive, unless we can gain some sense of what these costs are, compared to other processes, and the rate of successful launching of funded change initiatives. The drafting of the initial proposal requirements for the pool of entrants is a significant task, but at the same time, the daunting requirements should shrink the potential pool of applicants, thus reducing the number of reviewed applications. In addition, the second stage acts as an iterative real screen, and likely serves to detect any remaining disguised innovative teams. Thus, one may safely assume that the payoffs for task orders in the iterative two-stage process have probabilities of success that are significantly higher than the two-stage model, and far higher than a one-stage model.

▶ Conclusion

The models strongly suggest that when private foundations or government agencies determine on a course to encourage social change

innovations, the common two-stage grant-making model should always be employed. Further research that assesses the resource costs and success rates of both the common two-stage model and the iterated two-stage model would need to be conducted to determine the efficiency gains of employing the iterated two-stage model over the common two-stage model. The potential for the iterative two-stage model seems large; however, research aimed at teasing out the circumstances when such a model can be used over the common two-stage model would need to be performed before attempting to employ it beyond its sole current use: the AHRQ ACTION process.

Two Types of Change Agents: Lessons from Applying Decision-Theoretic Models

It is arguable that social change agent grant-makers fall into two categories: (1) those that focus on specific communities over time (regardless of the issue area focus) and (2) those that focus time on specific issues over time (regardless of the location of the grant-ees). Social change grant-makers that focus on specific communities over time would appear more likely to face applications and also to fund from a limited set of agencies and organizations (and a limited set of collections of the same). Social change grant-makers facing this environment would be best served by using multiple versions of the single-stage decision model, one for each potential applicant and collection of applicants. Over time, the grant-maker could refine the probabilities for each model based on prior outcomes using Bayesian information updating methods. This would be accomplished by identifying the lead person (or persons) for each project funded and assessing the success of the project to achieve the desired social change objective. Within a few cycles of grant-making, the foundation could substantially improve the predictive power of this single-stage model. It is entirely possible that for foundations that focus over long periods of time within specific communities that the predictive power of the single-stage model would surpass the power of a two-stage model. This makes intuitive sense, as the iteration of funding within specific communities would provide a wealth of information enabling the repeated updating of the probabilities for each model.

For social change grant-makers that focus on a specific issue but not on specific communities, a two-stage grant-making model would seem most appropriate in all cases. Grant-makers of this type will not regularly accumulate information on specific applicant agencies, organizations, or collectives of the same. The use of a screening process (as described earlier) would greatly improve the chances of successfully achieving the desired social change innovations.

At least one federal agency, the AHRQ, appears to have merged these two types of grant-making—perhaps arriving at the same conclusions regarding the identification of entrepreneurially led collectives. The AHRQ develops some large social change innovation projects using first a two-stage application process. Upon completion of the two-stage process, however, there is no grant awarded. Instead, the two-stage process identifies a pool of applicants to whom—over a period of several years—various social change innovation funding opportunities are sent. Using this process, the AHRQ has effectively used BOTH a two-stage model and iterative one-stage models that can be updated over time.

Summary

Innovative, change-focused projects and programs in the healthcare context are generally high-risk and high resource endeavors. Change agent grant processes are strong evidence of this and provide useful clues into the ingredients of success for such endeavors. They require identifying communities ready for change and entrepreneurial leadership for the projects to have a realistic probability of success. This look at modeling grant-making suggests that single-stage grant-making processes for social change efforts, which appear to be abandoned by all large grant-makers (both foundations and federal agencies), **should be** abandoned by **all** grant-makers. Few practitioners, researchers, and/or funders would argue that the readiness of communities for change combined with entrepreneurial leadership is the primary key to success. However, little effort has been made to systematically identify these elements, and then use this guidance to design models of grant-making processes that can help reduce the risk of failure and maximize the use of resources in these processes. There have been voices calling for a "rethink" of the overall strategy of grant-making, incorporating much of the what has been discussed here, and more. Further research along these lines will provide additional empirical support to those making such arguments.

Appendix

The Patient Protection and Affordable Care Act (PL 111-148 & 111-152), signed into law on March 23, 2010, is a comprehensive health reform act with 10 titles (PL 111-148):

- I Quality, Affordable Health Care for All Americans;
- II Role of Public Programs;
- III Improving the Quality and Efficiency of Health Care;
- IV Prevention of Chronic Disease and Improving Public Health;
- V Health Care Workforce;
- VI Transparency and Program Integrity;
- VII Improving Access to Innovative Medical Therapies;
- VIII Class Act;
- IX Revenue Provision; and
- X Strengthening Quality, Affordable Health Care for All Americans.

and two titles (PL 111-152):

- I Coverage, Medicare, Medicaid, and Revenues and
- II Education and Health.

All 12 titles will be briefly discussed later. It is noteworthy that this bill builds on the themes of increased access, increased quality, and decreased costs. Remarkably little, if anything, in this bill has not been vetted and in many cases tried at the state or local level.

Title I, Quality, Affordable Health Care for All Americans is an extensive section consisting of 7 subtitles and 72 sections. *Part A, Individual and Group Market Reforms* includes sections such as no annual lifetime limits (Sec. 2711) that disallows insurance company limits

frequently set a 1 to 2 million dollars, prohibition of rescission (Sec. 2712) that disallows the cancellation of health insurance coverage when claims get "too high," and coverage of preventive health services (Sec. 2713) that requires coverage of immunizations and preventative screenings endorsed by the U.S. Preventive Services Task Force and the Health Resources and Services Administration. All three of these sections are examples of actions taken by health insurance companies to limit their costs and exposure to financial loss while inhibiting patient access to care.

Section 2717, "Ensuring Quality of Care" is a lengthy section that lists many of the reporting requirements familiar to current health leaders, such as increased case management, decreased hospital readmissions, care coordination, and extensive discharge planning. These topics and many similar topics all fall under the umbrella of increasing quality of care delivery while holding providers responsible for patient care outcomes and cost of care delivery. Section 2718, "Bringing Down the Costs of Health Care Coverage," follows the above quality of care section with a section on insurance company accountability for ensuring that funds are directed toward patient care and that patients receive value (high quality at the lowest possible cost) for their premiums. Section 2719, "Appeals Process," requires a transparent appeals process for insurance coverage disputes. Finally, in this part are sections 1002–1003 that ensure provision of consumer information, establishment of an ombudsman office at the state level to assist consumers, and a process for premium rate reviews.

Subtitle B, Immediate Actions to Preserve and Expand Coverage includes Sections 1101–1105 that address development of temporary pools for high-risk individuals and early retirees and establishment of a website for state residents to identify affordable health insurance options.

Subtitle C, Quality Health Insurance Coverage for All Americans has two parts that include: Part I, Health Insurance Market Reforms, and II, Other Provisions. Part I disallows any form of discrimination, including participation in a wellness plan (sections 2704, 2705, & 2706); establishes premium rate variance by (1) individual or family coverage, (2) rating area, (3) age, with rate variance limited to 3:1, and (4) tobacco use, with rate variance limited to 1.5:1 (section 2701); and requires comprehensive coverage as defined by ACA essential benefits (section 2707), guaranteed issuance (section 2702) and renewability (section 2703), and no waiting periods (section 2708). Part II, Other Provisions has two sections ensuring the right to maintain existing coverage (section 1251) and that any rate reforms must apply to all plans (section 1252).

Subtitle D, Available Coverage Choices for All Americans has five parts that include: Part I, "Establishment of Qualified Health Plans"; Part II, "Consumer Choices and Insurance Competition Through Health Benefit Exchanges"; Part III, "State Flexibility Relating to Exchanges"; Part IV, "State Flexibility to Establish Alternative Programs"; and Part V, "Reinsurance and Risk Adjustment." Part I, Section 1301 provides criteria for CO-OP and insurance company qualification including certification and provision of essential benefits and offers insurance company criteria stating the company (1) is licensed and in good standing, (2) offers one silver and one gold plan, (3) provides the same premiums for plans on or off the exchange, and (4) complies with established regulations. Section 1302 establishes essential health requirements as limited cost-sharing; actuarially defines plans as bronze (60%), silver (70%),

gold (80%), and platinum (90%); and includes (1) ambulatory patient services, (2) emergency services, (3) hospitalization, (4) maternity and newborn care, (5) mental health and substance abuse care, (6) prescription drugs, (7) rehabilitation and habilitation care, (8) laboratory services, (9) chronic care, preventive and wellness services, and (10) pediatric care, including oral and vision care. This section also provides direction for periodic evaluation and promulgation of necessary changes limitations on deductions. Section 1303 prohibits use of public funds for abortions, an assurance of having at least one health plan per region, and conscious rationale for providers not participating in abortions. Finally, section 1304 defines large employers as greater than 100 employees and small employers as equal to or less than 100 employees.

Subtitle D, Part II, Section 1311 establishes the authority for the HHS Secretary to ensure that "American Health Benefit Exchanges" are established offering qualified health plans to eligible individual and small business consumers. It additionally provides an Exchange template and technical assistance from HHS to the states in developing Exchanges. The next section establishes the option and criteria for individuals and employers to enroll in qualified health plans (1312) and standard plan financial integrity criteria (section 1313).

Part III allows HHS to establish and operate an Exchange if the State fails to do so (section 1321), provides criteria for development and operation of a "Consumer Oriented and Operated Plan" (CO-OP) (section 1322), "Community Health Insurance Option" (section 1323), State flexibility to establish alternative qualified health plans for low-income individuals not eligible for Medicaid (section 1331), defines a waiver process for developing alternative qualified plans (section 1332), and provisions for offering plans in more than one state (section 1333).

Part IV provides criteria for contracting with reinsurers to ensure financial stability of transitional high-risk pools (section 1341), the establishment of transitional high-risk corridors for calendar years 2014–2016 (section 1342), and risk-adjustment criteria (section 1343).

Subtitle E, Affordable Coverage Choices for All Americans, Part I, Subpart A, Premium Tax Credits and Cost-Sharing Reductions amends the Internal Revenue Code of 1986 with Section 36B Refundable Credit for Coverage Under a Qualified Health Plan. This defines the

- Refundable tax credit (e.g., adjustable monthly premium of the second lowest silver plan),
- Applicable taxpayer as one whose household income is between 100% and 400% of the federal poverty level,
- Exemption from coverage whose plan exceeds 9.8% of household income, and
- Provides as scale for reduction of cost-sharing based on poverty level, from 100%–199% of poverty level receiving 90% cost-sharing to 300%–400% of poverty level receiving 70% cost-sharing.

Subpart B, Eligibility Determinant establishes the requirements for demographic information and citizenship attestation (section 1411), guarantees payment to insurers based on an individual's household income the previous tax year (section 1412), ensures that those eligible for Medicaid or CHIP are excluded from the Exchange (section 1413), amends the Internal Revenue Code of 1986 allowing the Secretary of Treasury to share tax return information with HHS officials (section 1414), and directs that tax payments to an insurer cannot be counted as income and any cost-sharing payments are counted as being made to the health plan (section 1415).

Part II, Small Business Tax Credit, Section 1421 amends the Internal Revenue Code of 1986 with *Section 45R "Employee Health Insurance Expense of Small Employers"* providing details for the amount of premium that can be withheld for nonelective benefits and additional criteria for small employer tax credits.

Subtitle F, Shared Responsibility for Health Care, Part I, Individual Responsibility (sections 1501 and 1502) details individual responsibility for having and maintaining qualified health coverage, a penalty structure for violating the coverage mandate, exemptions for low income, and reporting requirements for employers. Part II, Employer Responsibilities details an employer's responsibility to provide qualified health coverage automatic enrollment (section 1511); communicate coverage options (section 1512); offer a qualified health plan for firms with at least 50 employees, defining full-time employee as working an average of 30 hours per week (section 1513); report as a responsibility (section 1515); and offer qualified health plans (section 1516). Part II consists of amendments to either the Fair Labor Act of 1938 or Internal Revenue Code of 1986.

Subtitle G, Miscellaneous Provisions provides a variety of definitions of and assurances against discrimination (sections 1551–1560), information technology requirements for electronic enrollment in federal and state programs including correlation of data records (section 1561), conforming amendments (section 1562) that cover a number of technical amendments not covered in the earlier sections, and savings anticipated due to statute implementation (section 1563).

Title II, Role of Public Programs has 12 subtitles and 42 sections that focus on increased and improved Medicaid and CHIP access. *Subtitle A, Improved Access to Medicaid* provides eligibility requirements, federal fund assistance, and mental health parity requirements (section 2001), detailing:

- Income requirements based on modified gross income (section 2002),
- Requirements for premium assistance for employer-sponsored insurance (section 2003),

- Medicaid coverage to children in foster care for greater than 6 months and less than 25 years age (section 2004),
- Payments to territories increasing 30% per year (section 2005),
- Increase of Federal Assistance Matching Program (FAMP) for states recovering from a natural disaster (section 2006), and
- Rescinding of unused funds (section 2007).

Subtitle B, Enhanced Support for the Children's Health Insurance Program increases FAMP by at least 23% (section 2101) and provides technical corrections to the CHIP Reauthorization Act of 2009 (section 2102).

Subtitle C, Medicaid and CHIP Enrollment Simplification amends Title XIX of the Social Security Act detailing enrollment simplification and coordination with Exchanges for those not meeting enrollment requirements (section 2201) and allows hospitals to make presumptive eligibility determination (section 2202).

Subtitle D, Improving Medicaid Services allows for payment to freestanding birth centers (section 2301), concurrent care and payment for children under hospice care (section 2302), and payment to non-physician providers (section 2303).

Subtitle E, New Options for States to Provide Long-Term Services and Supports amends section 1915 of the Social Security Act allowing states to provide home- and community-based care to eligible individuals through the State Plan (section 2401); allowing states to provide home- and community-based care based on changing needs under a 1115 waiver and to targeted populations (section 2402); amending the Deficit Reduction Act of 2005 extending the Money Follows the Person Rebalancing Act through 2016 and reducing the 90-day institutional requirement (section 2403); allowing for otherwise eligible recipients to receive home and community care while avoiding spousal impoverishment (section 2404); providing an additional $10,000,000 to fund State Agency and Disability Resource Centers for FY 2010 and FY 2014 (section 2405); and calling for Congress to act on the recommendations for the Pepper Commission Call to Action for elder care (1990) and Olmstead v. L.C., 527 U.S. 581 (1999) that calls for increased home- and community-based care options for the disabled and elder-disabled (section 2406).

Subtitle F, Medicaid Prescription Drug Coverage amends the Social Security Act to increase the minimum pharmaceutical rebate for single source and innovator drugs and all other drugs, require Medicaid MCOs to extend prescription drug rebates to enrollees, provide for additional rebates of reformulations of existing drugs, and set a maximum rebate amount (section 2501); amends the Social Security Act to add a list of drugs that are nonexcludable (section 2502); and establishes the upper limit of pharmaceutical payment as 175% of the weighted average of the average monthly price and excludes from the average monthly price any prompt pay provisions (section 2506).

Subtitle G, Medicaid Disproportionate Share Hospital (DSH) Payments provides rationale for calculating the reduction in DSH payments based on the reduction of the insured (section 2551).

Subtitle H, Improved Coordination for Dual-Eligible Beneficiaries amends the Social Security Act to provide for demonstration projects lasting 5 years with an additional 5-year extension provided the project demonstrated improvements during the first 5-year period and defines dual-eligible beneficiaries as those individuals qualifying for both Medicare and Medicaid (section 2601) and provides for the establishment of a CMS Federal Coordinated Health Care Office with the responsibility of integrating and improving coordination of care between Medicare and Medicaid for the benefit of dual-eligible beneficiaries (section 2602).

Subtitle I, Improving the Quality of Medicaid for Patients and Providers amends Title XI of the Social Security Act by inserting *Section 1139A Adult Health Quality Measures* instructing the Secretary of HHS to develop a core set of health quality measures for adult Medicaid recipients and a "Medicaid Quality Measurement Program" (section 2701); requires the Secretary to identify state practices that prohibit payment for healthcare acquired conditions and incorporate these practices at the federal level (section 2702); amends Title XIX of the Social Security Act with *Section 1945, State Option to Provide Coordinated Care Through A Health Home For Individuals With Chronic Conditions* including definitions, payment methodologies, such as alternative payment models, planning grant options, and implementation, and evaluation reports (section 2703); provides for a 4-year demonstration project evaluating bundled payment for integrated care of hospitalized Medicare beneficiaries (section 2704); provides for a 2-year demonstration project for the adjustment of payment to an eligible safety net hospital from fee-for-service to a capitated global payment (section 2705); provides for the establishment of a 4-year Pediatric ACO demonstration project that ensures maintenance of quality of care delivery; establishes savings targets and provides incentive payments for meeting savings targets (section 2706); and provides for a 3-year demonstration project of "Medicaid Emergency Inpatient Psychiatric" access, discharge planning, assessment of the project's impact on the full cost of mental health care, and recommendations for whether to continue the program (section 2707).

Subtitle J, Improvements to the Medicaid and CHIP Payment and Access Commission (MACPAC) revises for MACPAC membership, review and evaluation topics, utilization,

and financial performance and requires coordination, as appropriate, with the Medicare Payment Advisory Commission (MEDPAC) (section 2801).

Subtitle K, Protections for American Indians and Alaska Natives provides for zero cost-sharing for Indians at or below 300% of the poverty level in qualified health plans, states that Indian-specific health programs are the payer of last resort and provides express enrollment of Indians in Medicaid and CHIP (section 2901), and makes permanent Indian hospital and clinic full reimbursement for Medicare Part B services (section 2902).

Subtitle L, Maternal and Child Health Services amends Title V of the Social Security Act with *Section 511, Maternal, Infant, and Early Childhood Home Visiting Program* that provides grants for the development of childhood home visitation programs including all eligibility and evaluation requirements (section 2951), provides for the continuation of research including grant provisions on postpartum depression (section 2952), amends Title V of the Social Security Act with *Section 513 Personal Responsibility Education* providing grant funding for adolescent-targeted sexually transmitted disease and pregnancy prevention programs (section 2953), restores funding for abstinence training (section 2954), and provides for the execution of a healthcare power of attorney for youths aging out of the foster care system (section 2955).

Title III, Improving the Quality and Efficiency of Health Care has 7 subtitles and 95 sections that focus on linking access and quality of care to payment for services. *Subtitle A, Transforming the Health Care Delivery System,* Part I, Linking Payment to Quality Outcomes Under the Medicare Program through amendments for the appropriate sections of the Social Security Act. This provides a directive for the Secretary of HHS to establish a hospital value-based purchasing program effective

FY 2013 (section 3001). This is to be revenue neutral through fiscal incentives limitation being equal to the total amount of the reduced payments for all hospitals. The program criteria include at least quality improvement measurements of acute myocardial infarction, heart failure, pneumonia, surgical care improvement project, healthcare-acquired infections, Hospital Consumer Assessment of Healthcare Providers and Systems (HCAHPS), and efficiency (Medicare spending per beneficiary). The section provides additional guidance for program exclusion, implementation, and evaluation. This includes improvements in the physician quality reporting program including integration of the physician quality reporting program with meaningful use and additional criteria for inclusions, exclusions, waivers, implementation, and evaluation (section 3002). It directs the Secretary of HHS to improve the physician feedback program through the use of claims data to measure the resources necessary for care, develops an episode grouper that combines clinically related items and services into the episode of care, and provides guidance on utilization review and data analysis (section 3003). It also provides:

- Quality reporting guidance for long-term care hospitals, rehabilitation inpatient units, and hospices with payment reductions of 2% beginning in 2014 for not reporting (section 3004);
- Quality reporting criteria for PPS-exempt cancer hospitals beginning FY2014 (section 3005);
- Criteria for the Secretary of HHS to use in the development of a value-based purchasing program for skilled nursing facilities and home health agencies (section 3006);
- Criteria for development of a risk-adjusted value-based payment modifier providing a differential for the quality of care delivered to patients by physicians or physician groups (section 3007); and

- Criteria for risk-adjusted reduction in payment to hospitals of up to 99% for hospital-acquired infections beginning FY 2015 (section 3008).

Part II, National Strategy to Improve Health Care Quality amends Title III of the Public Health Service Act with *Part S, Health Care Quality Programs, Subpart I, National Strategy for Quality Improvement in Health Care, Sec. 399HH*. This directs:

- The Secretary of HHS "to establish a national strategy to improve the delivery of patient care services, patient health outcomes, and population health" (section 3011) and
- The president to convene an Interagency Working Group on Health Care Quality to ensure coordination, collaboration, and communication to reduce and align quality improvement efforts (section 3012).

It then amends Title IX of the Public Health Service Act with *Part D, Health Care Quality Improvement, Subpart I, Quality Measure Development, Sec. 931*. This directs the Secretary of HHS on:

- Developing a process for the development and continual evaluation of quality measures (section 3013) and
- Developing and using a multi-stakeholder group for the selection of quality measurements and improvement in population health and the implementation of the national health strategy (section 3014).

It amends Title III of the Public Health Service Act with *Sec. 399II, Collection and Analysis of Data for Quality and Resource Use Measures*. It directs the Secretary of HHS to collect, aggregate, and analyze quality data from a broad range of patient populations, providers, and geographic areas. The Secretary is allowed to provide grants and enter into contracts to provide the aggregation and analysis of these data and is provided with direction of the public reporting of these data analytic results (section 3015).

Part III, "Encouraging Development of New Patient Care Models":

- Amends Title XI of the Social Security Act to appropriate funds for the establishment by CMS of an innovation center to test payment and care delivery models that enhance the effective and efficient coordination and delivery of care in a cost-effective manner (section 3021);

- Amends Title XVIII of the Social Security Act to establish a shared savings program for ACOs providing cost-effective, coordinated care with demonstrated quality outcomes (section 3022);

- Amends Title XVIII of the Social Security Act with a new section National Pilot Program on Payment Bundling that provides criteria for the establishment of a bundled payment program focused on integrating care, reducing hospital readmissions, and improving patient-centered care and patient outcomes within a 3-day episode (section 3023);

- Amends Title XVIII of the Social Security Act with a new section, Independence at Home Medical Practice Demonstration Program, which provides criteria for the establishment and evaluation of home care provided by a physician-led team caring for frail patients with 2 or more chronic conditions resulting in a reduced use of hospital resources, improved patient outcomes, and increased efficiency of care (section 3024);

- Amends Section 1886 of the Social Security Act and provides criteria for the reduction of payments to hospitals that demonstrate an excessive number of hospital admissions and readmissions (section 3025);

- Provides criteria for the establishment of community care transition programs that seek to reduce readmissions and improve the quality of care for frail individuals with mental health concerns, multiple readmissions, and other chronic illnesses (section 3026); and

- Provides extensions for existing gainsharing programs (section 3027).

Subtitle B, Improving Medicare for Patients and Providers, Part I, Ensuring Beneficiary Access to Physician Care and Other Services:

- Amends several sections of the Social Security Act providing technical corrections and extensions;

- Provides an updated conversion factor for physician payment of 0.5% for 2010 (section 3101);

- Provides for the geographic adjustment of practice expenses (section 3102);

- Provides technical corrections for physician pathology payment (section 3104);

- Provides technical language changes for ground, air, and super rural ambulances (section 3105);

- Provides technical changes for payment to long-term care hospitals (section 3106);

- Provides for an extension of physician payment for mental health services (section 3107), the ordering of post-hospitalization services by physician assistants (section 3108), the exemption of certain pharmacies from quality improvement accreditation requirements (section 3109), a special enrollment period for disabled Tricare beneficiaries (section 3110), and the payment of bone density tests (section 3111) and brings to zero the amount in the Medicare Improvement Fund (section 3112);

- Provides for the payment of complex laboratory tests such as gene protein expression, topographical genotyping, or cancer sensitivity testing (section 3113); and

- Increases access to certified nurse midwife services (section 3114).

Part II, Rural Protections, extends:

- Hold harmless outpatient provisions to rural hospitals and sole community hospitals (section 3121),
- Certain Medicare reasonable clinical diagnostic laboratory payments for certain rural hospitals (section 3122),
- The Rural Community Hospital demonstration project by 1 year and increases the numbers of states and hospitals eligible to participate in the program (section 3123), and
- By 1 year the Medicare-Dependent Hospital program (section 3124).

It also:

- Provides inpatient hospital payment improvements and criteria for low-volume hospitals (section 3125);
- Increases the number of counties and physician offices eligible for participation in the Community Health Integration Models project (section 3126);
- Directs MEDPAC to conduct a study including analysis of payment adjustments to providers and suppliers in rural areas, access by Medicare beneficiaries in rural areas to items and services, adequacy of rural provider payments, and quality of care furnished in rural areas and report findings and recommendations to Congress within 1 year (section 3127);
- Provides for a technical cost correction for critical access hospitals (section 3128); and
- Extends innovative and advanced payment models to rural hospitals (section 3129).

Part III, Improving Payment Accuracy provides the following criteria:

- The development of payment improvements to home health agencies (section 3131);
- Assessing and improving payments to hospices (section (3132);

- Reduction of DSH payments to hospitals, including 25% of previous payments, plus the inclusion of three additional factors based on current and anticipated payments, changes in the uninsured rate, and changes in uncompensated care (section 3133);
- Increasing payment for advanced imaging and reduces for multiple imaging procedures (section 3135); and
- Increasing the payment for power-driven wheelchairs (section 3136).

This section directs the Secretary of HHS to:

- Revalue physician payment codes that have demonstrated high growth, substantial changes in practice expenses, new technologies or services, various bundles of codes, and codes that have not been revalued since the implementation of RVRBS (section 3134) and to use the MEDPAC criteria to reestablish the hospital wage index to a less volatile standard (section 3137);
- Conduct a study of how cancer treatment hospital costs compare to costs incurred by other hospitals and to make appropriate adjustments if the cancer treatment hospitals are found to incur higher costs (section 3138), define biosimilar products, and provide a payment algorithm (section 3139);
- Conduct a 3-year demonstration project providing Medicare beneficiaries enrolled in hospice programs services normally paid for by Medicare and provide Congress an evaluation report on how this combination of benefits affected patient care, quality of life, and cost-effectiveness of care delivery (section 3140);
- Apply budget neutrality when calculating Medicare Hospital Wage Index Floor (section 3141);
- Conduct a study on the need for additional payments to urban Medicare-dependent

hospitals, whether to include rural Medicare dependent hospitals, and only to include those hospitals in the study that receive no other additional payments (section 3142); and

- Ensure that no provisions in the Act shall result in the reduction of benefits to home health services provided to Medicare beneficiaries (section 3143).

Subtitle C, Provisions Relating to Part C, provides the Secretary of HHS:

- Detailed instructions on how to calculate payments to Medicare Advantage plans (section 3201),
- Decreased and predictable cost-sharing by beneficiaries and provisions for rebates and performance bonuses (section 3202), and
- The authority to conduct an analysis of coding accuracy and incorporate findings into risk adjustments beginning in 2011 (section 3203).

It also:

- Allows beneficiaries to disenroll from Medicare Part C plans during the first 45 days of the year and only enroll in traditional Medicare for the remainder of the year (section 3204),
- Provides for specialized Medicare Advantage plans for frail PACE-like beneficiaries (section 3205),
- Extends reasonable costs contracts (section 3206),
- Extends the Medicare Advantage 2008 waiver plan to Medicare Advantage fee-for-service coordinated care plans that contract directly with the Secretary of HHS (section 3207),
- Establishes as permanent the Medicare Advantage Senior Housing Plan (section 3208) and provides the Secretary of HHS with the authority to reject Medicare Advantage or Medicare Part C bids

that propose significant increases in cost or decreases in benefits (section 3209), and

- Updates standards for Medigap plans to include a cost-sharing provision (section 3210).

Subtitle D, Medicare Part D Improvements for Prescription Drug Plans and MA-PD Plans includes several amendments to the Social Security Act. These provide:

- Criteria for the Secretary of HHS to negotiate and contract for discounts with pharmaceutical manufacturers supplying drugs to Medicare Prescription Drug plans (section 3301);
- Clarity on determination of the Medicare Part D low income benchmark premium (section 3302); and
- The Secretary of HHS the authority to grant a waiver of a *de minimis* premium, auto enroll beneficiaries in plans that wave *de minimis* premiums (section 3303,) and extend the eligibility time for individuals whose spouse has died during the eligibility year by 1 year (section 3304).

It directs that the Secretary of HHS shall provide individuals re-assigned to drug plans information on formulary differences and the right to request a coverage determination exception (section 3305). It also provides:

- The Secretary of HHS with appropriated funding for low-income program and outreach activities (section 3306),
- For categories of drugs to be included in formularies of Medicare Prescription Drug Plans (section 3307),
- Criteria for reducing Part D premium subsidy for high-income individuals based on modified adjusted income (section 3308), and
- The elimination of cost-sharing for institutionalized dual eligible (section 3309).

The Secretary of HHS is directed to:

- Work with appropriate stakeholders to establish prescription drug dispensing regimens that reduce the waste associated with 30-day dispensing (section 3310),
- Develop and maintain a prescription drug complaint process (section 3311), and
- Establish a uniform appeal for determination of prescription drug coverage program (section 3312).

It also directs the Inspector General of HHS to study to determine the commonality of drugs used by beneficiaries in Medicare Prescription Drug plans compared to those used by full-benefit dual eligible including pricing and pricing discrepancies (section 3313), along with updated criteria for costs paid by support programs to be included as out-of-pocket costs (section (3314).

Subtitle E, Ensuring Medicare Sustainability adds several amendments to the Social Security Act, providing:

- Criteria for organizational and program-specific market basket updates (section 3401);
- Adjustments of the Part B premium calculator through 2019 (section 3402); and
- An Independent Medicare Advisory Board to provide recommendations on maintaining the solvency of Medicare, reducing its costs, and maintaining or increasing the quality of care delivered to Medicare beneficiaries (section 3403).

Subtitle F, Health Care Quality Improvements amends the Public Health Service Act. It provides for the establishment and funding of:

- Healthcare delivery system research seeking to determine processes and approaches to improve patient care delivery and outcomes, and increase patient safety (section 3501);
- High-quality, organized community care delivery for primary care and

patient-centered medical homes (section 3502);
- Medical management teams (section 3503);
- Regional emergency response systems and emergency care research (section 3504);
- Qualified nonprofit Indian Health Service, Indian tribal, urban Indian trauma centers and public or nonprofit, safety net, or hospitals in underserved areas providing trauma services (section 3505);
- Collaborative patient care decision processes that take into consideration treatment options, scientific evidence, and patient circumstances, beliefs, and preferences (section 3506);
- The integration of patient safety and quality improvement training in health professional education programs (section 3508);
- An Office of Women's Health that oversees the promotion, treatment, and research in all aspects of women's health (section 3509); and
- Four years of qualified patient navigator programs (section 3510).

It also directs the Secretary of HHS to consult with the FDA Commissioner to determine the best way to display quantitative drug benefit information on promotional literature and advertising that will improve consumer decision-making (section 3507).

Subtitle G, Protecting and Improving Guaranteed Medicare Benefits ensures that Medicare benefits will not be reduced and that Medicare solvency will be maintained while improving access and quality of care and reducing costs (section 3601), while also protecting Medicare Advantage beneficiaries from any program reductions or eliminations (section 3602).

Title IV, Prevention of Chronic Disease and Improving Public Health. *Subtitle A, Modernizing Disease Prevention and Public Health Systems*, established the National Prevention, Health Promotion and Public Health Council chaired by the Surgeon General and consisting of federal agency heads and the Advisory Group on Prevention, Health Promotion, and Integrative and Public Health chaired by the Surgeon General and consisting of licensed professionals. The purpose of both of these councils are to make recommendations on preventative health, chronic disease prevention and management, integrative practices, and health promotion to the president and Congress (section 4001). Appropriates additional funding beginning FY 2010 for prevention and public health programs focused on improving public health and restraining the growth in private and public health costs (section 4002). It directs the:

- Director of CDC to establish a Community Preventive Services Task Force composed of individuals with expert knowledge to review scientific evidence related to the effectiveness, appropriateness, and cost effectiveness of preventive interventions (section 4003) and
- Secretary of HHS to establish a public-private partnership for the development and implementation of a public health education and outreach campaign that, among other techniques, may include the use of humor (section 4004).

Subtitle B, Increasing Access to Clinical Preventive Services provides:

- Criteria for awarding grants for the establishment of school-based health centers that provide comprehensive primary physical and mental care services to underserved populations experiencing barrier to care (section 4101);
- An amendment of the Public Health Service Act directing the Secretary of Health and Human Services and Director of CDC to consult with oral health professional and establish a 5-year oral health prevention campaign and providing grant funds to providers of services to underserved populations for research demonstrating

the effectiveness of dental caries disease management (section 4102);

- Criteria and funding for an annual wellness visit and establishment of a personalized health plan for Medicare beneficiaries (section 4103);
- A definition of preventive health and removing any beneficiary cost associated with preventive health services (section 4104);
- For the inclusion of preventive services to Medicaid recipients including those assigned grade A or B by the U.S. Preventive Services Task Force, vaccines approved and recommended by the Advisory Committee on Immunization Practices, and physician or licensed practitioner medical or remedial services at no cost to the recipient (section 4106);
- For no cost comprehensive smoking cessation services for pregnant women receiving Medicaid benefits (section 4107); and
- Grant funding for the development of preventive health programs for Medicaid beneficiaries focusing on tobacco use cessation, weight control or reduction, cholesterol reduction, blood pressure production, and avoidance or improved management of diabetes (section 4108).

Directs the Secretary of HHS to modify and align preventive services with those recommended by the U.S. Preventive Services Task Force at no cost to the beneficiary (section 4105).

Subtitle C, Creating Healthier Communities provides:

- Grant funding for governmental and community agencies providing community-wide transformational programs focused on weight reduction, proper nutrition, increased physical activity, decrease in tobacco prevalence, improvement in emotional well-being and mental health, other community-specific factors from the BRFSS, and factors deemed appropriate by the Secretary (section 4201);

- Criteria and grant funding for governmental agencies to provide public health interventions, screenings, and clinical referrals focused on improving the health of individuals between 55 and 64 years of age including evaluation of reduction of health risks, improved chronic condition management, and reduced use of health services (section 4202);
- A requirement for barrier free diagnostic and medical office equipment for disabled individuals (section 4203);
- The Secretary of HHS to negotiate contracts with vaccine providers that states can then purchase upon submitting a state plan assessment, education, cost reduction, and promotion (section 4204); and
- Labeling standards for restaurants with 20 or more establishments that include explicit display of item calories and percent of daily caloric intake and, upon request, nutritional content of food item (section 4205).

It also directs the Secretary of HHS to conduct a demonstration project at 10 community health centers to determine if the provision of wellness plans will reduce health risks for individuals using these services (section 4206) and requires employers of more than 50 employees to provide nursing mothers a private area to express breast milk for up to 1 year without required compensation for time off work to do so (section 4207).

Subtitle D, Support for Prevention and Public Health Innovation directs the Secretary of HHS to conduct research on evidence-based practices regarding areas identified by the Secretary of the National Preventive Strategy of *Healthy People 2020*, analyze how academic interventions translate into application, and strategize for the organization, financing, and

delivery of public health services (section 4301). It also provides:

- Criteria for a comprehensive approach to data collection on disparities in access to healthcare services based on demographic characteristics and disabilities (section 4302),
- The support and evaluation of employer-based wellness programs (section 4303),
- Grants for laboratories to increase surveillance and reporting of infectious disease data (section 4304), and
- Appropriations for a childhood obesity demonstration project (section 4306).

Lastly, it directs the Secretary of HHS to work with the National Academies to convene a Conference on Pain, encourages the Director of NIH to continue an aggressive program of pain research, directs the Secretary to establish the Interagency Pain Research Coordinating Committee, and directs the Secretary to award grants for training and education on the treatment and management of pain (section 4305).

Subtitle E, Miscellaneous Provisions establishes the sense of the Senate and Congress of the need to work with CBO on scoring preventive programs due to the difficulty of measuring such programs (section 4401) and directs the Secretary of HHS to conduct and evaluation of federal health and wellness initiatives (section 4402).

Title V, Health Care Workforce. Under *Subtitle A, Purpose and Definitions*, this section addresses how to assess the need for an increased healthcare workforce to meet the need of underserved areas and populations, improve access and delivery of healthcare services for all populations through an increase in the supply of qualified healthcare workers, enhance healthcare delivery for all through improved healthcare workforce education and training, and support the means necessary for the existing healthcare workforce to improve access and delivery of services (section 5001). To do this, it provides:

- A series of definitions, including health workers and educational requirements, healthcare delivery facilities, and topical health care terms (section 5002).

Subtitle B, Innovations in the Health Care Workforce, provides:

- The establishment for a National Health Care Workforce Commission with the primary purpose of the need for healthcare workers, educational requirements, how to provide training and regulations allowing healthcare professionals to practice at the highest level of their license (section 5101);
- Grant funding to states for planning and other related activities leading to comprehensive healthcare workforce development strategies (section 5102); and
- The development of a National Center for Health Care Workforce Analysis to provide workforce analytic information to the National Health Care Workforce Commission (section 5103).

Subtitle C, Increasing the Supply of the Health Care Workforce. This revises the payback requirement for medical school and primary care provider loans to include a 10-year payback period, including residency or until the loan is repaid. If not repaid within 10 years, interest will accrue at 2% annually (section 5201). It also:

- Increases the amounts nursing students may borrow (section 5202);
- Provides for loan payment of up to $35,000 per year for no more than 3 years to providers providing pediatric specialty or subspecialty services to children and adolescents in or from underserved areas (section 5203);
- Appropriates funds for a Public Health Workforce Loan Repayment Program

administered by the Secretary of HHS for a period of equal to or greater than 3 years and includes payment not to exceed $35,000 and 1/3 of a $105,000 loan (section 5204);
- Establishes an Allied Health Workforce Recruitment and Retention program (section 5205);
- Enables the Secretary of HHS to provide grants to educational entities providing public health degree or professional training to mid-career public health professionals (section 5206);
- Establishes appropriations for the National Health Service Corps (section 5207).
- Provides grant funding for Nurse-Managed Primary Care Health Clinics that have at least one advanced practice nurse, are managed by an advanced practice nurse, and are associated with an educational or nonprofit organization (section 5208);
- Eliminates the cap on the National Health Services Corps (section 5209); and
- Provides criteria for the establishment of a Ready Reserve Corps of the National Health Service Corps for service in times of national emergency (section 5210).

Subtitle D, Enhancing Health Care Workforce Education and Training. Provides appropriation authority and establishes criteria for:

- The establishment and support of primary care training programs (section 5301);
- Grant funding to institutions of higher education providing training to direct caregivers preparing to work in long-term care facilities, skilled nursing facilities, assisted living facilities, intermediate care facilities for individuals with mental retardation, and home- and community-based settings (section 5302);
- The planning and provision of dental education preparing dentists and oral

hygienists preparing for careers in general, pediatric, or public health dentistry (section 5303);

- The Secretary of HHS to award up to 15 demonstration project grants for training and employment of alternative dental providers with the purpose of increasing access to primary dental care (section 5304);
- Grant funding to educational institutions and individuals ranging from physicians to family caregivers to enhance and increase educational training in care of the elderly (section 5305); and
- Grants to institutions of higher education for undergraduate and graduate education support and recruitment of students preparing for careers in mental health and behavioral health (section 5306).

Additionally, it directs the Secretary of HHS to collaborate with experts to develop and disseminate curricula increasing public health proficiency, cultural competency, and increased aptitude for working with individuals with disabilities (section 5307); makes technical updates to the nurse-midwifery program criteria (section 5308); and authorizes and appropriates funds for the Secretary of HHS to award grants for advancement of non-baccalaureate prepared nursing personnel to advance to the baccalaureate level, increase nurse retention, and improve patient quality (section 5309).

Parts B–D of **Title VIII** (section 5312) requires:

- The Director of CDC to promote positive health behaviors and outcomes through the use of community health workers focusing on areas with high numbers of insured eligible yet uninsured individuals, high percentage of chronic diseases, and high infant mortality rate (section 5313);
- The Secretary of HHS to provide fellowships to address shortages in state and

local public health units of epidemiologists, laboratory, and informatics staff (section 5314); and

- The Surgeon General to establish a U.S. Public Health Track to include all levels of health professionals and provide educational experiences ranging from supporting professional education and post-doctoral fellowships to CME units with the goal of increasing the public health workforce (section 5315).

Lastly, it also provides technical corrections for loan payments to nurse faculty teaching in an accredited nursing school (section 5310) and updated criteria for the nurse student loan payment program (section 5311).

Subtitle E, Supporting the Existing Health Care Workforce provides:

- The Secretary of HHS with authorization, appropriations, and disbursement criteria used to establish Health Care Centers of Excellence (section 5401) and
- Appropriations for loan repayment programs for fellowships and faculty, scholarships, and educational assistance for students from disadvantaged backgrounds (section 5402).

It further authorizes the Secretary of HHS to provide grant funding to:

- Capable existing or future health education programs and the improvement and modification of existing health education programs (section 5403),
- Programs that allow associate and diploma nurses to enter into bridge or degree completion programs and into other accelerated nursing completion programs (section 5404), and
- Appropriations and authorization for primary care extended educational program (section 5405).

Subtitle F, Strengthening Primary Care and Other Workforce Improvements. This provides:

- A 10% incentive payment to primary care and general surgical providers (section 5501),
- Criteria for the redistribution of primary care and general surgery resident positions (section 5503),
- Adjustments in how the hours of a resident count toward an FTE including time spent in a nonprofit setting provided the hospital pays the resident's stipend and fringe (section 5504),
- Criteria for counting non-patient care activities such as didactic and conference time to resident FTE (section 5505), and
- Criteria for how to redistribute resident positions when a hospital closes, with those in the most immediate area having the first option to increase the residency cap to absorb residents displaced by the closure and then moving geographically outward (section 5506).

It also directs the Secretary of HHS to:

- Establish and evaluate use of a prospective payment system for Federally Qualified Health Centers (section 5502),
- Collaborate with the Secretary of Labor to award grants for the development and implementation of healthcare educational programs resulting in appropriate numbers of healthcare workers per geographic area (section 5507),
- Award grants for development of new or expansion of existing primary care residency training programs (section 5508), and
- Establish an advanced practice nurse demonstration program paying hospitals for the training of advanced practice nurses (section 5509).

Subtitle G, Improving Access to Health Care Services. This provides:

- Additional appropriations for Federally Qualified Health Centers and criteria for

contracting with health centers and hospitals serving low-income patients (5601) and criteria for the establishment of the Commission on Key National Indicators that is directed to work closely with the National Academy of Sciences to establish and monitor key national indicators (section 5605).

In addition, it directs the Secretary of HHS to collaborate with appropriate stakeholders and, using the rules process, define medically underserved populations and health professions shortage areas (section 5602). Lastly, it provides two authorizations: reauthorizing the Wakefield Emergency Medical Services for Children program for two additional years and providing appropriations for current plus future years (section 5603) and authorizing the Secretary of HHS to award grants and cooperative agreements as a demonstration project for primary and specialty care practices to locate with community mental health providers for the provision of integrated care (section 5604).

Subtitle H, General Provisions directs the Secretary of HHS to require reports from those entities receiving funds under this title on an annual basis and to provide reports to the appropriate congressional committees on an annual basis (section 5701).

Title VI, Transparency and Program Integrity. *Subtitle A, Physician Ownership and Other Transparency*. This provides:

- Transparency and conflict of interest criteria for physician owners and other investor owners of hospitals, requiring hospitals to gain physician acknowledgement if admitted when no physician is present, and criteria for facility expansion (section 6001);
- Criteria for reporting any transfer of value to a physician by any healthcare-related entity or business including civil monetary penalties for non-reporting (section 6002);

- Criteria for reporting use of drug samples by physicians (section 6004).

Lastly, it requires physicians providing diagnostic services in-office to provide patients with a list of alternative providers (section 6003) and establishes PBM reporting requirements for annual reports submitted to the Secretary of HHS (section 6005).

Subtitle B, Nursing Home Transparency and Improvement. Part I, Improving Transparency of Information. This provides:

- Detailed criteria for reporting any type of ownership or potential conflict of interest by director, officer, or manager (section 6101);
- Criteria for SNF development of a comprehensive compliance and ethics program and direction for the implementation of a quality assurance and process improvement program (section 6102);
- Criteria for the development and maintenance of a Nursing Home Compare Website, including required information and tools to interpret information (section 6103);
- Criteria for costs reports (section 6104); and
- Criteria for reporting staffing, employee turnover, and census data (section 6106).

It also directs the Secretary of HHS to develop a standardized complaint and resolution process (section 6105) and the U.S. Comptroller General to conduct a study of the 5-star nursing home rating system, including implementation, system or implementation problems, and improvements (section 6107).

Part II, Targeting Enforcement. This section provides the Secretary of HHS with guidelines for the reduction of civil monetary penalties for self-reporting deficiencies with a plan for resolution and a process for dispute resolution and collection of civil monetary penalties (section 6111). It also directs the Secretary in consultation with the Inspector General of HHS to conduct a 2-year demonstration project development and evaluation of an independent monitoring program to monitor the performance of interstate and large interstate chains of skilled nursing facilities (section 6112) and to conduct two demonstration projects not to exceed 3 years, seeking best practices for SNF and facility culture change and use of information technology (section 6114). Lastly, it establishes a notification and transfer process to follow when a facility is closed, including civil and monetary penalties for failure to follow the process (section 6113).

Part III, Improving Staff Training makes a technical addition, including agency and contract personnel, in the requirement for ongoing, dementia management, and patient abuse training (section 6121).

Subtitle C, Nationwide Program for National and State Background Checks on Direct Patient Access Employees of Long-term Care Facilities and Providers, provides the Secretary of HHS with criteria for the development of a background check program for all caregivers coming in direct contact with long-term care patients and directs the Inspector General of HHS to conduct an evaluation of the program (section 6201).

Subtitle D, Patient-Centered Outcomes Research, authorizes the establishment of the Patient-Centered Outcomes Research Institute as a nonprofit organization for the purpose of conducting patient-centered outcomes research, funded through the Patient-Centered Outcomes Research Trust Fund; establishes criteria used to manage the research conducted under its authority; and provides criteria for the Secretary of HHS to use in the development of Medicare and Medicaid payment for results of Patient-Centered Effective Research (section 6301). It also terminates the Federal Coordinating Council for Comparative Effectiveness Research, established under the American Recovery and Reinvestment Act, upon enactment of this Act (section 6302).

Subtitle E, Medicare, Medicaid, and CHIP Program Integrity Provisions, focuses on enhancing existing integrity measures and adding new measures for better measurement of quality while also protecting against fraud, waste and abuse. It directs:

- (And provides criteria for) the Secretary under consultation with the Inspector General of HHS to screen all providers and suppliers to Medicare, Medicaid, and CHIP, enhanced oversight for new providers and suppliers, state disclosure requirements, temporary enrollment moratoria, and establishment of a compliance program (section 6401);
- Inclusion in the CMS Integrated Data Repository of claims and payment data from all federal government-sponsored health programs for the purpose of matching for the identification of potential fraud, waste, and abuse, including detailed criteria for self-reporting, reporting, civil and monetary penalties; performance statistics; and annual evaluations for Medicare and Medicaid (section 6402);
- The Secretary to maintain a national healthcare fraud and abuse data collection program and to cease operation of the Healthcare Integrity and Protection Data Bank, transferring all data within the data bank to the National Practitioner Data as the sole source of healthcare fraud and abuse data (section 6403);
- To level penalties of $50,000 for each fraudulent act or connection with a fraudulent act, plus $15,000 per day for any delays in providing requested clinical documentation (section 6408);
- To establish a Self-Referral Disclosure Protocol for any actual or potential violation of the Social Security Act within 6 months of the occurrence of the actual or potential violation and provide the Secretary with the discretion of reducing the penalty (section 6409);

- To expand the Recovery Audit Contractor plan to Medicaid (section 6411).
- To reduce the maximum time for submitting Medicare claims from 1 year to 3 years (section 6404);
- To require physicians or other health professionals who order items on Medicare-covered recipients be enrolled as Medicare-eligible physicians or providers (section 6405);
- To allow the Secretary of HHS to revoke physician or supplier enrollment for not more than 1 year for each incidence of refusal to provide documentation or orders for durable equipment, home health services, or referrals to other services (section 6406);
- To require that a physician or mid-level practitioner have a face-to-face encounter with a patient (including through telehealth means) within 6 months prior to ordering durable medical equipment or home health services (section 6407); and
- To adjust the competitive bidding process for durable medical equipment, prosthetics, and orthotics to the 21 most populous metropolitan statistical areas (section 6410).

Subtitle F, Additional Medicaid Program Integrity Provisions. This subtitle strengthened integrity rules for Medicaid to bring these rules closer to those of Medicare. This included:

- Terminating providers from Medicaid if terminated from Medicare or any other state plan (section 6501) and
- Requiring the Secretary of HHS to exclude any individual or entity from Medicaid if the individual or entity owns, manages, is controlled by, or is in any other way associated with such individual or entity that has unpaid overpayments or is excluded from participation (section 6502) as well as any agent, clearinghouse, or alternate payee submitting claims on behalf of a

healthcare provider (section 6503) and extending the time for collection of overpayments from 60 days to 1 year (section 6506), and

- Prohibiting payments for items or services provided to any institution outside the United States (section 6505).

It directs the Secretary of HHS to expand the Medicaid Management Information System required data reporting elements (section 6504) and require use of the National Correct Coding Initiative or other similar programs. (section 6507).

Subtitle G, Additional Program Integrity Provisions. This section focused on strengthening ERISA integrity provisions by:

- Amending ERISA to prohibit anyone associated with an employer welfare arrangement regarding the financial condition; benefits provided; regulatory status governing collective bargaining, labor management relations, or intern union affairs; or regulatory status of a plan regarding exemption from state regulatory authority (section 6601) other small clarifications (section 6602);
- By directing a request that the National Association of Insurance Commissioners develop a national uniform fraud and abuse reporting format (section 6603).

This subtitle strengthened the Secretary of HHS by:

- Providing the ability to promulgate regulations, for the purpose of combating fraud and abuse, requiring providers of multiple employer welfare arrangement abide by the state laws of the state they are operating in (section 6604);
- Providing the authority to order cease and desist of multiple employer welfare plans that are fraudulent; create an immediate danger to public safety or welfare; or are causing or can be reasonably expected to

cause significant, imminent, and irreparable public injury (section 6605); and

- Requiring multiple employer welfare plans to register with the Secretary of HHS (section 6606) and providing evidentiary privilege for national or state departments appropriate for the enforcement of this title (section 6607).

Subtitle H, Elder Justice Act. Cited as the "Elder Justice Act of 2009" (section 6701 and 6702), it provides several definitions; establishes an Elder Justice Coordinating Council for the purpose of advising the Secretary of HHS on issues relating to elder abuse, neglect, exploitation, and other crimes against elders; establishes an Advisory Board on Elder Abuse, Neglect, and Exploitation to make recommendations to the Elder Justice Coordinating Council; establishes Elder Abuse, Neglect, and Exploitation Forensic Centers; provides grant funding to enhance long-term care staff training and to offset HER purchase expenses; and establishes the evaluation of Elder Justice Programs (section 6703).

Subtitle I, Sense of the Senate Regarding Medical Malpractice. The Senate recognizes this is a prime time to address malpractice concerns and encourages the states to experiment with potential national solutions (section 6801).

Title VII, Improving Access to Innovative Medical Therapies

Subtitle A, Biologics Price Competition and Innovation. Formally cited as the "Biologics Price Competition and Innovation Act of 2009," it gave a sense for the Senate that the biosimilars pathway should be established (section 7001) by providing criteria for submission and evaluation of a biosimilar licensure and patent (section 7002). It also requires the Secretaries of Treasury and HHS to determine the savings associated with enactment of this title and use such savings for deficit reduction (section 7003).

Subtitle B, More Affordable Medicines for Children and Underserved Communities expands the option for use of the 340B program to previously excluded children's hospitals, free-standing cancer hospitals, critical access hospitals, rural referral centers, or sole community hospitals; and disallows 340B discounts through group purchasing arrangements for outpatient drugs (section 7101). It also authorizes the Secretary of HHS to improve manufacturer compliance with drug pricing for preventing overcharges and other discount pricing requirements and with criteria for violation of 340B regulations penalties (section 7102), while also requiring the U.S. Comptroller to have evaluated the 340B program 18 months following the enactment of these regulations to determine if there is a need to expand the program (section 7103).

Title VIII, CLASS Act

Title VIII can be cited as either the "Community Living Assistance Services and Supports Act" or the "CLASS Act" (section 8001) and provides criteria for establishment of a national voluntary program for the purchase of long-term care insurance that allows individuals with functional limitations to secure necessary care while maintaining financial independence and priced based on actuarial analysis (section 8002).

Title IX, Revenue Provisions

Subtitle A, Revenue Offset Provisions focused on generating additional revenue. To do this it:

- Provided for a 40% excise tax of excess benefit (a.k.a. Cadillac) health plans including detailed criteria for calculating excess benefit and a long list of exclusions (section 9001) and for the distributions from a variety of pretax savings accounts for prescribed medicines and insulin (section 9003);
- Updated the inclusion of employer-sponsored coverage costs on W-2 forms with the exception salary reduction to a flexible spending account (section 9002) while increasing the tax on HSAs and Archer HSAs not used for qualified medical expenses to 20% and 15% respectively (section 9004) and placing a $2500 limit on deductions to flexible spending accounts that are part of cafeteria plans (section 9005);
- Updated information taxable corporations must report to IRS (section 9006); and
- Formalized in law administrative rules increasing IRS reporting requirements for charitable hospitals, including completing a community health needs assessment and acting on the identified needs, has a financial assistance policy, provision without discrimination of emergency care, limits the amount charged to uninsured individuals requiring emergency care to the lowest amount charged those with insurance, and does not use extraordinary collection actions until the hospital has taken reasonable actions to determine if the individual qualifies for financial assistance including a monetary of $50,000 for noncompliance with the above policies and a triannual review of community benefit activities by the Secretary of the Treasury (section 9007).

Annual fee criteria had criteria provided:

- To companies providing branded pharmaceuticals and imported pharmaceuticals (9008),
- To companies providing durable medical equipment and imported durable medical equipment (9009), and
- To providers of health insurance (9010).

Direct tax law changes included:

- For tax years 2013–2018 (ending 2019), reducing the amount of deductible medical expenses to 7.5% from 10% for taxpayers and spouses aged 65 years or greater (section 9013);

- Disallowing tax deduction for remuneration to any health insurance employee in excess of $500,000 (section 9014);
- Imposing 0.5% tax on any joint filing greater than or equal to $250,000 or in any other case $200,000 (section 9015);
- Modifying the tax treatment for health insurers who spend less than 85% of premium proceed of reimbursement for clinical services (section 9016); and
- Imposing a 5% tax on any cosmetic surgery that is not reconstructive (section 9017).

Lastly, it directed the Secretary of Veterans Affairs to conduct a study on the effect of the previous three sections on the cost of care to veterans and access to branded drugs and medical devices by veterans (section 9011) and eliminate the Medicare Part D deduction for subsidy expenses (section 9012).

Subtitle B, Other Provisions. This subtitle provides criteria for:

- Exemption benefits provided by any Indian tribal government (section 9021),
- The establishment of cafeteria plans by small employers (section 9022), and
- Qualified therapeutic discovery tax credit of 50% of the annual investment (section 9023).

Title X, Strengthening Quality, Affordable Health Care for All Americans

Subtitle A, Provisions Relating to **Title I** includes the following amendments to *Subtitle A* of the Public Health Service Act or Internal Revenue Code:

- Disallows lifetime monetary limits to covered benefit after January 1, 2014 with the exception of specific pre-2014 essential benefit restrictions;
- Requires group health plans to provide the Secretary of HHS and the state with requested information;

- Prohibits group insurance plans from discriminating against highly compensated individuals and collection of information on firearms ownership by any entity;
- Requires insurers to provide value to customers through the measurement of the risk loss adjustment of 85% for large insurers and 80% for small insurers, with any amounts less than these values rebated to customers, and requires hospitals to annually provide a list of standard charges.
- Provides criteria for the establishment of an appeals process by health insurers;
- Ensures that plan participants may choose a participating primary care provider;
- Provides for unrestricted access to emergency care and allows for the use of pediatricians as primary care providers for children;
- Allows women to seek care from a participating OB/GYN physician without referral or authorization; and
- Provides for the establishment of a data center for the establishment and publication of fee schedules (section 10101).

Subtitle B amended only the requirement for the establishment of a website where consumers and small businesses can find information on health insurance plan options (section 10102).

Subtitle C amendments provide for the non-investigative insurance coverage of beneficiaries involved in clinical trials and requires an annual report to be complied by the Secretary of Labor on self-insured plans and provides criteria for the Secretary of HHS to conduct a study of self-insured plans (section 10103).

Subtitle D amendments include provisions for co-op plans, patient-centered medical homes, premium rating variances based on rating area, and payments to federally qualified health centers, including no funding for abortion services; and provides detailed criteria for oversight of multi-state qualified health insurance plans by the Director of the Office or Personnel Management (section 10104).

Subtitle E amendments include multiple technical amendments to the Internal Revenue Code and direct the Secretary of HHS to conduct a study of the federal poverty level to determine if geographic variations to the federal poverty level are necessary based on geographic variations in the cost of living (section 10105).

Subtitle F amendments include an economic summary of the effects from the U.S. fractured healthcare system, provide criteria for penalties due to lack of purchasing health insurance, and provide criteria for the imposition of a $600 fine per employee of a large employer who has to wait greater than 60 days for health insurance coverage (section 10106).

Subtitle G amendments include criteria for and directs the Comptroller General of the United States to conduct a study of the incidence of denials of medical service and health insurance coverage (section 10107) and criteria for employers to offer free choice vouchers to employees for the purchase of minimal essential coverage on the health exchange for cost to the employee greater than 8% but not greater than 9.8% of adjusted gross income (section 10108). It also directs the Secretary of HHS to solicit and develop administrative and operative standards focused on increasing efficiency and reducing administrative health system costs (section 10109).

Subtitle B, Provisions Relating to **Title II**. *Part I, Medicaid and CHIP* provides for the extension of Medicaid or CHIP to young adults up to age 26 years who were in the foster care system and on Medicaid or CHIP while in the foster care system; provides criteria for the distribution of funds to the states; provides criteria for the conduct, evaluation, and reporting of Medicaid and CHIP demonstration projects; and directs the Comptroller General

of the United States to conduct a study of quality and payment actions taken under this act (section 10201). It also provides criteria for incentives to states that provide up to 50% on long-term care service in non-institutional settings, such as home or community settings (section 10202), and authorizes and appropriates CHIP funding through 2015 (section 10203).

Part II, Support for Pregnant and Parenting Teens and Women defines accompaniment, eligible institution of higher education, community service center, intervention service, Secretary, state, supportive social services, and violence (section 10211); establishes a Pregnancy Assistance Fund under direction of the Secretaries of HHS and Education (section 10212); provides criteria for use of Pregnancy Assistance Fund supporting pregnant women and parents of children obtaining education through an institution of higher learning (section 10213); and appropriates $25 million per year for the Pregnancy Assistance Fund FY 2010–FY 2014 (section 10214).

Part III, Indian Health Care Improvement. Allows for the use of a Certified Dental Therapist or Mid-level Dental Health Provider in place of a Certified Dentist when allowed under state law (section 10221).

Subtitle C, Provisions Relating to **Title III** provides criteria for the establishment of an Ambulatory Surgical Center Value-Based Purchasing program (section 10301); provides a technical revision to the National Strategy for Quality Improvement in Health Care (section 10302); provides criteria for the development of outcomes measures for the five most chronic, resource-intense diagnoses and primary preventive care (section 10303); revises Sections 1890(b)(7) and 1890A of the Social Security Act by replacing "quality" with "quality and efficiency" (section 10304); directs the Secretary of HHS to establish a strategic framework for the public reporting of health data to support healthcare delivery (section

10305); allows the Secretary of HHS to limit testing of payment models to defined geographic areas, criteria for the use of telehealth for medically underserved areas or the Indian Health Service, and selecting of quality measures that reflect national priorities (section 10306); provides the Secretary of HHS the authority to use a partial ACO model or any other model deemed appropriate resulting in no additional expenditures (section 10307); provides the Secretary of HHS the authority to expand the pilot program after January 1, 2016 if the pilot program reduces spending without reducing quality of care or improves the quality of care and reduces spending (section 10108); provides a technical revision reducing payments to hospitals for the Readmissions Reduction Program (section 10309); repeals the physician payment update (section 10310); includes technical revisions to ground and air ambulance extensions (section 10311); extends payment rules for long-term care hospitals from 4 to 5 years and continues the moratorium on certain hospitals and facilities (section 10312); provides the Secretary of HHS the authority to extend the Rural Community Hospital demonstration project for an additional 5 years (section 10313); increases the number of discharges to low-volume hospital provisions from 1500 to 1600 (section 10314); directs the Secretary of HHS to conduct a study of low income Medicare beneficiaries and to make payment adjustments as necessary (section 10315); provides technical corrections to Medicare DSH payments (section 10316); provides for revisions and extensions to the Hospital Wage Index (section 10317); revises transnational extra benefits under Medicare Advantage by inserting 2009 (section 10318); revises hospital market basket adjustment by 0.5% for FY 2011 and 0.1% for FY 2012–FY 2014 (section 10319); broadens the reporting requirements and responsibilities of the Independent Payment Advisory Board (section 19320); revises community health teams to

include other primary care providers (section 10321); reduces the annual update for psychiatric hospitals that fail to report quality data by 0.2% (section 10322); provides detailed screening and qualifying criteria for individuals exposed to environmental health hazards allowing them to enroll in Medicare Parts A and B (section 10323); defines frontier state and county providing that neither of these geographic areas shall have a hospital inpatient or outpatient area wage index or practice expense index of less than 1.0 (section 10324); delays implementation of Resource Group Utilization IV (Prospective Payment and Consolidated Billing for SNF) and implementation of specific RUG-IV changes with a lookback period to ensure only services furnished post-SNF admission are used to calculate case mix index (section 10325); directs the Secretary of HHS to conduct pilot test of value-based payment at psychiatric hospitals, long-term care hospitals, rehabilitation hospitals, PPS-exempt cancer hospitals, and hospice programs, directs that all payments shall be revenue neutral, and provides the Secretary authority to expand the duration and scope of the program if the expansion is expected to reduce spending without reducing quality of care or improve quality of care without reducing spending (section 10326); provides for an increase in physician quality reporting of 0.5%, provided detailed criteria are met (section 10327); requires prescription drug plan sponsors to offer medication therapy management to criteria targeted beneficiaries (section 10328); directs the Secretary of HHS to consult with stakeholders and develop a methodology to measure health plan value (section 10329); directs the Secretary of HHS to develop a plan and budget to modernize the CMS computers and data systems to support improvements in health care delivery (section 10330); directs the Secretary of HHS to develop a Physician Compare website with criteria for required data elements, develop methodologies ensuring that these data are reliable and accurate, and determine when to transition physicians to value-based purchasing payments (section 10331); provides criteria for the use of Medicare data for program evaluation purposes (section 10332); authorizes the Secretary of HHS to provide grants to community-based collaborative networks that work as a consortium of healthcare providers providing coordinated and integrated care to low-income populations (section 10333); establishes a CMS Office of Minority Health focused on improving minority health, improving the quality of healthcare minorities receive, and eliminating racial and ethnic disparities (section 10334); provides a technical correction for the hospital value-based purchasing program (section 10335); directs the U.S. Comptroller General to conduct a study of the impact on Medicare beneficiaries receiving high-quality dialysis services, including oral drugs furnished during treatment (section 10336).

Subtitle D, Provisions Relating to **Title V** amends *Subtitle A* by replacing "2010" with "2020," "research and health screenings" with "research, health screenings, and initiatives," and "for preventive" with "regarding preventive" (section 10401). It amends *Subtitle B* by inserting "and vision" after "oral" and with a section detailing annual wellness physical requirements (section 10402). Amendments to *Subtitle C* include language to ensure the inclusion of rural and frontier areas (section 10403). Amendments to *Subtitle D* replace "by ensuring" with "and ensuring" (section 10404). It amends *Subtitle E* by striking section 4401 (section 10405). It also rescinds the need for coinsurance for coverage of preventive services and provides 100% coverage of grade A and B preventive services recommended by the U.S Preventive Task Force (section 10406); directs the Secretary of HS and Director of CDC to develop a biannual report on diabetes care (section 10407); authorizes the Secretary of HHS to provide small businesses grants for the development of comprehensive wellness programs based on criteria established in this section (section 10408); provides the Director of NIH the criteria for establishment of a Cures Accelerated Network, providing grants for development and production of biopharmaceutical and medical products that would not be feasible in the commercial market (section 10409); provides the Secretary of HHS criteria for the development of national centers of excellence for the treatment of depression and authority to award grants to healthcare organizations developing and implementing these centers (section 10410); authorizes the Secretary of HHS through the Director of CDC to develop a national congenital disease surveillance system, including detailed criteria to be included in the development of such system and the authority to award grants for its development (section 10411); provides technical revisions to the Automated Defibrillation in Adam's Memory Act (section 10412), and provides criteria and grant funding for the development of a program for young women's breast health awareness and support of young women diagnoses with breast cancer (section 10413).

Subtitle E, Provisions Relating to **Title V**. Amendments to the Public Health Service Act, Social Security Act, and **Title V** of this act include (section 10501):

- Including after employers, representatives of small business and self-employed individuals;
- Providing for the elimination of barriers to entering and staying in primary care;
- Inserting optometrists and ophthalmologists after occupational therapists;
- Establishing the Interagency Access to Health Care in Alaska Task Force to assess access by federal beneficiaries and provide strategies for improved delivery of healthcare services;
- Directing the Secretary of HHS to establish a training demonstration program for

training of family nurse practitioners and a 1-year primary care training program for current nurse practitioners;

- Directing the Secretary of HHS to collaborate with the Director of CDC to establish a National Diabetes Prevention Program to include (1) grants for community-based diabetes prevention model sites, (2) a program eligibility program within the CDC, (3) a training and outreach program for lifestyle intervention instructors, (4) CDC evaluation, monitoring, and technical assistance, and (5) establishment of a prospective payment system for FQHCs providing these services;
- Providing for grants to providers treating a high percentage of medically underserved individuals;
- Directing the Secretary of HHS to collaborate with HRSA to provide grants for the recruitment of students most likely to practice in underserved rural communities, provide rural-focused training and experience, and increase the number of medical graduates practicing in underserved rural communities;
- Directing the Secretary of HHS to collaborate with HRSA and CDC to award grants or contracts for the provision of preventive medical specialty training to graduate medical residents;
- Appropriating $100,00,00 for FY 2010 for debt service on construction or renovation of an inpatient care or outpatient service at a U.S. public university that contains the state's sole public academic medical and dental school;
- Providing for the establishment of a Community Health Center Fund administered by the Secretary of HHS for the expansion and sustainment of community health centers; and
- Directing the Secretary of HHS to collaborate with HRSA to establish a 3-year demonstration project for the provision of comprehensive healthcare services to the uninsured at reduced fees.

Subtitle F, Provisions Relating to **Title VI** extends time limits by 6 months to Medicare exceptions to the prohibition on certain physician referrals for hospitals (section 10601); clarifies access and use of data for patient-centered outcomes research and members of outcomes review council (10602); strikes provisions relating to individual provider application fees (section 10603); makes technical corrections to section 6405 regarding services provided in collaboration with a physician (section 10604); allows nurse practitioners, nurse clinical specialists, nurse midwives, and physician assistants working in collaboration with a physician to make home face-to-face health visits (section 10605); increases the penalties for convictions of healthcare fraud to "... reflect the serious harms associated with healthcare fraud and the need for aggressive and appropriate law enforcement action to prevent such fraud ..." and provides the Attorney General or designee subpoena authority for evidence relating to healthcare fraud (section 10606); provides the Secretary of HHS the authorization to award grants for a period not to exceed 5 years to states to develop, implement, and evaluate alternatives to current medical tort litigation with the goals of dispute resolution over injuries and reduction of healthcare errors through the collection and analysis of patient safety data plus additional criteria for awarding and evaluating grant proposals and outcomes (section 10607); extends medical malpractice coverage to any individual providing services to or through a free clinic (section 10608); and provides for labeled drugs that undergo labeling changes due to this act to not be considered mislabeled or, if it is determined that the labeling negatively impacts the drug use, the drug will not be eligible for approval (section 10609).

Subtitle G, Provisions Relating to **Title VIII** provides several technical language changes to program information (section 10801).

Subtitle H, Provisions relating to **Title IX** includes longshoremen as employees engaged in high-risk professions (section 10901); provides for limitation and inflation adjustment on healthcare cafeteria plans (section 10902); modifies the limitation fs charges by charitable hospitals by replacing "the lowest amounts charged" with "the amounts generally charged" (section 10903); modifies the annual fee on medical device manufacturers and importers (section 10904); provides criteria for the modification of annual fee on health insurance providers (section 10905); increases FICA or SECA on high-income taxpayers from 0.5% to 0.9% (section 10906); imposes a 10% tax on indoor tanning services (section 10907); excludes from gross income any amount received under any federal or state repayment program that intends to increase healthcare services to underserved or health professional shortage areas (section 10908); and increases the adoption or adoption assistance credit limit from $10,000 to $13,170 and provides for an annual cost of living adjustment (section 10909).

▶ PL 111-152 Health Care and Education Reconciliation Act of 2010.[1]

Title I, Coverage, Medicare, Medicaid, and Revenues

Subtitle A, Coverage.

■ Technical correction for healthcare insurance premium tax credits (section 1001)

■ Technical revisions to criteria for individual responsibility income and penalties (section 1002).

■ Criteria for how to calculate the number of full-time employees attributed to large employers (section 1003).

■ Definition of modified adjusted gross income, required health exchange information, exclusion of amounts expended for medical care, self-employed health insurance deduction, coverage under self-employed deduction, benefits provided to members of a voluntary employees' beneficiary association and their dependents, and medical and other benefits for retired employees (section 1004).

■ Establishes the Health Insurance Reform Implementation Fund (section 1005).

Subtitle B, Medicare.

■ Provides a $250 rebate to individuals who have exceeded the individual coverage in their Medicare Part D plan, closes the Medicare Part D donut hole, coverage for generic drugs, and reduces the growth rate of out-of-pocket costs (section 1101).

■ Repeals sections 3201 and 3203 of the Patient Protection and Affordable Care Act.

■ Establishes criteria for the phase in of modified benchmarks, quality determinants, beneficiary rebates, and coding intensity adjustment (section 1102).

■ Requires a health plan medical loss ratio of at least 85% and authorizes the Secretary of HHS to cancel the plan if a plan fails to maintain a medical loss ratio of less than or equal to 85% for 5 consecutive years (section 1103).

■ Decrease DSH payments by 0.1 percentage points for fiscal year 2014 and 0.2 percentage points for fiscal years 2015, 2016, and 2017 (section 1104).

---

1 This law is a "clean-up" law passed in the absence of an available conference reconciliation process.

- Provides for market basket updates of 0.3 percentage point for FY 2014; 0.2 percentage point for FY 2015 and 2016; and 0.75 percentage point for FY 2017, 2018, and 2019 (section 1105).
- Redefines physician hospital ownership, provider agreement, and high Medicaid facility (section 1106).
- Revises the utilization rate for expensive imaging equipment to 75% instead of the rate in the final rule (section 1107).
- Decreases the physician geographic practice cost index (GPCI) from 0.75 to 0.5 (section 1108).
- Provides for payment to qualifying hospitals and defines hospitals located in a county that rates in the lowest quartile of such counties in the United States based on its rankings of age, sex, and race adjusted benefit spending on parts A and B (section 1009).

Subtitle C, Medicaid.

- Defines federal funding levels for states that agreed to expand Medicaid, ranging from 100% for FY 2014–FY 2016 to 90% for FY 2020 and thereafter (section 1201).
- Defines primary care physician and pays physicians at not less than 100% of the applicable payment rate for service furnished in FY 2013 and FY 2014 (section 1202).
- Provides criteria for the reduction of DSH payments to states for distribution to hospitals for fiscal years 2014–2020 (section 1203).
- Provides funding criteria for the territories to support health exchange subsidies and Medicaid expansion (section 1204).
- Delays the Community First Choice Option by 1 year (section 1205).
- Provides criteria for rebates of new formulations of existing drugs (section 1206).

Subtitle D, Reducing Fraud, Waste, and Abuse.

- Provides technical language revisions expanding the reach of community health centers (section 1301).
- Repeals Medicare payment review limitations (section 1302).
- Provides additional funding to fight fraud, waste, and abuse (section 1303).
- Allows the Secretary of HS to hold DME payments for 90 days if there is a determination of the potential of fraudulent activity (section 1304).

Subtitle E, Provisions Relating to Revenue.

- Provides several technical revisions and adjustments regarding multiemployer plans and costing adjustments (section 1401).
- Inserts a new chapter following *Subtitle A, Chapter 2A, Unearned Income Medicare Contribution* that imposes a 3.8% tax on net investment income or the excess of modified adjusted gross income over the threshold amount ($250,000 for married couples and $200,000 for individuals) on individual, estate, and trust income plus criteria defining various types of income (section 1402).
- Delays limitation on health flexible spending arrangement under cafeteria plan 1 year or until 2013 (section 1403).
- Amends Section 9008 of PL 111-148 by delaying action by 1 year until 2010 and striking $2,300,000,000 and providing a table with annually adjusted amounts through 2019 and thereafter (section 1404).
- Amends Chapter 32 of the Internal Revenue Code by inserting *Subchapter E, Medical Devices* that imposes a 2.3% tax on the sale of any medical device and provides criteria for the definition and exemption of medical devices (section 1405).
- Amends Sections 9010 and 10905 of PL 111-148 regarding health insurance providers by delaying implementation by

3 years or until 2013 and provides revised criteria for determination of applicable net income (section 1406).

- Delays elimination of deduction for expenses allocable to Medicare Part D subsidy by 2 years or until 2012 (section 1407).
- Eliminates unintended application of cellulosic biofuel producer credit (section 1408) and codifies economic substance doctrine penalties (section 1409).
- Increases the estimated corporate tax by 15.75% (section 1410).

Subtitle F, Other Provisions. Establishes grants for community colleges and career training programs (section 1501).

Title II, Education and Health

Subtitle A, Education Parts I and II address student loans and loan repayment options.

Subtitle B, Health.

- Adds provisions regarding excessive waiting periods, lifetime limits, and extension of dependent coverage to grandfathered health insurance plans (section 2301).
- Technical correction striking "covered drugs" and inserting "covered outpatient drugs" (section 2302).
- Amends Section 10503(b)(1) of PL 111-148 regarding community health centers by increasing dollars amounts available (section 2304).

Index

Note: Page numbers followed by *f* or *t* indicate material in figures or tables, respectively.

P